How to
Survive
and Maybe Even Love
Health
Professions
School

Retention and Career Placement Guide

Dedication

This book is dedicated to all students who want to change their lives and make a difference in the world.

I want you to know,

You Can Do It!

This book will be your guide.

Arlene M. Muller

Special Note to Students

Dear New Student:

If you are reading this book, you have made the commitment to study and learn new skills for a health professions career. My congratulations to you! I salute your courage to learn about a new career path. Not everyone has your courage. You should feel proud of yourself right now, and others will feel proud of you when they see you at graduation.

One of the best things about the journey you are about to undertake is that you just need to follow the plan set before you and concentrate on one day at a time. You cannot live tomorrow until it is here. So relax and approach today with 100% of your time and energy, whether you are learning in the classroom, completing your assignments, or studying with a group.

Achieving your dreams will require you to put in a lot of hard work and make some sacrifices, but those challenges will make your achievement all the greater in the end. The objective of this book is to prepare you to do the following:

- Balance the challenges of work, family, and school
- Learn how to study and take a test
- Create a professional resume
- Plan how to network and market yourself
- Conduct a professional interview
- Understand the challenges of a new position

This book will act as your guide to your new career and assist you in making your dream of a new career into a reality.

Arlene M. Muller

Preface

Purpose

The purpose of this book is to be a motivating tool that will help to keep you on the path to graduation. This book goes beyond discussing normal classroom skills and instead helps students to develop the skills that they need to face the real-life challenges of returning to school; juggling school, family, and other responsibilities; making it to graduation; conducting a career search; and beginning a new career. It offers answers, advice, suggestions, tools, and the motivation necessary to resolve the common challenges that students face as they proceed toward graduation and begin work as a health-care professional.

Organization

The book is divided into two parts. The chapters in **Part 1, Going Back to School,** focus on helping you to create a new attitude for success that will guide you to achieve your goal of graduation. Along your journey, you are likely to encounter several challenges inside and outside the classroom, including adjusting to school, overcoming personal challenges at home and work, and learning or remembering how to study and take tests. Part 1 offers guidance that will realistically answer your questions, help you develop coping skills, and put you on the right path to becoming a graduate and starting a new career.

Part 2, Preparing to Be Successful in Your New Career, prepares you to be able to develop the marketing, networking, and interviewing skills you will need to make new contacts in the health-care field and present your skills to prospective employers. In addition, these chapters answer questions you might have about developing and formatting a resume, answering interview questions, and managing a career search. The book takes you even further, though, with the final chapter, Survival Guide for the New Graduate, which offers guidance on surviving the first day in your new position and becoming successful in your new career.

Features

The book has been designed to include an array of features that will help you to accomplish your goals. Its comprehensive coverage takes you from your first day of school to graduation and beyond, stopping along the way to discuss potential challenges and offer suggested solutions. The clear and simple approach of this book will help you to address these real student issues head-on.

Throughout each chapter, you will find three very special features that are intended to keep you on the right path to graduation by providing instruction, advice, and motivation:

- **On Track** exercises help to keep you engaged with the text, gauge your understanding of the information, and help you to apply the information to your own life.
- **Mentor Moments** are real-life accounts of other students' experiences that can help you to understand how to handle common challenges and realize possible solutions.
- **Motivational Moments** are words of inspiration from people of different backgrounds who believed in their dreams and made a difference in the world.

At the end of each chapter, you will also find **Success Journal** questions that will help to bring all of the chapter content together for you. These exercises serve as the building blocks for the tools you will need to make it to graduation and succeed in your new career.

How to Use this Book

Allow this book to be your guide on your new journey in health professions school. If you keep an open mind, this book will continue to motivate and inspire you to achieve your goals throughout your journey. **YOU CAN DO IT!**

Reviewers

Delena K. Austin, BTIS, CMA (AAMA)
Program Coordinator
Medical Assisting
Macomb Community College
Clinton Township, Michigan

Kaye F. Bathe, BSHA, CMA (AAMA)
Program Coordinator
Medical Assisting
Tri County Technical College
Pendleton, South Carolina

Terri Brame, MBA, CPC-GENSG,
CPC-H, CPC-I
Administrator
Clinical Revenue and Compliance
University of Washington
Seattle, Washington

Mary Elizabeth W. Browder, BA,
CMA (AAMA)
Assistant Professor
Medical Assisting
University of Cincinnati, Raymond
Walters College
Cincinnati, Ohio

Judith Cabanban, RHIT
Instructor
Health Information Management
Portland Community College
Portland, Oregon

Sheryl S. Chambers, CBCS
Medical Instructor
Education
Indiana Business College
Indianapolis, IN

Clintonette Garrison, MHA, RRT,
CPT, CHE
Allied Health Director
Regulatory Affairs
YTI Career Institute
York, Pennsylvania

Laura A. Gilpin, RN
Educator
Health Sciences
Cumberland County High School
Crossville, Tennessee

Cheri Goretti, MA, MT (ASCP),
CMA (AAMA)
Professor and Program Coordinator
Medical Assisting and Allied
Health
Quinebaug Valley Community
College
Danielson, Connecticut

Liana Gunakan
Instructor
Alhambra High School
Alhambra, California

Dolly R. Horton, MEd, CMA (AAMA)
Coordinator
Medical Assisting
Mayland Community College
Spruce Pine, North Carolina

Joy Hurst, MFS, MATL, CMA (AAMA)
Professor
Medical Assisting
Kaplan College
Frederick, Maryland

Judith L. Lichtenberger, CMT, FAAMT
Adjunct Faculty
Office Administration
Northampton Community College
Bethlehem, Pennsylvania

Melissa Nieto, LVN
Instructor
Medical Assisting
Texas State Technical College
Harlingen, Texas

Amy Sager, RN, BSN, MS
Program Coordinator
Medical Assisting
Seward County Community
  College/Area Technical School
Liberal, Kansas

Nanette B. Sayles, EDD, RHIA, CCS, CHPS, FAHIMA
Program Director and Associate
  Professor
Health Information Management
Macon State College
Warner Robins, Georgia

Beth A. Stewart, RN
Teacher
Evans High School
Evans, Georgia

Kari Williams, BS, DC
Program Director
Medical Office Technology
Front Range Community College
Longmont, Colorado

Acknowledgments

I want to acknowledge the contributions made by Joanne Leming, LPN, who worked with me to create the table of contents that was the basis for this book. Her ideas were an inspiration for the early chapters.

I also want to acknowledge Dr. Flora Velsco for her contributions to the medical information related to surgical technology and other allied health areas, as well as Teri Erhardt and JM Financial for their knowledge and research, which was used to establish the financial section as a guide for the reader.

Contents in Brief

Tables and Figures

Contents

Going Back to School

Yes, You Can Do It!

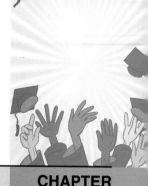

Learning Outcomes

After reading this chapter, the student will be able to:

1. Define and set goals toward a commitment to a new career.
2. Understand the importance of commitment to achieving at least 90% attendance.
3. Understand and discuss how a positive attitude can help to meet challenges and break down "brick walls."

Going Back to School

Welcome to the beginning of an exciting new career in the health professions field. Whether you have decided to return to school to pursue a career as a medical assistant, dental hygienist, medical biller, or some other health professional, the schooling that lies ahead of you is designed to give you the knowledge, vocabulary, clinical lab skills, and customer service skills that are appropriate for the field you have chosen. However, the education you will receive from your classes is just the first step on your journey. You will continue to learn each day as you work at your profession. In addition, as the health professions field changes, you will have to adapt to those changes, learning new skills and information that accompany new processes and procedures.

As you probably already know, the road that lies ahead of you might not be easy. Along with the typical challenges of returning to school, such as test taking, doing homework, and learning medical terminology, processes, and procedures for your particular profession, you will face many other challenges, both professionally and personally. One of those challenges will be the need to become more organized to create quality study time in your already busy schedule. One way to successfully overcome these challenges is to prepare yourself for them as much as you can. And you need not face these challenges alone. This book will act as your guide to a successful journey through your education and on to graduation. So, let's start by answering some basic questions that you might be asking yourself right now as you begin your program.

Motivational Moment

66 Show me someone who has done something worthwhile, and I'll show you someone who has overcome adversity. 99

Lou Holtz, former Notre Dame football coach

How Did I Get Here?

Mentor Moment

I never graduated from high school, so afterward, when people I went to school with went on to college, I found myself working two part-time jobs just to make ends meet. It wasn't easy, and I wasn't sure what I wanted to do with my life. Then I saw a commercial on television for a school that trained people for careers in the health professions field. I was curious about learning more about those careers, so

Mentor Moment (continued)

I called to get more information. The admissions representative I spoke with helped me to realize that a career as a surgical technologist was right for me.

Janice from Flagstaff, AZ

So, let's start at the beginning. Sometime in your recent past, you decided to take on this new venture. Stop and think of what led you to return to school. What were your goals? Some possible goals include the following:

- Having a career
- Helping your children
- Helping your parents
- Making more money
- Having medical insurance
- Having a better place to live
- Owning a car that does not need to be fixed every 3 months

Whatever your goals, they inspired you to make a change in your life. Maybe you even hit a breaking point when you decided that you just could not take it anymore—that you needed to turn your life around or do something different with it. At the time, maybe you were not even sure what that change would be. Somehow, though, you heard about the exciting opportunities available to you in the health professions field. Maybe you heard about them from a television commercial or from a coworker or friend. However it happened, you courageously began the journey of investigation and found out how easy it would be to get started on your new career path—one that would allow you to finally fulfill your lifelong dreams.

Now that you have enrolled in an educational institution, chosen your career path, and are about to begin your education, you may be wondering why you decided to face this challenge at all. Keep in mind that you wanted to make a change in your life and that education is the path to create that change. Jobs are everywhere, but careers, such as those in the health professions field, are best found when you have an education. The good news is that the effort you put forth toward your education will pay off. In general, careers offer greater stability and longevity, not to mention personal satisfaction, than do most jobs. Also, you are sure to be proud of the career you have chosen in the health professions field. Health professionals play an important role in society, and careers in the health professions will always be necessary as long as people continue to get sick and need health care. In fact, the demand for professionals in the health-care field is expected to increase due to the baby boomer population. As this generation ages, their need for health care will continue to grow, creating more employment opportunities for people like you who are interested in careers in the health-care field.

How Do I Get to Graduation and My Career?

Now that you have been accepted to a program, you might be wondering what it will actually take for you to complete it. One answer is focus, focus, and more focus. You will need to set goals; make a plan to achieve those goals and work that plan; keep your mental motivation going morning, noon, and night; and identify a support system. Your success starts with your commitment to reach your goal.

Of course, such a major life alteration will require adjustment, change, and sacrifice. Each of these components is defined not by using the word "easy" but by using the word "courage." Although this might sound overwhelming, you have already proven yourself to have this courage, as well as the personal skills and other strengths required to succeed, when you made the call to inquire about your health professions program. Overcoming challenges will also require you to "think outside the box" and stretch yourself beyond your comfort zone. Although it will not be easy, each step you take will not only get you closer to your goal but will also build your confidence, self-esteem, and self-worth. For this reason, you should remember to say "thank you" along the way for the things that move you one step closer to your goal. Appreciating the challenges that you will overcome will help you be more grateful when you finally achieve that goal.

What else will it take for you to get to graduation? The path to graduation is paved with class attendance. Whether the classes you are taking are online or at a campus facility, if you are not in class, you cannot learn. In fact, class attendance is the most important way to ensure that you stay on the path to graduation. In high school, you may have been absent often or consistently tardy. However, when you enroll in a program at an educational institution, your daily attendance is required. This is not a drop-in atmosphere. Here you will be held accountable for the material covered each day in class, whether you are in attendance or not. Attendance might also be a part of your grade. Do not give away attendance and grade points just because you are not motivated to go to class on a particular day. Instead, find your motivation. No matter what issues are in front of you, keep the end result in mind: you are going to graduate and begin a new career! Attending class and being prepared for each day by completing your homework the night before show your dedication to your goal of becoming a health professional. Finding the time to do this may be hard, but being prepared for and attending class will play a huge role in your overall success and learning in health professions school.

Given all that it will take for you to get to graduation, maybe you are wondering if you can really do it. One thing is certain: you *can* do this and *want* to do this, or you would not be here right now. You would not have already taken the steps that you have taken if you did not want to be here. It is important for you to keep this in mind, along with all of the other accomplishments you will gain, to maintain the motivation you will need to complete the program.

Mentor Moment

When I first got accepted to my medical assistant program, I had no idea how hard it would actually be. Sure, I knew going back to school after so long would be a challenge, but I don't think I was prepared for everything that went along with juggling school, work, and my two kids at home. I mean, it had been years since I studied for a test! But by learning to manage my time and continuing to attend class and study hard, I did it! I earned good grades and reached graduation. I actually did it!

Lila from Fayetteville, NC

Can I *Really* Do This?

When you first decided to go back to school, was your decision challenged by others? Did some of your friends, family, or coworkers tell you that you were crazy to try to go back to school and start a new career? Maybe they said that you would never be able to finish the program. Maybe they said that you were too old to start something new. Maybe they said that you could not afford to go back to school. Maybe you even had some of these same thoughts yourself. Throughout the process of deciding to go back to school, you probably had several conversations with the "little voice in your head" about whether you could be successful in this new journey. Those types of doubts probably left you wondering whether you had made the right decision and whether you really could get your diploma or degree and make a new career for yourself. Well, the answer is you can—*and you will*! Remember that you have already taken some of the hardest steps by seeking out this new opportunity and applying and getting accepted to your program.

Finding a way to silence the negativity of others—and yourself—is important. You should be able to silence the doubts that you have by reminding yourself each day that you *are* doing this. You have what it takes to be a success in your health professions program or you would not have qualified to be here. Focus on your achievements rather than your failures, and turn negativity into positivity. Make sure that the little voice in your head no longer casts doubts on your ability to succeed but rather cheers you on as you accomplish your goals. With the right guidance and mind-set, you can do anything you want to do.

Silencing the negativity of others can be easy, too. The first step is to avoid people who are not supportive of your goals. This might include friends, family, or coworkers. Anyone who expresses doubt or tells you that you cannot succeed will only contribute to negative ways of thinking. Some people will selfishly cast doubt and negativity on your ability to succeed simply because they are afraid to try themselves. Others may be jealous that you possess the strength, courage, and determination to better your life when they do not. They may fear being left behind when you accomplish your goals. Steer clear of these people as much as possible. If you cannot avoid them (e.g., if you live with your family and your family is not supportive), then try to avoid discussing your goals with them. Such conversations open the doorway to your own negative thinking.

Most likely, as you progress through your education, you will face hard times, and the doubts that you have had will return to challenge you. However, you cannot let them stop you from focusing on your goal. No matter how hard it gets and what others might say, remember that you *can* do this! You must take the negativity and use it to fuel your determination to accomplish your goal and get to graduation.

O N   T R A C K

Be sure to take time each day—in fact, take time right now—to stop and say to yourself, "Yes, I can do it!" Repeat this positive affirmation three times each day, even if you think it is silly or unnecessary, and do it with positivity, sincerity, and conviction. Reminding yourself each day that you can do it will help you stay on track toward achieving your goals.

"I can do it!" These four small words can help you manage the negative thoughts that will try to stop you from moving forward. Believing these words is as simple and as difficult as believing in yourself. Of course, you might find believing in yourself a difficult task. Maybe you have failed in or given up on previous efforts, or maybe you were always just told by others that you would never be successful. If so, don't worry. Remember that now is the time to stop listening to those voices and to start building your self-confidence in the belief that you can do this.

You have probably already realized it, but this new journey will be unlike your previous school experiences. Even if you took advantage of vocational classes and programs in high school, you will find the experience of attending a health professions school different for many reasons. And remember that the path that got you here is different as well. You choose to take these classes in order to fulfill your dream of having a career. Knowing that you choose to embark on this journey should help keep you motivated and should make it easier for you to remember your dream and why you wanted to be in class in the first place.

Overcoming Challenges

Mentor Moment

While I was in school, I faced a huge hardship: my father died. Being the oldest child, I found that my family was really looking to me to take a leadership role in making the funeral arrangements. I didn't think that I had time because I was already struggling to find time to study and do my homework, and I was already working all the time. But my mom was a mess and didn't speak English very well, and my brother and sister lived too far away, so I had no choice but to take on this one more thing. I almost withdrew from school. What stopped me was that I thought about my dad. I remembered how proud he was of me for returning to school to become a medical biller and coder. The loss of my dad was a huge obstacle, but I was able to overcome it because I knew that he was still there, supporting me and cheering me on.

Marian from Somerset, NJ

Facing Your Brick Walls

Standing at the beginning of your journey to your new career and looking at the path that lies ahead of you, you might feel overwhelmed by all that you will need to accomplish to achieve your goal. Remember to take this journey one step at a time. Health professions programs are broken down into small parts for you, called "courses" or "modules." Today, just look at your first course, your first chapter, or your first week. This should help to keep you from feeling overwhelmed. It will also help you to focus on the immediate tasks at hand, making them more manageable and achievable.

As you know, this new endeavor will also force you to overcome many challenges. Like Randy Pausch, a former professor at Carnegie Mellon University, you might find it useful to think of these challenges as "brick walls." Pausch was a middle-aged married man with three young boys when he ran into his biggest brick wall: he was diagnosed with terminal pancreatic cancer. After many doctors' appointments and treatments, Pausch made a decision not to let this brick wall stop him; instead, he choose to overcome his obstacle by continuing to have fun and living his life to the fullest. The key to his success was a positive attitude. Despite having an illness that he knew would kill him, Pausch was filled with optimism and a zest for life. His experience is a testament to what a person can do if he or she has the right mind-set.

Pausch talks about his experience in his famous lecture, entitled "Really Achieving Your Childhood Dreams" (available at www.thelastlecture.com), and in his book, *The Last Lecture*. This inspirational lecture might be a good place for you to start to build your own positive mind-set. It provides a unique perspective on what a person can do when he or she has a driven attitude, even in the face of the greatest adversity.

Motivational Moment

66 Brick walls are there for a reason. They let us prove how badly we want something. They are there to stop anyone who doesn't want it badly enough to break through. They let us show our dedication. 99

Randy Pausch, professor and author of **The Last Lecture**[1]

Although not every brick wall is as serious as Pausch's life-threatening illness, most of us have hit at least one brick wall along our journey through life; in fact, most of us hit them all the time. Some people have faced brick walls when their parents got divorced, when they were the victim of a bully, when they received poor grades, when a friend betrayed them, or when they lost someone who was close to them. Each wall is different. Some are serious and can only be overcome with major life changes, whereas others are more like stumbling blocks that require only a little courage, fortitude, and determination to overcome. Even the same issue is different for each person because of the personal circumstances. But each person can manage the circumstances if he or she has a plan. Brick walls you may encounter along this journey include balancing time between your family, work, and school; finding time to study; and overcoming negativity. How these brick walls affect you depends on you. With the right attitude and a proper plan, you can and will overcome each of the brick walls you will face along this new journey.

O N   T R A C K

You are on track if you can answer the questions Randy Pausch answered in his book *The Last Lecture*[1]:

What was your childhood dream? _____

_____

_____

What did you want to be when you grew up? _____

_____

_____

Give examples of one to three "heroes" in your life. _____

_____

_____

Building the Proper Mind-set

You will need a certain amount of strength and determination to overcome the obstacles that lie ahead of you, but you can do it. The first step toward this success is to put yourself in the right mind-set by creating a positive attitude. Most likely, this task will be the first brick wall you need to overcome, and doing so will not be easy. It will require you to forgive yourself for the times in the past that you have let your brick walls get the best of you. Perhaps you let go of your dreams too easily before or gave up on certain projects when the going got tough. That's okay. It's human nature to take the easiest path when challenged, and letting go of these past "failures" is an important step toward moving forward and overcoming your own self-doubt.

Think about how a real brick wall is built; it takes time for such a wall to be built because each brick must receive a smear of the mortar that holds the wall together. Remember that when you think about your own brick walls. For example, it took you a while to place each brick in the wall you know as "self-doubt." Over time, the "I can't because . . ." brick, the "They told me it wouldn't work" brick, the "It's not the right time for me" brick, and many others were each set in place, held securely together with the mortar you have accepted as truth: a lack of self-confidence that may have grown from the discouraging words spoken to you by previous teachers, family, friends, and sometimes complete strangers. But also remember how quickly a brick wall can be taken apart. One firm impact and the wall can come crumbling down. Today is the day to start taking your brick wall apart so that you can move forward with what you want to do. All you need to destroy your wall of self-doubt is the right amount of self-confidence in your ability to succeed. Sometimes it is hard to knock down a brick wall because we fear the unknown; remember, however, that success can also be in the realm of the unknown. Think of this new opportunity you are about to begin as a chance to start fresh, to become a new version of yourself, to change how people see you and how you see yourself. Do not be afraid to create this new path for your life, one that leads to graduation and your new career. Remember, you can do it!

Motivational Moment

66 Nothing is hard if you break it into small parts. 99

Henry Ford, founder of Ford Motor Company

Once you have overcome that wall, you will be ready to move on and take the next steps that will get you to graduation. Keeping in mind Pausch's determination to have a positive outlook and live life to the fullest should remind you of the importance of maintaining a good mind-set. Remembering each of the brick walls that you have already broken down will also help to build your self-esteem and self-confidence. Take a few minutes to reflect on some of those brick walls. You have probably overcome more obstacles than you give yourself credit for because you are used to listening to the negative voice in your head. Perhaps one brick wall was going back to school. Maybe you had a great conversation with the little voice in your head about that decision; however, you wanted a career badly enough to break through the wall and sign up for classes. Do not forget to give yourself the proper credit for great achievements such as this.

Motivational Moment

66 Luck is what happens when preparation meets opportunity. 99

Seneca, Roman philosopher

A positive attitude is like a favorite pair of jeans: you put it on and it makes you feel great. In some ways, having a positive attitude is as easy as believing that you have one. After all, you are the only person who feeds your mind. Therefore, to have a positive attitude, you need to ensure that what you are feeding your mind is a diet of only positive thoughts. So try on a positive attitude and see how it makes you feel. Start building your positive attitude with the suggestions on this list and later add your own items:

- Start building your positive attitude before your feet hit the floor in the morning. Say "thank you" for the day that you are about to experience, and know that you are going to have a great day.
- Say "good morning" with a smile to everyone in the house. Even if it seems silly, try doing this for a week and see what happens. The good feeling

becomes contagious. Your family might even turn it into a contest to see who can say "good morning" first.

- Make sure to eat breakfast each morning. It is hard to keep a positive attitude on an empty, growling stomach. Even eating something small, such as an apple or a breakfast bar, can make a big difference in how your day goes.
- Get yourself, and everyone else in your household, ready for the day by preparing the night before. For example, performing the following simple tasks the night before can help you avoid stress at the start of your day.
  - Select your clothes the night before to prevent having to stand at your closet in the morning trying to decide what to wear.
  - Gather work papers, homework, and book bags together in one place the night before to make going out the door easier.
  - Put your keys and wallet in a safe place so that you will know where they are and so that you will not forget them when you leave in the morning.
- Smile at the first person you meet after you leave the house. You might not realize this, but smiling uses only 17 muscles and frowning uses 43, so you are really using less energy when you smile. Plus, the good feeling you get from this small energy expenditure will be well worth it!
- Once you are in the car, train, or bus, turn off the negative voice in your head. A key way to do it is to say "thank you" each time you realize that there is something wonderful ahead in your day. Even the not-so-wonderful can be diminished with a "thank you"; do not give your obstacles power over you. Send them packing with a positive "thank you"!

Mentor Moment

Talk about "brick walls." I feel like I was raised by the first single mother in the world. My parents divorced in the 1950s, when the term "single mother" had not even been invented yet. I worked to get good grades because my mother's entire focus during my upbringing was on education, a gift I will never forget and will continue to share with whomever will listen. Tuition was $50 a semester in 1961, and I needed a scholarship in order to pay it. I later graduated and was recognized in *Who's Who Among Students in American Universities and Colleges*. I went on to teach in high school, adult education, and later, vocational schools and colleges. Being poor was a circumstance, not a life-threatening illness, and I overcame it with great success.

Arlene (author) from Fullerton, CA

Once you start kicking your brick walls down, take those bricks and start laying them for your new path to graduation. What better use for the obstacles that have held you back than to put them beneath your feet to remind you each day that you did overcome them and you are a success!

Finding Your "Cheerleaders"

Most likely, you cannot forget the people who have cast doubt on your ability to accomplish your goal of completing your program in the health professions field. But have you taken the time to think about the people who are cheering you on, the ones who know you can finish and are willing to help you every step of the way? As much as you can, you should distance yourself from the people in your life who have caused you to doubt yourself, and you should surround yourself with friends, family members, and others who have been supportive of your decision to pursue this new career. These "cheerleaders" will believe in you and encourage you to keep going, even when you face your brick walls.

Mentor Moment

When students come to me and tell me that they have to quit school because of one problem or another, I tell them about a student I once advised named Maria. Maria had five children. As you can imagine, juggling school and children was quite a challenge for Maria. She came to me one day and told me that she needed to withdraw from her program. When I asked why, she confided that her husband wasn't much help when he came home from work, so she found it difficult to find time to study, complete her homework, and even go to class. I advised Maria to explain to her husband that her classes were not just a hobby and that her new career would make life better for the entire family, but that she needed his support in order to be successful. I was delighted when both Maria and her husband came in to see me and told me that Maria was going to stay in school. In the end, she earned all A's and was one of the best students who ever made her way through our program. So I tell other students, "If Maria could do it, so can you!"

Luisa, a student services director from El Paso, TX

Take some time now and think about who your "biggest fan" is when it comes to your new dreams and goals. Maybe it is your mother or a favorite aunt. This person does not have to be a family member, though; in fact, it might be best to have someone outside that close circle as your best supporter. How do you find that person who truly supports you? Tell your family and friends that you are going back to school and then listen to their questions and comments; their responses will help you find the one person who truly shares and supports your dream. You are about to ask this person to be your "head cheerleader" through this challenging experience, the person you can go to when times get tough and you need a "high five" for encouragement. This person must be someone who will always tell you the truth, not what you want to hear in the moment. He or she must be someone who will give you *constructive* criticism, not just criticism. Be honest with yourself about who this person is. Listen to your heart, and you will know who will support you when you need to hear the truth or words of encouragement or when you need to brag because you have taken a major step that kicked another brick out of your wall. When you graduate, that person will be the first on the invitation list for the graduation ceremony, the first person you call to invite to come see you walk in your cap and gown on graduation day.

O N   T R A C K

Write the names of friends and family members who could be your "cheerleaders." Come back to this list to remind yourself of these supporters when you are facing a brick wall and need to get back on track.

_____

_____

_____

If you feel right now that you do not have enough "cheerleaders" in your life, do not get discouraged and do not feel alone. You will find a strong support system in health professions school. School administrators, including the campus director, director of education, and staff from student services and career services, will support you on your journey to graduation. Your instructors will be concerned about how you learn, what resources you will need to learn, and, of course, whether you attend classes. You will also find other students in your classes who will become part of your support group. Many of these classmates share your goals, and you will be surprised by how many of them are overcoming some of the same challenges and brick walls that you are. The experiences that you share during your education and the accomplishments that you achieve together during your program can become the foundations for new, lifelong friendships. And knowing that you are not alone on this journey will help keep you focused on and motivated toward graduation.

Mentor Moment

My fourth grade teacher taught me that the word "TEAM" stood for "Together Everyone Accomplishes More." This always stuck with me, but it was never more true than when I went to health professions school. I made so many new friends at school, and these new friends became study partners who helped me pass the most challenging tests and learn the most complicated procedures. I was always happy, and grateful, to be a part of that wonderful team.

Ranisha from St. Paul, MN

Support can come from many other sources as well. Until you find your head cheerleader, you might find support in a movie that inspires you, a book that motivates you, or even a CD or YouTube video that gets you excited about life.

Planning Ahead
Understanding the Difference Between a Job and a Career

Do you remember when you were a child and you watched your parents get ready to go to work? Maybe you were even able to tag along with each of them for a day. If so, depending on what kind of work your parents did, you might have been exposed to the differences between a job and a career early on, even though you probably did not know it.

Jobs are just that—they are work, a way for a person to make money. They generally do not require any lengthy training or formal education. Some examples of common jobs include waitress, maintenance worker, and construction laborer. Most likely, you have had a job such as this in your past; maybe you are even working at a job like this now. Jobs such as these are important to keep society functioning. Unfortunately, however, the fact that they do not require a lot of training also means that the people who perform these jobs are commonly paid less than people who have careers. Think of the word "job" as an acronym for "Just Over Broke," meaning that jobs can require a lot of hard work that does not really lead you anywhere.

Careers, on the other hand, lead you down a path that is created by you, your dreams, and your goals. They usually require special training and allow you to build your skills and experience over time. The payoff for this is generally a higher salary and benefits. In some cases, careers are also accompanied by greater security, flexibility, and responsibility. People who enjoy their careers find a sense of personal satisfaction in what they do. Careers offer people the opportunity to challenge themselves, nurture their personal growth, and feel they have made a difference in the world. (See Box 1.1.)

Considering these differences, it might become clear to you why your decision to pursue a career in the health professions field is so important. A career creates a passion that gets you up in the morning and makes you happy at the end of the day. Even more, a career in the health professions field allows you to feel the personal satisfaction of helping others every day. When you feel like you are making a difference in the world, your life has purpose. The joy you will get from helping a baby get well or escorting an elderly person to his room will be

BOX 1.1   JOBS VERSUS CAREERS

This list gives some examples of common jobs, as well as examples of careers in the health professions field. Compare and contrast the examples so that you can better understand the difference between a job and a career.

Common Jobs

- Food service worker
- Cook
- Security guard
- Construction worker
- Janitor
- Telemarketer
- Fast food employee
- Car wash attendant
- Personal care assistant
- Child care helper

Examples of Careers in the Health Professions

- Dental assistant
- Massage therapist
- Medical assistant
- Surgical technologist
- Radiologist technician
- Occupational therapist assistant
- Pharmacy technician
- Physical therapy assistant
- Medical biller and coder
- Hospital admissions clerk
- Health information management professional

its own reward. When you get home at the end of the day and someone asks you how your day was, you will feel great when you are able to smile and respond, "My day was great. I helped someone have a better quality of life."

A health professions education will help open the doors to this new career. What's more, a health professions education opens the opportunity for a career path that will be available to you no matter where you live. Everytown, U.S.A., has clinics, hospitals, and the need for medical personnel. In addition, the careers in this field are growing. As the large population of baby boomers grows older and requires more health care, the need for health professionals will continue to increase. Unlike other jobs, health-care positions continue to be available and grow, even during most economic downturns.

If personal satisfaction is not your only goal, there is no denying that money talks. As previously mentioned, the difference in the pay rate between a job and a career is significant. To illustrate this wide gap in income potential, take, for example, the popular job of food service. According to statistics from the U.S. Department of Labor, Bureau of Labor Statistics, waiters and waitresses make an average of $9.41 per hour.[2] For a person working full-time, that translates to approximately $19,580 annually. Compare that to the average annual incomes made by some common health professions:

- Medical assisting: $29,060
- Medical records and health information (a diverse field that includes the medical insurance billing and coding field): $32,960
- Dental assistant: $33,170
- Massage therapy: $39,850
- Surgical technology: $40,070.

Although these salaries vary with experience and the demographics of your geographic area, this example clearly illustrates the higher income potential that will be available to you with your new career.

Motivational Moment

ff People with goals succeed because they know where they are going . . . it's as simple as that. 99

Earl Nightingale, motivational speaker and author

Visualizing the Future

Now that you know how you got here and how to overcome some of the challenges that lie ahead of you, you can start to focus on your future. Visualizing that future will help keep you on the right path toward achieving your goal. Along the way, you must remember that the only person who feeds your brain is you! Your brain does not know the difference between real and imagined; it only knows the last impression you leave behind. Therefore, visualization is a good way to head in the right direction and stay on track toward meeting your goal— and making sure that you do it all with a positive attitude!

There are lots of ways you can use visualization to keep yourself on track. For example, you can help to create your winning mind-set by envisioning yourself as an "academic athlete." Think of your program as an obstacle course. Now think of all the tests you will have to take, chapters you will have to read, homework you will have to complete, and challenges you will have to overcome as hurdles on that obstacle course. Picture yourself running the course and jumping over each hurdle, one at a time, until you reach the finish line. Imagining yourself at the end of your forthcoming journey should put a huge smile on your face.

Now let's take that visualization one step further. Imagine how you are going to feel on graduation day. Getting your diploma or degree at graduation will make you feel like an Olympic champion receiving a gold medal. Imagine how the scenario will play out, considering all of the details. See yourself on the stage in your cap and gown receiving your diploma. Listen to your crowd of family and friends cheering for you and your success. Picture yourself having your photo taken with your fellow graduates to put in your scrapbook. Imagine the sense of accomplishment you will have as you leave the ceremony and head to your new career, knowing that the future of your family looks brighter because of your efforts to be an "academic athlete." Now keep this visualization in your mind as a vision of the goal you are seeking to achieve.

Another way to keep your goal in mind is to find a picture that represents your future and put it some place where you will be able to see it every day. For example, find a picture of someone performing the duties of your future career and keep that picture on your refrigerator, bathroom mirror, or car dashboard. Then look at the picture or think about it whenever you begin to doubt yourself. It should help to remind you of what your goal is and what it means to you. You can even take this exercise a step further by pasting a small picture of yourself into the image to make the visualization personal. The more lifelike you make the visual, the easier it will be for your brain to see it as reality.

Although the thought of pasting yourself into a picture might sound silly, many athletes, businesspeople, and others who have accomplished great feats have used visualization for years as a technique to improve their performance and achieve their goals. Olympic swimmers see the pool and feel the wall on their hands as they imagine reaching the end of the lap. Professional baseball players feel the ball striking the bat in their hands as they imagine hitting a home run.

Using visualization to succeed is not a secret; you just might not have used it to be successful. However, this process can work for you if you make it a part of your daily habit. For example, take just a couple of minutes each morning to visualize the day ahead of you and anticipate some of the brick walls you will face. See each day as you want it to happen; don't just let it happen. Take control by planning the day in your head and seeing yourself overcome the day's challenges. Of course, you will have days when your old habits return and sabotage your schedule, but keep visualizing. It takes time to ingrain any new habit, so practice, practice, and then practice some more. Once you are able to visualize your future accomplishments in detail, you will be able to call upon the positive energy that those visualizations bring whenever you need to overcome a brick wall.

One way to make the most out of your visualizations is to keep them positive and in the present moment. When you feed your brain its daily diet of positive thoughts, talk about yourself in the present tense, as if you have already accomplished your dream career. Do not use the phrases "I will . . ." or "I am going to . . ." to begin your thoughts; say them as if they have already happened. For example, "I am a successful pharmacy technician." Framing your visualizations in this way helps your mind to see this future as reality.

O N   T R A C K

Go over this checklist to see if you are on track toward your new career. Check off each accomplishment you have already achieved (we've even provided some examples to help you along!):

___ Courage: You showed courage when you picked up the phone to call the school for an appointment to discuss enrollment.

___ Goal: Your goal to make a difference in your life by helping others is clear in your mind.

___ Plan: Your plan is to attend a health professions school to receive the education you need to reach your career.

___ Support system: You have selected family and friends who you know will be honest with you and support your dream each day.

___ Visual: You have selected a picture of your career goal and posted it where you will see it every day.

___ Change and sacrifice: You are willing to change and sacrifice today so that you can achieve your goal tomorrow.

BOX 1.2 TEN PHRASES FOR POSITIVE THINKING

Here are some examples of phrases you can use to feed your brain its daily diet of positive thoughts:

1. I am a successful _____. (insert your profession)
2. I make good money.
3. I provide for my family.
4. I have a job with benefits.
5. I am preparing for a great retirement.
6. I live in my new house.
7. I am driving my new car.
8. I have new clothes.
9. I am going on a vacation.
10. I am getting a promotion.

Marketing Yourself

Now that you are on a path to success, you should start to think about how you will market yourself so that you can find your new career. What does it mean to "market yourself"? It means to communicate to the world who you are and let them know that you will soon be searching for a new career in the health professions field. Just like other forms of marketing, marketing yourself is a way to get your product's name (in this case, you) out there so that people know you exist and will remember you when they have a need to fill a position in your field. When it comes to marketing yourself, you also want to let people know about the skills you possess, your educational background, and your experience. The most common way to do this is via a resume (see Chapter 8 for more information on how to write a resume), but marketing yourself can take place in many different ways and at almost any time (see Chapter 7 for more information on marketing and networking).

Mentor Moment

One day I was standing in line at the grocery store, waiting to check out. I was wearing my medical scrubs because I had just come from class. A woman who was standing in front of me in line turned around and asked me where I was working. I explained that I was still a student. After a short and pleasant conversation, the woman gave me her business card and told me to give her a call when I graduated— she worked at a local medical office. Can you believe it? I called the woman and ended up working at that office after I graduated!

Tanya from San Diego, CA

You should not wait until you are almost finished with your program before you begin your marketing strategy. Start to develop and implement a marketing plan for yourself now so that you can take the time necessary to create a strong foundation for your career search. As you near the end of your program, you will be concerned with studying for exams and passing your national certification. Having a solid marketing plan already in place will decrease some of the stress you would otherwise encounter during this stage of your program. In addition, marketing yourself early could help you land a position even before you graduate. The reality is that you probably have taken out federal loans to help pay for school; in this case, your first payment on those loans is due 6 months after you graduate. That does not leave you a lot of time to find a job. Even if you do not have student loans, the ideal situation is for you to search for positions and interview 1 to 2 months before you graduate. Then you can decide which job you want, complete the new employee paperwork, and begin working right after you graduate.

A good way to begin marketing yourself is to create your own business card. Making a business card is easy. Your school might even have a service that can provide a student business card for you. If not, many common software programs, such as Microsoft Word and Publisher, offer templates that help you to create and print your own business card right on your home computer. If you have a software program such as this, or have access to one in your school's computer lab, just type the words "business card" into the program's help box and then follow the directions provided. When you are ready to print your cards, you can find already perforated card stock, which is relatively inexpensive, anywhere office supplies are sold. A good tip for creating your business card is to keep it simple. For example, see Figure 1.1.

Marketing yourself will also require you to network with other health-care professionals. Once you learn how to recognize them, you will find opportunities to network around every corner. For example, you might network with other professionals in the field when you complete your practicum (see Chapter 11) or at professional society meetings. Many times, practicums help students find their first positions in the health professions field. Your new business card will open the doorway for you for these networking opportunities.

One way to keep track of the details you will need to successfully market yourself is to create a "daily success journal." Just as visualization is a technique you can use to see yourself reaching your goals, journaling is a technique you can use to express and record your ideas, feelings, and planning steps to your goals. If you have never tried expressing your thoughts on paper, journal writing might seem difficult or silly. You might feel like you have nothing to say or that you do not express yourself well. But if you try to write down a little something each day, you will probably find that it becomes easier the more you do it. You can focus your journal writing on your personal experiences or on your hopes and dreams for your future. The best part about journaling is that there is no wrong way to do it. You should write down whatever you are thinking about or feeling.

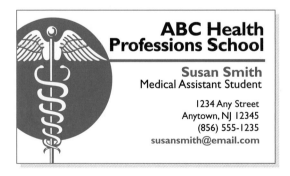

FIGURE 1.1 Sample business card.

Here are some items that you can write about in your daily success journal:

- Your goals
- Your accomplishments
- Your fears
- An experience that made you happy
- A summary of your day at school
- Contact information of people you meet in the field when networking
- Details about yourself that you will need to successfully market yourself.

Putting these items in your daily success journal frees up your mind to focus on other daily tasks, such as completing homework and getting your kids off to school. It also brings all of the elements of your life together in one place, a place to which you can return when you need to be inspired or reminded why you have taken on such a challenging task.

O N   T R A C K

Keep your networking on track by listing three medical offices you or your family members have visited in the last 6 months. Include the name of the doctor, the telephone and fax numbers of the office, the office manager's name, and any other staff members you might know by name. Use this list as the start of your networking list, which you should also include in your daily success journal.

1. _____

_____

_____

2. _____

_____

_____

3. _____

_____

_____

Like personal journals and diaries, your daily success journal should be private so you can write about your dreams, goals, and aspirations without worrying about someone else criticizing you. Remember, your success journal is all about—and all for—you! You should feel free to write about whatever you want in your journal. Free-form writing is the best way to get all of your ideas out. In other words, do not think; just write. You can always review what you have written later. What does not make sense right now may become more logical later in school or in your career.

Rest assured, these exercises are not designed to be hard or easy; they are designed to help you establish, visualize, and accomplish your goals. These assignments could be homework or evaluation questions. Try not to be critical of the assignments because doing so will only waste your time and energy—not to mention put you in a negative frame of mind. Instead, put that time and energy into thinking about and answering the questions as best you can. Also, do not skip assignments because they are often linked together, with one assignment building on the next. If you complete these exercises with true commitment, by the time you reach the end of your program, you will have a resume, reference page, portfolio, and more that you can use for your career search.

Success Journal

1. List all of your current skills in the following categories. Remember to include skills from your daily life, not just your jobs. For example, under "Cash management," you might write "Pay monthly household bills."

Cash management

_____

_____

_____

Computers

_____

_____

_____

Customer service

_____

_____

_____

Problem solving

_____

_____

_____

Supervision

_____

_____

_____

(continues on page 26)

Success Journal (continued)

Telephone

_____

_____

_____

General office

_____

_____

_____

Medical or laboratory

_____

_____

_____

Writing

_____

_____

_____

Specialty

_____

_____

_____

2. Think about what your life is like right now. Now list three reasons that you decided to attend health professions school.

1._____

2._____

3._____

3. Think about what you would like your life to be like after you graduate. List three dreams that you have for what your life will be like with your new career.

1._____

2._____

3._____

4. Using the sample provided in text as an example, create a business card for yourself.

5. Complete the following employment application to the best of your ability. Do not worry if there are sections that you cannot complete. This book is designed to help you build on those gaps as you progress through your program.

APPLICATION FOR EMPLOYMENT

PERSONAL INFORMATION

Date: _____

Name: _____

Address: _____

City: _____ State: _____ Zip: _____

Phone # (H): _____ (W): _____ (C): _____

Email: _____

Social Security #: _____

Are you at least 18?   Yes   No

Are you a U.S. citizen?   Yes   No

If you are not a citizen of the United States, are you eligible for
employment in this country?   Yes   No

Position applying for: _____

_____ in the field of health professions

_____ Full Time
_____ Part Time (include hours available) _____
_____ Temporary

Approximate salary desired: $_____ /year

If employed, when can you start? _____

Have you ever been convicted of a felony?   Yes   No
If yes, please explain the circumstances:

_____
_____

Are you related to anyone employed here?   Yes   No
If so, who? _____

Were you previously employed here or at another division of this company? Yes   No
If yes, where? _____

FIGURE 1.2 Sample employment application.

EDUCATION HISTORY

List any educational instruction, past and present, including business, trade, technical, or vocational school; and extension, correspondence, or evening courses.

Name and Address	Major Course of Study	Diploma/ Degree	Date Attended From	Date Attended To
High School				
Business or Trade School				
College or University				
Graduate/Professional				
Other				

Specialized training:_____
_____
_____
_____

Apprenticeships and skills:_____
_____
_____
_____

Extracurricular activities:_____
_____
_____
_____

Honors received: _____
_____
_____
_____

FIGURE 1.2—cont'd

Continued

REFERENCES

Please provide contact information for three personal references (for example, coworkers, teachers, professional acquaintances).

Name and Address	Occupation	Telephone # and Email Address	Years Known	Relationship	May We Contact This Person?
					Yes No
					Yes No
					Yes No

Submit an extra page to state additional information you feel would be helpful in considering your application, such as your interest in this company and any special experiences, skills, and community service.

EMPLOYMENT HISTORY

Employer name_____ Phone #_____

Address _____

Job title _____ Supervisor _____

Reason for leaving _____

Responsibilities _____

Employed   From_____ To _____ Hourly rate/Salary_____

Employer name_____ Phone #_____

Address _____

Job title _____ Supervisor _____

Reason for leaving _____

Responsibilities _____

Employed   From_____ To _____ Hourly rate/Salary_____

May we contact the employers listed above? Yes   No
If no, which employer do you wish us not to contact? _____
_____

FIGURE 1.2—cont'd

BIBLIOGRAPHY

1. Pausch, R., with Zaslow, J. (2008). *The Last Lecture*. New York: Hyperion.
2. U.S. Department of Labor, Bureau of Labor Statistics. (2009). *May 2008 National Occupational Employment and Wage Estimates, United States*. Retrieved August 24, 2009, from http://www.bls.gov/oes/2008/may/oes_nat.htm#b35-0000

Guidelines for Success

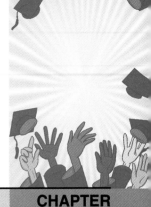

Learning Outcomes

After reading this chapter, the student will be able to:

1. Understand how to create a winning attitude.
2. List and prioritize the new responsibilities associated with starting school.
3. Identify that organization, prioritization, and attendance are the major factors that contribute to being successful in school.

Creating a Winning Attitude

Success in your new career begins with success in your new program. This exciting endeavor is an opportunity to work on increasing your self-esteem, learning new skills, and becoming ready for the reality of a health-care career. No matter what your past experiences have been, this experience is a new opportunity for you to be successful.

Your new education plan has a picture of success at the end. That picture is of you in your cap and gown at graduation surrounded by family and friends. How are you going to make it down that road to graduation? You will take it one step at a time. In conjunction with the other textbooks and resources your school offers you, this book will offer the skills you need to stay in school and succeed. This chapter has been designed to take your brain cells on an adventurous trip that will provide ideas on how to develop a winning attitude, solve problems, and create opportunities for a successful career. All you need to do is to be open to the suggestions you find; try them on once or twice and see how they work for you. Not all of the suggestions provided will work for everyone, but you will not know which ones will work for you unless you try them. So, starting now, tell your brain to open the door to the suggestions in this textbook and enjoy the adventure that they will bring. Some of the information will be refreshing, exciting, and, maybe, a little confusing the first time you read it. In addition, each student will face his or her own challenges along the way. Following certain principles can help improve your chances of success and make the journey to graduation a little smoother. The first guideline for success is to have a winning attitude—and the first step toward having a winning attitude is to think positively!

Motivational Moment

66 It's not whether you get knocked down; it's whether you get up. 99

Vince Lombardi, former NFL football coach

Feeding Your Mind a Diet of Positive Thoughts

To be successful, you must have faith in yourself. If you believe in what you want to accomplish, you are much more likely to achieve those goals with a positive attitude. As mentioned in Chapter 1, your mind knows only what you tell it. Therefore, you must be sure to tell it that you are going to be successful in your new career. The importance of having a positive outlook cannot be stressed enough. A direct correlation exists between the amount of positive energy you have and the success you will achieve in your program. Think of it this way: If you have a positive outlook on what you are trying to accomplish, you are more likely to believe that you can do it: this means that you will spend less time coming up with reasons why you will not be able to do it and fretting about how you are going to feel when you fail. Negativity requires a lot of energy, as it keeps you constantly thinking and being afraid. That same energy can be better spent accomplishing the tasks that will assist you in reaching your career goal.

Positive thinking could even be good for your health. Optimists are more likely to live longer, happier, and healthier lives. They are also less stressed and more successful and productive in life. Positive thinking can energize you, whereas a negative attitude can fog your head in a "cloud of depression" that prevents you from meeting your daily tasks, not to mention your long-term goals. A can-do attitude creates momentum that can help you to move through your day with ease and even overcome the difficult parts of your day.

For some people, having a positive attitude is hard work. Even if you could just buy a positive attitude for 5 cents, you would *still* find people who would tell you they could not afford a positive attitude. People have a tendency to get themselves stuck in ruts of negative thinking, especially when they do not get the support they need or are surrounded by the negative attitudes of family and friends. But what does that negative thinking accomplish? How many times have you had a negative thought and found soon after that it had become reality? You thought, "I feel like I am getting sick," and then you did get sick. Or you thought, "I know I am going to fail," and then it happened. In these instances, your negative mind was controlling your actions and producing the outcomes that you expected. Why not take this opportunity to reverse those thoughts and instead say, "I am healthy, and I can live a life where I am successful"? This type of thought can assist you in being successful. If you find it difficult to turn off the negative thoughts, remember that a positive attitude is something you create. It takes practice and a lot of focus, but once you get the hang of it, you will no longer find it to be hard work. Instead, you will be stuck in a rut of positive thinking, where the only downside will be that you cannot help but feel good and happy. What a concept!

When you believe that you can succeed, you have already overcome one of the hardest hurdles. Henry Ford said it best: "If you think you can, you are right; if you think you can't, you are right." When you do not believe in yourself, you set yourself up for failure by not attempting to accomplish new goals and by not trying your hardest when you do. Believing in yourself and your ability to succeed will also help to motivate you. Think of this change of mind-set as a "mental makeover" that will make the new life that awaits you all the more attainable.

Motivational Moment

66 Every possibility begins with the courage to imagine. 99

Mary Anne Radmacher, American writer and artist

Your mind will believe what you tell it. Now is the time to open up your mind and believe that you can do it. If you have not done so already, now is the time to start saying, "Yes, I can do it!" This phrase was the positive affirmation, or mantra, suggested in Chapter 1. However, if that does not work for you, try the phrase, "I **am** going to graduation!" When negative thoughts return, shout this phrase in your mind: "I **am** going to graduation!" Keep in mind that these phrases are only suggestions. Your positive affirmations are a key element of creating a winning attitude, so you should try to come up with statements that apply and make the most sense to you. It's important to remember, however, to state your affirmations in the present tense and in a positive way. The more you can repeat these positive affirmations to yourself, the better off you will be. Think of it this way: if you are constantly feeding your mind positive thoughts, the negative ones do not have a chance to get in.

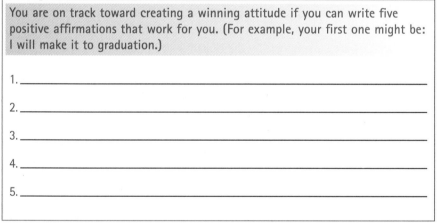

O N   T R A C K

You are on track toward creating a winning attitude if you can write five positive affirmations that work for you. (For example, your first one might be: I will make it to graduation.)

1. _____

2. _____

3. _____

4. _____

5. _____

The key to making the most of this opportunity is to not choose failure. Why pick failure when successfully reaching your goals has a much better feeling and reward? In fact, take this approach instead: failure is not an option. You cannot allow yourself to fail for so many reasons.

- You need to prove to yourself that you can do it.
- You need to show others that you can do it.
- You have already invested so much that it is not wise to turn back.

Failure is not an option. Knowing this, you have no choice except to go forward with a winning, positive attitude. Tell your mind that this is the path that you are choosing to take—the path to success. Start creating your new attitude by saying, "Yes, I can do it!" and visualizing your success now. Visualizing where you want to be and having a plan for how you are going to achieve it will definitely keep you on track.

O N   T R A C K

You are on track if you can make the visualization of your future real by creating a vision board. A vision board is a visual representation of what you want to accomplish. In other words, it is a collage of pictures and items that, to you, represent your commitment to reach graduation and your new career. Start with a piece of poster board and a glue stick. Then find pictures and other items that represent your future:

• Your success in school (such as some letter *As*)

• Your future career (for example, write yourself your first paycheck)

• Your future life (such as a picture of a new house or car).

Have fun, and do not limit your thinking. Remember, positive thoughts generate positive energy and events.
   See Figure 2.1 for a sample vision board.

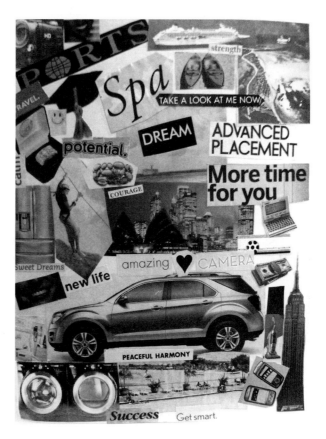

FIGURE 2.1 Sample vision board.

Motivational Moment

66 Every thought we think is creating our future. 99

Louise L. Hay, motivational author

Remember that your success does not end at your graduation. Rather, graduation is the beginning of your new lifetime of success. In your new career, you will receive praise for the great job that you do, for the responsibilities that you take on, and for the lives that you change. Your self-esteem will reach new heights in your new career.

Mentor Moment

My vision board looks a little bit like the game board for The Game of Life. It has the road that I plan to travel along. I started out with pictures of books because I knew that I would need to focus hard on my studies to make the rest of my vision board come true. Then I make my way to graduation. A graduation cap flying high in the air said it all for me. From there, I plotted out all of the wonderful things my new career will bring me and my family, like a new apartment where my kids can have their own bedrooms and, later, a new home with a big garage where I can park my brand new car!

Jennifer from Staten Island, NY

Positive thinking not only benefits you, it could also benefit the other members of your family. If you have children, you should remember that they are learning from your example. A poor attitude commonly rears its ugly head as low self-esteem, which is likely to rub off on your children. In addition to the daily affirmations that you give yourself, be sure to encourage your children to reach for their goals. Give praise at the dinner table or when you tuck your kids into bed. Praise goes a long way in building self-esteem. The praise you give and the example you set will be catalysts that will help your whole family choose success over failure moving forward.

Motivational Moment

66 Setting an example is not the main means of influencing another; it is the only means. 99

Albert Einstein, German physicist and Nobel Prize winner

Setting Realistic Goals

In this new journey, you will be challenged to be the best you can be and have the opportunity to set higher standards in your life. In the classroom, you will be graded on your performance—not your potential. Everything you learn will assist you in obtaining the skills that you will need to qualify for your new career in the health professions field. Remember, this new endeavor is an opportunity for you to recreate yourself and achieve all of the goals that you never thought you could. For example, at a vocational institution or community college, you might find that you can achieve good grades for the first time in your life. Success is an opportunity that is available to everyone.

The key to being successful throughout this process is remembering that you are now in control. You selected this new career field, which allows you to set higher standards for your own achievement. Although you should aim for your highest potential, you should also remember to set realistic goals that will keep you motivated with positive energy and will keep you from disappointing yourself. Remember that you do not need to be perfect. Setting your expectations too high is usually bound to lead to disappointment. If you are realistic about the goals that you set for yourself, you are more likely to achieve them. Do not set yourself up for failure. Understand your own personal limits, but know that it is possible to achieve your highest potential. When you do your best, you will feel great, which will feed your positive attitude and give you energy to accomplish more in life. Once you experience the excitement of achieving your goals, such as getting good grades and achieving new accomplishments, you will not want to stop. The sky is the limit for you when you perform like a winner.

Mentor Moment

I was a horrible student in high school. I graduated, but just barely. After being out of school for a while and working at a dead-end job, I decided to enroll in a vocational school. I didn't expect much and was surprised when I earned my first A. That motivated me to keep earning good grades, and I was amazed at how well I did. You never know what you can do until you study in a program you chose and like.

Sylvia from Myrtle Beach, SC

To understand how to set realistic goals, you must first understand that there are two types of goals:

1. **Short-term goals:** Short-term goals can be defined as immediate tasks that you want to accomplish.
2. **Long-term goals:** Long-term goals are the tasks that you want to accomplish in the future, perhaps 1 year or 3 years from now.

These goals are closely intertwined, and long-term goals cannot be achieved without successful focus on and completion of short-term goals. Short-term goals help you decide what you must accomplish each day, for example, "For homework, I must read Chapter 2 of *How to Survive and Maybe Even Love Health Professions School.*" Accomplishing this short-term goal is just one part of the necessary steps you will need to take to accomplish your long-term goal of graduation. Long-term goals give you purpose and direction, whereas short-term goals direct your immediate plans and actions and serve as the means for arriving at your long-term goals.

A goal, long-term or short-term, should have four major components. It should

1. be a statement of what you want to have, be, or do;
2. be realistic . . . something you can achieve;
3. be specific; and
4. be measurable.

You have the responsibility to define with realistic detail the goals you want to accomplish.

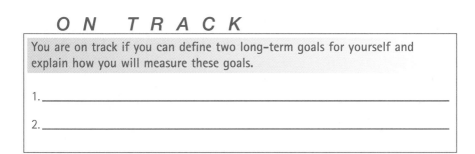

ON TRACK

You are on track if you can define two long-term goals for yourself and explain how you will measure these goals.

1. _____

2. _____

Getting Back on Track

Although feeding your mind a diet of positive thoughts will go a long way toward helping you achieve your goals, you must remember that things do not always turn out as expected. No matter how much you try, unpredicted obstacles are bound to occur. So what happens, for instance, when you fall off your diet and let negative thoughts into your mind? The answer is that you must simply pick yourself up and get back on track again. You must put aside those worries, tell yourself to think positively, and renew your faith in yourself. Even if you don't believe it at first, continuing to tell yourself to think positively will cause it to be true. However, there's no denying that this might be difficult for you. Like stopping most other bad habits, turning off negative thoughts is not easy. If it were *easy*, more people would have a positive attitude.

Positive thinking does not mean that you will always expect everything to work out or go your way. Anticipating that things are going to go wrong makes the situation more manageable when they do. However, having a positive outlook can help you to better prepare yourself for those negative events and keep you from dwelling on them afterward. Overcoming the challenge quickly is a key to staying on a positive track.

Something positive can come from every situation, so the other thing you should remember to do when something does not work out as planned is to put a positive spin on the situation. One way to do this is to add an "at least" statement to the situation. For example:

- I did not get all of the questions correct on my quiz, but *at least* I know which areas I need to review more closely for the exam.
- I did not receive all As, but *at least* my attendance is perfect.
- I do not have much money this week, but *at least* I have groceries for the week.
- I really need to do the wash, but *at least* my family has clean underwear for the next 2 days.
- I was late for school today, but *at least* I made it to class.

A good positive thinker can be realistic about a situation and at the same time not get too down about it, realizing that the experience offers a chance to learn how to do better the next time and creates a better, stronger person in the end. Your positive attitude will also become the foundation for the next attitude you will need in the health professions field—discipline.

Perhaps you are already wondering, "How can I think positive thoughts when I worry about going to school, taking care of my family, working, completing my homework, and handling all the other events that life brings?" Start with the basics. First, pause and take a deep breath. Then, remind yourself that the process of creating and thinking positive thoughts begins by telling your mind each day that you will be successful. Choose one of your positive affirmations and, in a calm and disciplined manner, repeat it to yourself three times, focusing only on that affirmation and the positive energy it brings.

Another way to keep yourself on track mentally is to create for yourself a CD or playlist of inspiring or happy songs. Call it "Songs for Success" or "Songs that Make Me Smile." The song "I Will Survive" has gotten many a heartbroken woman (and man) through some terrible times. So start thinking about songs that inspire you, represent who you are, or just simply make you happy. Listening to these songs whenever you start to think negatively or feel down will help to distract you from the negativity and remind you of your goals.

Mentor Moment

My personal happy songs have gotten me through some tough times. "Higher and Higher" by Jackie Wilson, "If You Wanna Be Happy" by Jimmy Soul, "Your Smiling Face" by James Taylor, and "Ob-La-Di, Ob-La-Da" by the Beatles are among my favorites. I can't help but smile when I listen to these classics.

Jaime from Jenkintown, PA

O N   T R A C K

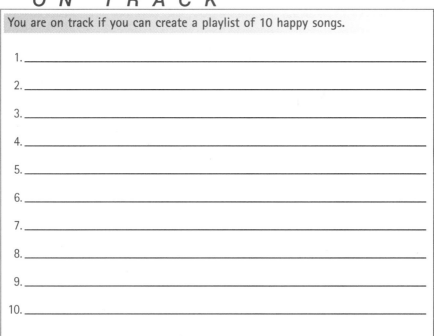

You are on track if you can create a playlist of 10 happy songs.

1. _____
2. _____
3. _____
4. _____
5. _____
6. _____
7. _____
8. _____
9. _____
10. _____

Combating the Negativity of Others

Depending on your situation, you might find as you begin your journey to graduation that you are surrounded by people who do not support your new goals. The negativity of others can confuse your mind and cause you to fall off track, especially if you listen to it and internalize it.

The truth is, not everyone sees the benefits of positive thinking. People who think negatively commonly believe they are being realistic about life and that positive thinkers are just lying to themselves. Even if you are surrounded by people who think like this, you must realize that thinking positively in any circumstance increases the chances that you will succeed. The longer you try and harder you work at a goal, the more likely you will succeed. That is just simple logic.

One simple step that will help you move toward your "mental makeover" is to be sure that you are surrounding yourself with people who believe in you and support you: your cheerleaders. Even more, you should surround yourself as much as possible with people who also have a generally positive outlook on life. Listening to the negativity of others can make you think negatively and feel inferior without even knowing that you are allowing it to happen. In some cases, others' negativity might not even be directed toward you, but surrounding yourself with such negativity still has a harmful impact on how you feel about yourself and your ability to change your life. Think of it like this: If you are on a diet but you surround yourself with junk food, most likely you are going to give in at some point and binge on that junk food, especially when you see everyone else eating it. You need your brain to keep focused on the diet of positive thoughts that you are feeding it. So, keep your cheerleaders on your sidelines and stay away from "opposing team members" as much as you can. If you find yourself surrounded by negativity, you might need to find new friends so that you surround yourself with positive and supportive people who fit your new lifestyle. (See Chapter 3 for more information on meeting new people.)

O N   T R A C K

You are on track if you are realizing that you must surround yourself with positivity. List three places or ways for you to meet new people.

1. _____

2. _____

3. _____

Of course, avoiding negativity is not always possible. That's why it is essential for you to combat this type of thinking with positive thoughts. You might not be able to do this all on your own, but don't worry; the pages of this book are filled with the inspiring words of many great motivators. Think of them as your own personal cheerleaders from now on. Also, many great minds have spent lots of time thinking of ways to help motivate people; you might find some of their approaches useful as well (see Box 2.1).

Another way to combat the negativity of others is to prove them wrong by showing them that you are successful. You have earned this chance, and when you achieve your successes, you should show them off. For example, post your test papers on the refrigerator for the entire family to see that you are achieving good grades. Keeping the A that you earn on your first exam in plain sight will help you prove to others and remind yourself that you are a success. Remember

---

BOX 2.1 THE GREAT MOTIVATORS

There are many great motivators, and each person has his or her own favorites. Here is a list of just a few, including some of the books that they have written:

- Rhonda Byrne
  - *The Secret*
  - *The Power*
- Dale Carnegie
  - *How to Win Friends and Influence People*
- Dr. Wayne W. Dyer
  - *How to Be a No-Limit Person*
  - *Inspiration: Your Ultimate Calling*
  - *Excuses Begone: How to Change Lifelong, Self-Defeating Thinking Habits*
- Spencer Johnson
  - *Who Moved My Cheese? An Amazing Way to Deal with Change in Your Work and in Your Life*
  - *The Present: The Gift that Makes You Happy and Successful at Work and in Life*
  - *Peaks and Valleys: Making Good and Bad Times Work for You*
- Eckhart Tolle
  - *The New Earth: Awakening to Your Life's Purpose*
  - *The Power of Now*
- Zig Ziglar
  - *Better than Good: Creating a Life You Can't Wait to Live*
  - *Conversations with My Dog*
  - *Something Else to Smile About: Encouragement and Inspiration for Life's Ups and Downs*

that each of these small accomplishments is also a step in disassembling your brick wall and creating a new path to graduation.

Motivational Moment

66 No one can make you feel inferior without your consent. 99

Eleanor Roosevelt, former First Lady of the United States

Preparing for New Beginnings and Responsibilities

Returning to school can be a tough assignment, and preparation is always the best way to approach an opportunity for change. You are about to become an "academic athlete." Start to prepare for that role by visualizing yourself as a star performer, reaching new heights academically to achieve your goals. Breaking old habits and learning new ones is part of your new job of being a health professions student. These changes will be necessary in order for you to succeed in this new venture and your future career. The first habit you must break, negative thinking, has already been discussed. However, you will experience many more changes along the way as well.

Have you ever seen the television program *The Biggest Loser*? This show deals with personal transformation and the personal sacrifice required to achieve that goal. The contestants all begin the program significantly overweight, with most weighing in between 250 and 400 lb. Over the course of the program, each contestant undergoes sweat, tears, and frustration as he or she tries to lose the greatest percentage of body fat. The contestants all enter the contest with a common goal: to lose weight and improve their lives. However, each contestant hits his or her own brick wall at some time during the program, feeling as if success cannot be reached. When this happens, another contestant always reaches out to give support. That other contestant encourages his or her teammate, and with the help of this new friend, the contestant does not give up and moves ahead toward his or her goal. The contestants' transformations are always amazing.

You are starting on a similar journey to transform yourself, and you will meet new friends, mentors, and teachers along the way who will give you the encouragement you need to complete your transformation. At some time during this journey, students will hit a personal brick wall that might leave them feeling as if their goals are out of reach. When that happens, another classmate, an instructor, or an administrator will be there to reach out and offer support. With the help of your new support system, you will continue to push on and move ahead toward graduation. These new allies become an integral part of the amazing transformation you are about to undergo. You just need to remember to be open to and accepting of this transformation because it will create the new positive attitude you need to help you to achieve your goals and stay on track toward graduation.

You might be worried that you are too old or set in your ways to undergo such an amazing transformation. If so, you would be wrong. In fact, you have already begun your transformation by enrolling in your health professions program. Now, you just need to work toward and be accepting of the other changes that go along with creating a positive attitude and becoming a success.

Dressing for Your New Role

Your process of change starts with presenting yourself in a professional manner. How you dress is an important part of your new professional life. Start to prepare for this transformation by doing some research:

- What do those in your new profession look like?
- What changes will you have to make?
- Will it require personal change?
- Are you ready for those changes?

Looking professional starts on the first day of school, when you dress to set the new standard for your future. Do not panic about this change. Your school will have specific guidelines about what you can and cannot wear. Following a dress code might even be a part of your grade. You will probably be expected to wear medical scrubs starting as early as orientation or by the end of your second week of class (see Figure 2.2). Your scrubs could be included as part of your tuition or you might be asked to buy them yourself, depending on the educational institution you are attending. Be sure you read your school's catalog to understand and ensure that you are complying with your educational institution's expectations regarding professional dress code requirements. (See Box 2.2). Taking a positive approach toward any modifications your school requires is the first step to becoming more professional for your new career. The best way for you to test your compliance is to ask your instructors. Most of them have probably been in the health professions field for years, and they can give you some wonderful real-life recommendations, examples, and references.

Although your educational institution's regulations may be stricter than those of your future new workplace, go with the flow. Your educational training will teach you the *highest* standards so you are prepared for the toughest settings. The medical profession can be a regimented arena that deals with helping people

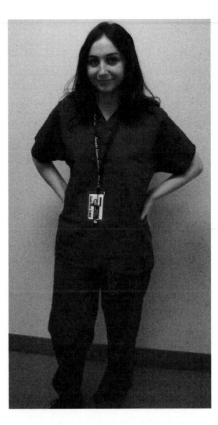

FIGURE 2.2 Scrubs.

BOX 2.2 WHAT TO WEAR AND WHAT NOT TO WEAR

Here are some general guidelines for what postsecondary educational institutions find acceptable and unacceptable for a professional appearance:

- **Jewelry:** Jewelry such as facial piercings, tongue rings, and large hoop earrings may be considered unprofessional and may pose safety threats to you or the patients for whom you will be caring. Prepare to remove these items before you begin your program, but remember that you can wear them when you are not in your scrubs.
- **Makeup:** Makeup should be applied in a way that makes you look healthy, attractive, and professional. That means applying it lightly and blending it in a way that enhances your natural features. Heavy or brightly colored makeup is not appropriate. If you are uncertain about whether your makeup is okay, ask yourself, "Do I look like I am ready to go out on a Saturday night?" If your answer is "yes," then your makeup is probably not appropriate for the health professions field. If you need help with your makeup, cosmetic departments in department stores commonly offer free makeup sessions by appointment.

(box continues on page 48)

BOX 2.2 WHAT TO WEAR AND WHAT NOT TO WEAR (continued)

- **Nails:** Keeping your nails neat, clean, and short will be a requirement in most medical offices where you work directly with patients. Dirt lives and breeds bacteria under your fingernails, and the only way to really keep them clean is with a fingernail brush. Some medical offices will provide a fingernail brush for you to use while washing your hands. Keep your nails no longer than fingertip or ¼ inch in length and avoid wearing acrylic nails.
- **Heavily scented perfumes:** Both men and women should avoid wearing heavily scented perfumes and colognes because they can be offensive, nauseating, and irritating, especially to people who have allergies. If you are going to wear perfume or scented lotion, be sure to use one that has a soft fragrance and use it only in moderation.
- **Personal care:** Although hygiene routines vary by culture, you should shower, brush your teeth, and use deodorant every day to look and feel fresh. During class, you may be asked to work closely with classmates. If you do not take care of your basic hygiene needs, you might produce an odor that offends your classmates and makes them avoid talking or working with you. Even if you are not aware of your own bad odors, your classmates might be. These practices are also important when you work in the health professions field because you will be working very closely with patients, sometimes reaching over and across them and getting very close face-to-face. Caring for your own personal hygiene on a daily basis promotes a comfortable school and work environment.

get well and caring for people in life-and-death emergencies. If you cannot follow the easiest of dress code rules, how will you be able to follow the other rules one must follow in the health professions field? The changes that your school asks you to make are to help you to complete your transformation and achieve your goals. In addition, many of the rules have patient safety issues behind them. For example, health-care providers wear scrubs because scrubs do not have buttons, zippers, or frills that can lead to accidents in the health professions field. Once you understand the reasons behind your educational institution's dress code rules, you are more likely to find it easier to comply with them. Furthermore, making small changes to your appearance, such as wearing scrubs and removing jewelry while in school or on the job, is a small price to pay to change your life. And remember, you still have the option to wear your jewelry when you are not in school or at work. Comply with your facility's regulations rather than creating a situation that puts you in an impractical uphill battle. The price for not complying with these straightforward requirements simply is not worth it. Sadly, your education may be put on hold if you do not comply with your institution's dress code.

Now is the time for you to undergo a mental makeover for the best reason you have ever had: to make a dramatic change in your life. Even if you change your appearance initially for the sake of your school, you will soon find that your new appearance will improve how you feel about yourself. Although it may be hard to believe, new clothes, different makeup, and a haircut can change people from the inside out. Just be sure that your dress is professional, and understand the differences between dressing for work and dressing for an evening out on the town.

Mentor Moment

When I met Malcolm, he really lacked confidence. Because he had a hearing problem, he was always quiet and never wanted to attract attention to himself. One day, however, he couldn't help it. He walked several blocks to school each day, and one rainy day he arrived soaked. His instructor stopped class when she saw that he was dripping wet. She brought in a dry pair of scrubs for him before returning to her lecture. Malcolm had never had anyone pay so much attention or show so much concern for him, and that simple gesture made a monumental impression on him. It increased his motivation to succeed in his program and transformed him from a quiet, shy student to someone who is now making a difference in the health professions field.

Teri, a campus director from Skokie, IL

You can expect this transformation to continue to occur throughout your education as you gain a better understanding of what is expected of you and what your new responsibilities are. With these changes also come new levels of self-confidence that you might not have expected. All of these changes will contribute to you being able to see yourself in the health professions field more clearly than before.

Preparing for the First Day of School

Believe it or not, the day will arrive when you are rushing to get things together for your first day of school. Most likely, you will feel a little nervous, wondering how your first day will go. If you have children, you already know what that first-day-of-school energy feels like. If you do not have children, maybe you can remember the feeling from your own childhood. It is a unique blend of nervousness, anxiety, and anticipation for the exciting new experience that awaits you.

Being prepared for that first day includes making sure that you have the normal back-to-school supplies, such as pens, pencils, paper, notebooks, and an appropriate backpack or book bag. Many different types of book bags are available. Think about which one will best fit your needs. For example, you might choose a bag on rollers that will help you to prevent straining your back. Also, be sure to choose one that is big enough to fit all of your books and that will help you to stay organized. Being able to keep everything in one place and organized can reduce stress.

Starting with the first day of school, you should also begin developing a routine that will help you to prepare for each day. Placing important items, such as your wallet, keys, homework, and books, in the same location each day will help to make getting out of the house easier. Depending on the time of your class, you might want to bring a snack or small meal. If you have children, just prepare something for yourself while you prepare their meals. Organizing yourself in this manner will save you time, not to mention preserve some of your sanity, because you will not waste time wondering if you have forgotten something.

One way to get through the first day of school is to remember that you are not alone. You will not be the only nervous person sitting in class. Think about the people you met at orientation. Today is the first day for everyone, and many people are nervous about the big changes they are making in their lives, just like you. Talking to other people as you wait for class to begin is a good way to keep your mind from worrying, not to mention a good way to meet new people. Who knows, the first few people you meet may become part of your new study or support group.

Getting to Know Your Instructors and the Classroom

One advantage of attending an educational institution like yours is that you have a complete faculty and staff ready to assist you in reaching your goals. The most prominent members of this staff in your education will be your instructors, who you will encounter 4 to 5 days each week, whether in class, online, or both. Most accreditation agencies require your instructors to have worked in the health professions field for a minimum of 3 years after their graduation. You will find that most instructors exceed that minimum, having returned to education after years of service to give back and help you graduate.

Your instructors have been hired to teach you the details of your new career. Some of the language, processes, and procedures will be new to you.

At times, it might seem as if your instructors are speaking a foreign language, and in fact, they are. This new language is the language of medical terminology. Before you can be successful in the health professions field, you must learn this language, which is spoken in medical offices, hospitals, and clinics. You will not only need to learn how to say the names of diseases, treatments, medications, and other medical terms, but you will also need to learn how to spell them and what each of them is.

- Medical assistants need to know diseases, disorders, signs and symptoms, and more because each patient's file contains a detailed medical history.
- Medical billers and coders must be familiar with surgical procedures so that they can correctly enter the procedure completed by the physician into the computer and generate an accurate bill.
- Dental technicians must know the names of each tooth as well as the names of diseases of the mouth and gums.

The concept of learning a new language might seem overwhelming, but keep in mind that everyone who works in the health professions field started out by learning medical terminology.

Motivational Moment

66 Take the attitude of a student: never be too big to ask questions, never know too much to learn something new. 99

Og Mandino, motivational speaker and author of
The Greatest Salesman in the World

To get the most from your time in class, have an open mind and a desire to learn. Remember that the time that you are spending in class is an *investment* that you are making in yourself. You must be sure to get the biggest possible return on your investment by taking your classes seriously. Take notes so that you can review the lecture information later on, such as when you are at home completing your homework. Also, do not be afraid to sit up front and ask questions. Asking questions is not a sign that you are stupid or do not belong in class. On the contrary, it shows your interest in the material and your desire to better yourself by understanding the information being presented. Even more, unanswered questions can lead to frustration after class when you are trying to do your homework. Asking the question of your instructor and getting a quick answer can be a timesaver when you go home to review the material. If you are too shy or do not have a chance to ask the instructor during class, you can also seek your instructor's advice before and after class. Making an appointment will ensure that you have quality one-on-one time.

Motivational Moment

66 The wise man doesn't give the right answers, he poses the right questions. 99

Claude Levi-Strauss, French anthropologist

But remember, even instructors do not always know *all* the answers. Certain issues and questions can best be addressed by other members of the staff (see Box 2.3). In addition, the health professions field is a wide one that is constantly changing, with new medications and treatments being developed and even new cures and diseases being discovered all the time. Keeping up with these developments will always be a part of your continuing education throughout your career.

BOX 2.3 FINDING HELP AROUND CAMPUS

Here is a directory of the departments and staff members who are available to help at most health professions schools:

- **Administration office**—Campus director/president: You might want to visit the administration office if you encounter a problem or have a concern that cannot be addressed by your instructor or the education department.
- **Admissions department**—Admissions director or manager: You should visit the admissions department if you need help completing the admissions process or encounter any issues with your admission process.
- **Business department**—Business manager: You might need to visit the business department to make your tuition payments and receive your books and scrubs, if these tasks are not handled by another department or office at your school. Many schools do not have business departments on campus.
- **Career services/placement department**—Career services director or manager/ placement director: This department can also assist you in developing and proofreading your resume, practicing your interviewing skills, and assist you in finding employment after graduation.
- **Education department**—Director of education (DOE)/academic dean; student services manager or director; registrar: This department consists of a number of staff who are available and willing to assist you with different concerns you might have during your education, including issues with attendance, transcripts, grades, and academic probation. The staff in this department is also able to help you cope with any personal challenges you might encounter while attending school, such as balancing school, family, and work schedules. When you have any issues that could prevent you from attending classes or making it to graduation, you should visit the education department. If you are required to complete a practicum as part of your program, you will need to visit the education department for assistance in finding a practicum. You will

BOX 2.3 (continued)

also direct any questions or concerns you have during your practicum and turn any practicum paperwork into this department as well. The DOE or academic dean coordinates and supervises the education department as well as the other campus faculty and staff.
- **Financial aid department**—Financial aid director or manager: If you have any questions concerning your school payments, financial aid, loans, or grants, you should visit the financial aid department.

Being Successful in School

At this point in your life, one of your long-term goals should be to graduate from your health professions program. Succeeding in school will require you to use your positive attitude to stay focused on your studies, attend class every day, and achieve good grades. You must understand the importance of and commit to achieving these short-term goals in order to put yourself on the path to success.

Sometimes people never reach their highest potential for a variety of reasons:

- They do not take charge of their time.
- They were never taught how to prioritize daily activities.
- They were always procrastinators.
- They are always helping others first.
- They make others more important than themselves.

If one or more of these situations applies to you, do not worry. There are skills that you can learn to move you past these brick walls. There is never a right age for learning how to create a better life for yourself, there is just a right time. *Now* is the right time! You have taken a major step in your life by enrolling in a program in the health professions field and deciding that graduation is now your major long-term goal. Now you must learn to do what it takes to achieve that goal.

Focusing on Your Studies

Achieving your goals will require you to keep yourself focused on your studies. Making your studies a priority in your daily life can be a hard task, especially if you have spent most of your life thinking about other people. Although you might find it difficult to do, you must put yourself first sometimes when you are going to school—and putting yourself first means taking time to focus on your studies. Doing so will probably require you to sacrifice some other activities. However, if you sacrifice now for your family, you will reach your goal of a new career. Remembering that you have reprioritized your goals for the time being in order to achieve something better for your entire family later on should help you to stay focused on your studies.

Learning to focus is not an art form; it is a form of organization. If you are organized and have your priorities in order, then you can study stress free and get the most out of your study time. You can use certain methods to keep your tasks organized and maintain your focus on the task at hand (see the section Making Time for School later in this chapter). However, keeping focused is no easy task no matter how organized you are during the day. It requires you to not only keep all of your tasks prioritized but also to keep your mind off other things when you should be focused on your studies.

As mentioned in Chapter 1, one way to unclutter your mind and keep yourself focused on your studies is by journaling. If you have never tried it, journaling can be refreshing. You will be surprised how thoughts just start pouring out of your mind once you give them an opportunity and have a space to write them down. First, you can write down any problems you are having. Putting these problems in your journal frees your mind from them, allowing you to focus on other tasks at hand. You can also "dump" any negative thoughts you have in your daily journal and then forget about them. Journaling also helps you to keep your goals in front of you. You can list your goals and then write why they are important to you. Last, you can use your journal to keep track of important people, places, and events. Putting these important parts of your life on paper will ensure that you do not have to worry about forgetting them. Daily journaling will allow you to start each day fresh and without unnecessary "mind baggage" pulling you down. By putting not only negative thoughts but also positive affirmations in your journal, you will also keep yourself on the path to developing a new positive attitude.

Motivational Moment

66 People often say that motivation doesn't last. Well, neither does bathing—that's why we recommend it daily. 99

Zig Ziglar, American author and salesman

Understanding the Importance of Attendance

If you take away only one thing from this chapter, it should be this: class attendance is crucial. Whether you are taking classes online or at a campus, you must attend class in order to learn the information that you need to succeed in the health professions field. Missing 1 day of class at a postsecondary educational institution is not like missing 1 day of class in high school. In high school, you had one class for 1 hour two or three times per week. However, in health professions school, you will attend class for 4 to 5 hours a day of concentrated lecture, computer lab, or clinical lab on one subject. It is thanks to this academic style of learning that you will graduate in months instead of years. However, also because of this, missing *1 day of class at a postsecondary educational institution is equal to missing 1 week of academic information.* That is a lot of information to fall behind on and have to make up, and trying to do so generally causes people to fall further behind. You must let your commitment to your education serve as a reminder that you must attend class every day.

Class attendance is important not only because you will need to learn the information covered but also because future employers may review your attendance record. Future employers know that educational institutions track your daily attendance, and they may look to your attendance record to learn more about what type of employee you will be. Being in class each day shows both the school and your future employer your level of commitment and dependability. A potential employer might even ask you about your attendance and follow up the conversation by verifying your attendance record with the school. If you regularly attend classes, your attendance record can be something to talk about with pride during your interview. It might even prove to be a deciding factor for employers hiring in a tough economy.

Class attendance requires you to not only show up for each class but also to be on time, pay attention, and stay for the entire class. Here are some suggestions for you to get the most out of your class attendance:

- Make it a habit to arrive to class on time—that means, arriving at least 5 minutes before class is scheduled to begin.
- Promptly return to the classroom after any breaks or lunch periods.
- Strive not to miss any classes. Instead, earn perfect attendance awards that you can add to your graduate portfolio.
- While you are in class, remember to stay focused on the lecture by freeing your mind from your other concerns.

Remember that you are attending class for you; it is no longer enough to show up simply to get the checkmark that you were there. You must take advantage of the knowledge that is being passed on to you in class by paying attention and maintaining focus.

The new habits that you develop with regard to class attendance will transfer to your new position in the health professions field. Instructors, employers, and supervisors are always looking for employees with a good record of accomplishments when it is time for awards, promotions, and even raises. They seldom reward individuals who were late, absent, or always leaving a few minutes early. Avoiding these poor habits will benefit you in school and in your career.

Perfect attendance should be your goal, but an occasional absence is sometimes necessary. If it is absolutely necessary for you to miss a class, you might need to do the following:

- Call the school beforehand to notify them of your absence.
- Notify your instructor beforehand and, if necessary, leave a message on voice mail.
- Call the registrar and explain why you will not be in school.
- Contact the school's website and get your lecture notes and homework.
- Review your lesson plan calendar for the material being covered in class.
- Call a classmate to confirm any material and class activities you missed.

Review your institution's catalog for the specific procedures you must follow if you need to be absent.

O N   T R A C K

You are on track if you realize attendance equals graduation. To show your commitment to attend class, read aloud the following attendance commitment pledge:

"I pledge to be on time to class each day and to stay for the full lecture, including clinical lab and computer skills, and to not leave until class is dismissed by the instructor."

Now write the above pledge in the space provided here and show your commitment to it by signing it with your full signature.

_____

_____

_____

_____

_____

_____

Getting Good Grades

The importance of getting good grades is obvious. Good grades show your instructors and future employers that you understand the information that you learned and can apply it to complete the tasks that are required of you in your new career. Your mastery of medical information, terminology, and laboratory skills is crucial in the health professions field because it will allow you to make a difference in other people's lives. Knowing that you will someday have such an important impact on others should be a strong motivating factor to get you up each morning with a positive attitude and keep you striving to get good grades.

It does not matter what your grades were like in high school. Each person brings with them past educational experiences that can be used to their benefit in a new health professions program.

- Maybe you sailed through high school. Learning just came easy to you because you were lucky to have wonderful teachers who taught you basic skills in your early education. You will need to continue to build on your basic skills to have continued success in your health professions program.
- Maybe you did well in high school, but you had to work hard for your diploma. People struggle with basic learning skills for different reasons. Maybe you were out sick in elementary school and never quite caught up. Maybe you needed glasses, but no one realized it until you were in third grade. Maybe you were just too shy or afraid to ask questions. If you had to work hard, that determination will continue to serve you well in your health professions program.
- Maybe you never finished high school and went back to earn your GED. You need to acknowledge that it took determination for you to complete that GED. Reach back and find that courage again to keep you focused on and committed to graduation. This is a new opportunity in which you have the chance to show yourself and others what you can do.
- Maybe you are an ability-to-benefit (ATB) student who does not have a high school diploma or a GED. You had to test for and qualify to enter your health professions program just like everyone else. Your courage is strong because you realize now that education is the only path to a career. Dramatic events in your life might have kept you from reaching your goal of a diploma, but you now have found the courage to improve your circumstances.

Whatever your past educational experiences were, health professions school is an opportunity for you to have a brand new start, where good grades and a positive attitude are within your grasp. You can do it! It will require hard work to achieve your goal of a new career, but everyone begins health professions school with a clean record that allows them to start over and make of it what they want.

Getting good grades starts with your attendance in class. You also cannot get good grades without studying for your quizzes and exams. Grades depend on not only devoting time to study but also ensuring that the study time you put in is *quality* study time. Spending some time to prioritize and organize your life is a way to start creating quality study time. Selecting the time and place to study is important and having your mind free to focus is even more important. Many students spend their study time "spinning their brain cells" and not really learning anything because their minds are not free to focus.

Your final grade might also be determined by your behavior and participation in class. The more you participate, the more you learn. This learning will also translate into good grades. Class participation involves paying attention in class, asking questions, and possibly even joining a study group. You will also be assigned class projects in which interaction with your classmates will be part of your grade. Creating a positive attitude toward these group experiences will give you a higher energy level that will help you to contribute most to and get the most out of them.

Remembering a new translation for your ABCs will provide you with a simple way to achieve grades that will make you feel proud:

- *Attitude:* As previously mentioned, you might need to give yourself a mental makeover to ease your transition to your new classroom environment. You need to think like a winner, an academic athlete, to reach your highest academic level ever. If you need a visual to complete your mental makeover, think about the Blue Angels, the U.S. Navy's flight demonstration team. They perform graceful aerobatic maneuvers at high speeds with only a few feet between each plane. One of the Blue Angels' sayings is "Attitude = Altitude." Your new attitude will take you to a new altitude of academic achievement. It is now time to aim for a high GPA.
- *Behavior:* Your behavior is considered a part of your classroom participation, and it usually counts as part of your grade, sometimes as much as one-third or one-fourth of your grade. Therefore, an easy way to improve your grade is to exhibit professional behavior and classroom participation. To understand why your behavior in class is so important and what kind of behavior your professors expect of you, stop and think about the medical offices you have visited. Professional behavior in these situations is about customer service—for example, how you were greeted and treated as a patient. Remember that as an employee, your responsibility will be to serve the customer, the patient. Respect is the main factor in good customer service. Start your customer service practice during your program by being respectful of your instructors and other classmates. (See Box 2.4 for some basic rules to follow while in class.)
- *Commitment:* Your level of commitment to your education is up to you. Because of the steps that you have already taken to get into your program and the sacrifices you have already made, that commitment to achieve your goals should be great. It should also be the same level of commitment that you give to your attendance in your new program. Why enroll in school, pay money for an education, and then not make a commitment to get the most out of every day? Doing so would be like ordering a five-course meal at a restaurant and then eating only part of it—you paid for the entire meal, so you should not just get up and walk away without enjoying dessert.

BOX 2.4   CLASSROOM RULES

Following these simple suggestions during class will help you not only get good grades but also prepare for and practice the behavior that will be expected of you in your new career:

- Be on time to class.
- Come to class prepared with paper and a pen to take notes.
- Participate and ask questions.
- Do not talk when the instructor is lecturing.
- Do not talk when another student is asking a question.
- Focus on taking notes.
- Be respectful of others in class and during breaks.
- Dress appropriately for class each day.
- Do not use foul language.
- Do not yell.

O N   T R A C K

You are on track if you have made a personal commitment to achieve a specific grade point average (GPA). A GPA of 4.0 means that you will get all A's; a 3.0 means all B's; and a 2.0 means all C's. Using your new interpretation of the ABCs as your guide, consider what GPA you are willing to work toward and write it here: _____.

Making Time for School

As discussed in the previous section, your ability to be successful in school depends on how well you can focus on your studies, how committed you are to attending class, and whether you can achieve good grades. And all of these factors, in turn, depend on how much time you are able to commit to your studies. Finding the time not only to attend class but also to study and complete homework outside of class will be challenging, especially if you have a family and are working full- or part-time. These tasks can be particularly challenging if you are taking online courses, which might require you to have an even greater sense of responsibility and commitment to your goals.

To find the proper time required for you to be successful in school, you will probably need to organize a schedule for yourself (and your family, if applicable) and create a routine that allows you to have quality study time. This planning step is a crucial part of your overall success. Proper planning reduces stress, helping you to improve your attitude and keeping you focused when you study. In addition, it will ensure that the time that you do get to spend with your family is quality time.

Organizing and Prioritizing

The best way to make time in your schedule for studying and to free yourself to truly focus while you are studying is to get yourself organized. From the time you wake up in the morning until your head hits the pillow, you should have your activities organized so that they maximize the time that you have—for yourself, with your family, and for your studies. When your personal life runs smoother, you can study stress-free and retain the information that you are studying, which helps to improve your scores on tests and quizzes.

There are several ways to organize and prioritize your daily activities:

- ***To-do list:*** At the end of each day, take time out to write yourself a "to-do list" for the next day. The list should include every goal that you want to accomplish that day, including chores such as shopping and homework that you need to complete. Remember, these are your short-term goals. You can keep your to-do list in a small notebook or on a 3" × 5" index card. You can organize your tasks either in order of their importance or in the order in which you will need to complete them during the day. For example, you might organize them under general time slot headings, such as the following:
  - Before work
  - During lunch
  - After work
  - After dinner

You should keep a copy of your list with you at all times so that you will remember what you need to get done and can cross off items as you complete them. Doing so will give you a feeling of accomplishment. Turn those moments into "Woo-Hoo moments" in your day. Acknowledging the importance of these moments and congratulating yourself for them will help keep you motivated for similar accomplishments. (See Figure 2.3 for sample to-do lists.)

Before work	During lunch	After work	After dinner
* Call Mom	* Buy bread	* Attend study	* Read Ch. 4
* Mail get-well	* Pick up clothes	group @ 2:30	* Do laundry
card to Aunt Lois	at cleaners	* Make cupcakes	
	* Make dentist	for Madison's class	
	appointment	* Write sick note	
		for Jason	

FIGURE 2.3 Sample to-do list

Motivational Moment

  66 The way to get started is to quit talking and begin doing. 99

Walt Disney, American animator, entertainer, and philanthropist

- *Call-Write-Do list (CWD list):* Another way to stay organized is by using a modified to-do list called a call-write-do list. Take a sheet of notebook or typing paper and fold it in thirds or draw two vertical lines to form three sections. Add headings to each section. The first, "Calls," will be for the people you need to call, anyone from a friend or classmate to a repairperson. The second section, "Write," is for anything you need to write, such as projects for school, letters, applications, and notes to the teacher. The final section, "Do," is for the things that you need to accomplish in the next day or the next week. List all of the things you must do to keep your life from getting out of control. Keep the paper with you in a folder or on a clipboard so that you can refer to it as you go through your day. And remember to cross off tasks as you complete them so that you can feel the sense of accomplishment you deserve. (See Figure 2.4.)
- *Daily planner:* Another way to stay organized is to use a daily planner. You can find daily planners at any office supply store or general merchandiser. In

Call
* Dentist to make appointment
* Mom

Write
* Sick note for Jason

Do
* Mail get-well card to Aunt Lois
* Attend study group @ 2:30
* Pick up clothes at cleaners
* Buy bread
* Wash laundry
* Read Ch. 4
* Make cupcakes for Madison's class

FIGURE 2.4 Sample call-write-do list

addition, many portable electronic devices, such as phones, now offer electronic planners that you can use to organize your time. Most are divided into either hour or half-hour time segments. You can use a planner to organize your time and create reminders of important events, such as test and quizzes, as well as the tasks that you need to accomplish each day. For example, you can sit down each night and list the things on your planner that need your attention the following day. Your list can be general or more detailed to meet your family's needs. If you find it helpful, list everything from getting yourself ready when you get up in the morning, to getting your kids ready for school, to attending class, to quality time with your family. You can indicate specific times to ensure that you stay on schedule or just allot certain time frames so that you know how much time during the day the task will take. Just remember to be realistic about your time if you have young children at home. Being this specific about your time will help you to see at a glance when you have too much going on and when you have free time that can be used for studying. (See Figure 2.5 for a sample daily planner entry.)

March 31 - April 6

31 Monday		1 Tuesday		2 Wednesday	
7:00		7:00		7:00	
7:30	Call Mom	7:30		7:30	
8:00	Mail get well-card to	8:00		8:00	
8:15	Aunt Lois	8:15		8:15	
8:30		8:30		8:30	
8:45		8:45		8:45	
9:00	Class	9:00	Class	9:00	Class
9:15		9:15		9:15	
9:30		9:30		9:30	
9:45		9:45		9:45	
10:00		10:00		10:00	
10:15		10:15		10:15	
10:30		10:30		10:30	
10:45		10:45		10:45	
11:00		11:00		11:00	
11:15		11:15		11:15	
11:30		11:30		11:30	
11:45		11:45		11:45	
12:00		12:00	Make dentist	12:00	
12:15		12:15	appointment	12:15	
12:30		12:30		12:30	
12:45		12:45		12:45	
1:00		1:00		1:00	
1:15		1:15		1:15	
1:30		1:30		1:30	
1:45		1:45		1:45	
2:00		2:00		2:00	
2:15		2:15		2:15	
2:30		2:30		2:30	Study group
2:45		2:45		2:45	
3:00		3:00	Pick up clothes at	3:00	
3:15		3:15	cleaners	3:15	
3:30		3:30		3:30	
3:45		3:45		3:45	
4:00	Buy bread	4:00		4:00	
4:15		4:15		4:15	
4:30		4:30		4:30	
4:45		4:45		4:45	
5:00		5:00		5:00	
5:15		5:15		5:15	
5:30	Dinner	5:30	Dinner	5:30	Dinner
5:45		5:45		5:45	
6:00		6:00		6:00	
6:15		6:15		6:15	
6:30		6:30		6:30	
6:45		6:45		6:45	
7:00	Write sick note for	7:00	Do laundry	7:00	Make cupcakes for
7:15	Jason	7:15		7:15	Madison's class
7:30		7:30		7:30	
7:45		7:45		7:45	
8:00	Read Chapter 4	8:00		8:00	
8:15		8:15		8:15	
8:30		8:30		8:30	
8:45		8:45		8:45	
9:00		9:00		9:00	

FIGURE 2.5 Sample daily planner entry

O N   T R A C K

You are on track if you can write down your activities for 1 day. Be sure to include school, work, and family activities.

6:00 a.m. _____

6:30 a.m. _____

7:00 a.m. _____

7:30 a.m. _____

8:00 a.m. _____

8:30 a.m. _____

9:00 a.m. _____

9:30 a.m. _____

10:00 a.m. _____

10:30 a.m. _____

11:00 a.m. _____

11:30 a.m. _____

12:00 p.m. _____

12:30 p.m. _____

1:00 p.m. _____

1:30 p.m. _____

2:00 p.m. _____

2:30 p.m. _____

3:00 p.m. _____

3:30 p.m. _____

4:00 p.m. _____

4:30 p.m. _____

5:00 p.m. _____

5:30 p.m. _____

6:00 p.m. _____

6:30 p.m. _____

7:00 p.m. _____

7:30 p.m. _____

8:00 p.m. _____

8:30 p.m. _____

9:00 p.m. _____

9:30 p.m. _____

10:00 p.m. _____

Although a daily planner is the best way to keep track of routine tasks, you might also find that you want to be able to see your commitments on a more long-term basis so that you know what is ahead of you. In this case, you might want to keep a weekly or monthly planner. Although these types of planners are not very useful for managing daily activities, they do allow you to keep track of more long-range goals and commitments, such as tests, quizzes, and reading assignments. At the beginning of your semester/ module, your instructor might even pass out a monthly calendar that indicates lectures, tests, quizzes, reading, and homework assignments. You can keep this calendar or you can transfer the important tasks to your daily, weekly, or monthly planner. No matter which type of planner you use, the goal will be the same: to keep track of all of the tasks you need to complete in order to make time to study.

- *Family boxes:* Another way to keep yourself organized that is especially help-ful if you have a family is to use "family boxes." Create a box for each of your children by labeling a shoebox or small basket with the child's name, or make the creation of the boxes a family event and let everyone design his or her own box. Then, make it part of your children's routine to put important papers that need your attention, such as permission forms, announcements, and teacher notices, in their boxes when they get home from school each day.

Keep the boxes in the kitchen or near the front door so that you will remember to take care of these items before you go to bed at night. After you have reviewed, signed, or placed your stamp of approval on each item, put them into the child's book bag. Remember to mark important events, such as class trips and talent shows, in your daily planner so that you will not forget them. This organization method will not only save you time, but it will also leave you feeling good knowing that you and your children are ready for each day.

Use these ideas for organizing yourself and prioritizing your daily activities as foundations upon which you can build, adding your own twists to meet your needs. They will help ensure that all of your tasks and chores get done, although maybe not at the same pace you would have completed them before you started your career program.

O N   T R A C K

You are on track if you can commit to choosing one of the organizational methods above and trying it out for the next week. You might find that the method you choose does not work for you, but do not worry. The next week, you can try a new method. The goal is to find a tool that will help you accomplish your goals by keeping you organized.

List two choices you would like to try:

1. _____

2. _____

Creating a Routine

When you are going to school, you will find it important to create a routine that will allow you to have some quality study time. Although you might not realize it, you probably already have a routine for certain times of the day. For example, your morning routine might involve waking up, brushing your teeth, showering, and eating breakfast. When you come home from work or school, your routine might involve checking your personal e-mail, making dinner, and working out. Your routine could be very casual, or it could be crammed full of household chores. Your new challenge is to fit quality study time into your normal routine.

Motivational Moment

66 Begin with the end in mind. 99

Steven Covey, author of **The Seven Habits of Highly Effective People**

If you have children, creating a routine will be even more important. In fact, you are probably already aware of how a routine can make your day go more smoothly and how unexpected events, such as a child getting sick, can make your whole world come to a stop. The trick for you will be to work your new school-related responsibilities into your routine if you have one. If you do not already have a routine, this is the time to create one. Developing a routine for your family will help you to establish some stability by having a schedule for meals, homework, bedtime, and even quality time. Even if your day still seems chaotic, rest assured that "organized chaos" is better on your nervous system because you always have a foundation to which you can return when things get out of control.

As applicable, plan a routine that works for both you and the other members of your family. Mornings are usually most hectic, so focus on this time first. By creating a routine, you can reduce some of the stress that goes with accomplishing morning activities and getting everyone out the door. The more organized you start your day, the more you can accomplish during your day. In addition, how you start your day will help to create the attitude you will carry with you for the rest of the day. If you have children, your attitude will also carry over to them and shape how their days will go. Knowing that everyone in your household is beginning their day with a positive outlook should give you the energy you need to make it through the day and also have enough energy left over to study when you get home!

Evenings are a close runner-up in terms of their hectic nature. Plan to keep evening chaos to a minimum by creating routines for homework, dinnertime, and bedtime. You might also consider making downtime a part of your routine by allowing yourself to watch one television show each night or by allowing your children a scheduled amount of time for using the computer, playing video games, watching television, talking on the phone, or texting after their homework is completed.

Dinnertime is probably one of the most important parts of your routine, especially if you have a family, because preparing for and eating dinner will probably consume a lot of the time you have when you get home from work or class. Consider making dinnertime special by gathering the entire family around the table. As a family, you can plan the next day or the upcoming weekend during the dinner conversation. You can also encourage everyone to talk about their days, the good and the bad. Make dinnertime a "safe" time to discuss problems as a family by establishing a rule that no one gets in trouble for sharing his or her day. Doing so will encourage your children to be forthcoming and honest and will also allow you to discuss family problems in a productive manner. If your children report that they got in trouble during the day for inappropriate behavior or something else, consider discussing the following:

- Why they behaved the way they did
- How they feel about their actions now
- Whether they are proud of their actions
- Whether they think you would be proud of how they behaved
- What other behavior they could have chosen under the circumstances
- What they will do the next time a similar situation occurs

This simple method of discussing problems and issues can benefit everyone in the family. Your children will feel good knowing that they will not get in trouble for sharing their days. Younger children will listen to the suggestions and learn from them as well. Everyone should get a good night's sleep feeling that family problems were shared and discussed in productive way. And all of this means that you will have less stress and more quiet, uninterrupted, quality time to study later on in the evening.

As previously mentioned, homework should be a priority for everyone in your family. Keeping up with your children's homework can seem like a major chore when your children need your attention and help. This is another area in which creating a routine can be helpful. Start with a homework schedule that works for everyone, setting time aside after school or after dinner for each child to complete his or her homework. Establish a routine that works for the entire family and for each individual child. After-school activities and the ages of your children will play a major role here.

One good idea is to have a homework session once everyone gets home. Your children can sit at the kitchen table or in their rooms and start on their homework while you get dinner ready. You can also use this time to address the items in your family boxes, reading school announcements and signing papers. After dinner and before bedtime, you can check your children's homework and go over it with them. Start with the youngest child first because he or she will have the earliest bedtime. You might want to make a family rule that no child can watch television, play computer games, or use cell phones until you have reviewed his or her homework.

Knowing that your children have completed their homework will give you a chance to study stress free later on. Make sure that you include uninterrupted study time into your daily routine. Although your routine will probably involve you focusing on your homework after everyone else has gone to bed, you might also be able to work small study sessions into your evening and nighttime routines. For example, you can review your flash cards or answer workbook questions while you are making dinner and your children are completing their homework. These small study sessions might not seem like a lot, but if you incorporate them into your routine, you will find that they add up. Just be sure to save activities that require more focus, such as reading assignments, for your uninterrupted study time, when the children are in bed or early in the morning before they get up.

O N   T R A C K

You are on track if you can agree to the following commitment to make study time a part of your routine:

I pledge to study for __ hours per day every day. I choose the following times during my day that work for me and my family to meet that commitment:

Signature: _____

Planning Meals

Creating quality study time will require you to be inventive when it comes to the other daily tasks and responsibilities that require your time. You need to squeeze as much time as possible from these activities. Saving time can start with meal planning, which really includes planning, shopping for, and cooking meals. These tasks can be time-consuming, even for a family of one. Proper meal planning can save you not only time but also money.

Motivational Moment

66 The most remarkable thing about my mother is that for 30 years she served the family nothing but leftovers. The original meal has never been found. 99

Calvin Trillin, American journalist

Planning

Start by creating a meal plan or menu, where you write down what you plan to make for meals each day. You can create this menu in a notebook or, better yet, put it on a calendar that is hanging where everyone in your family can see it.

Although planning a menu will require a little time, it will also save you time later on, and it will allow you to keep your mind focused on your other tasks during the day. For example, you will be able to focus on what your instructor is teaching in class instead of worrying about what you are going to make for dinner that night. Here are some suggestions for making the most of meal planning for each meal of the day.

Breakfast

As you have probably heard a million times, breakfast is the most important meal of the day. A healthy, well-balanced breakfast can set the stage for a focused and productive day that you approach with a positive attitude. Eating breakfast every morning can also help you fight off the "ten o'clock hunger monster," which commonly leads to consumption of nonnutritious, sugary snacks around midmorning.

Because breakfast is so important, it requires and deserves the same planning as dinner. When you have a plan for breakfast, you are able to start your day with just one less item on your "worry list." The peace of mind could also make your nighttime study time more productive because you will not be worried about how you are going to start your next day. Certain breakfast items, such as fresh fruit, can be prepared the night before to make your mornings less hectic. Based on your personal preferences, budget, and family situation, breakfast can range from homemade meals to unwrap-and-eat convenience items. (See Box 2.5.)

BOX 2.5   BREAKFAST IDEAS FOR ANY SCHEDULE

Quick Breakfasts

- Instant oatmeal
- Instant waffles
- Cold cereal
- Yogurt with fruit, nuts, or granola

On-the-Go Breakfasts

- Breakfast bars
- Nutrition bars
- Granola with dried fruit or nuts

Create-and-Freeze Breakfasts

- Scrambled egg burrito
- English muffin sandwich with fried egg and cheese
- Toasted waffle and jam sandwich

BOX 2.5 (continued)

Weekend or Slow-Morning Breakfasts

- Pancakes (add fruit for a special treat or add jam to create colored pancakes)
- Scrambled eggs with sausage or bacon
- Eggs in a basket (Cut a 1-inch round hole in the middle of a slice of bread, place it in a buttered pan, and then break an egg in the hole and fry it; add more butter and turn the bread over to finish cooking.)

Mentor Moment

Raising three children on my own meant that I needed to make mornings run as smooth as humanly possible. That was hard, though, because each of my children went to a different school. I decided to reduce my morning stress load and household chaos by organizing breakfast into a schedule:

- Monday started the week with cold cereal.
- Tuesday was toaster waffles.
- Wednesday was freshly scrambled eggs.
- Thursday was instant oatmeal.
- Friday was cold cereal.
- Saturday was pancakes.
- Sunday was a pick-your-favorite cereal day.

Planning breakfast in this way definitely saved me time because I always knew what was for breakfast and what I had to buy when I went shopping.

Lorrie from Albuquerque, NM

O N   T R A C K

You are on track if you can list five quick and easy breakfast ideas that will work for your family.

1. _____

2. _____

3. _____

4. _____

5. _____

Lunch

No one in your family can work or learn on a hungry stomach, so it is important that you continue building on the positive energy you create with your morning breakfast by planning a nutritious lunch. If your child's school has a lunch program, you might not have to worry as much about this meal, as the menu will be planned for you. If that's not the case, however, there are some things that you can do to make preparing lunches easier:

- Premake peanut butter and jelly sandwiches using a loaf of bread at a time, wrap the sandwiches individually, and freeze them. You can take a large glass and cut the crust away by placing the glass over the sandwich and pressing down hard until the crust falls away. They will look just like those Uncrustables sold in the stores. If you take them out of the freezer when you pack your children's lunches in the morning, they will thaw and be ready to eat by the time your kids have lunch at school.
- Take 1 hour during the week to prepare nutritious snacks to add to lunches. Cut up fruits and vegetables and then portion them and other snacks into snack bags. Spray with lemon juice to keep a fresh color.
- Prepare more than you need for dinner so that *you* have leftovers that you can pack for lunch.

The main focus of these ideas is to prepare as much as you can beforehand so that putting lunches together in the morning or at night is easy, which maximizes your study time.

Dinner

Meal planning for dinner can also help save you time and money. As with all of your meals, the key to successful dinner planning is to be creative. One suggestion for creative dinner planning is to plan a week of dinners based on one item. For example, for ground beef week, you can make burgers, tacos, spaghetti and meatballs, and chili mac and cheese. For chicken week, you can make baked, fried, and broiled chicken and chicken salad. Get the idea? Planning meals around a single main ingredient makes meal preparation and shopping easier.

One way to approach planning your menu is to browse the store ads to see what is on sale and base your meals around sale items. You would be surprised at how easily you can come up with new and interesting meals by looking at supermarket circulars to see what is on sale. If you have children, you should also always keep certain staple foods in the house, such as hot dogs, chicken nuggets, and grilled cheese ingredients. That way you will know that you always have something to make that your kids will eat. (See Figure 2.6.)

Monday	Tuesday	Wednesday	Thursday	Friday	Saturday	Sunday
	1 Tacos	2 Sloppy Joes	3 Pasta w/meat sauce and salad	4 Pizza	5 Nacho salad w/leftover taco meat	6 Mac & cheese with sausages/ hot dogs
7 Baked chicken breast w/spinach and potatoes	8 Roasted chicken legs w/rice and carrots	9 Chicken and spinach salad & grilled cheese sandwiches	10 Chicken burritos	11 Fast food	12 Chicken tacos	13 Hot dogs
14	15	16	17	18	19	20
21	22	23	24	25	26	27
28	29	30	31			

FIGURE 2.6 Sample dinner menu

Even if you plan meals around a single item or sale items, occasionally you will probably need a break from cooking some weeks. Do not be too hard on yourself if you find it necessary to buy some of the convenience foods offered at your supermarket. For example, many supermarkets now sell hot, prepared foods, such as roasted and fried chicken, macaroni and cheese, fried potatoes, and soups. Some even sell interesting prepared vegetables, such as creamed spinach and curried vegetables. Most have salad bars where you can create a healthy side salad to accompany your meal. Or you can pick up some pizza crusts with all of the fixings and make a fun evening out of it by including your children in the meal preparation. Making pizzas together not only makes meal preparation easier for you, but it also creates quality family time together. The possibilities for healthy, easy-to-make meals are endless. (See Box 2.6.)

Motivational Moment

66 What lies behind us, and what lies before us are small matters compared to what lies within us. 99

Ralph Waldo Emerson, American poet

BOX 2.6 EASY-TO-MAKE DINNERS

- Tacos with beef, chicken, turkey, or fish sticks
- Pinwheels (take buttermilk biscuits or crescent rolls and roll them like a cinnamon roll with leftover taco meat or spaghetti meat sauce)
- Pigs in a blanket (roll smoked sausages or mini hot dogs in crescent rolls)
- Frozen chicken nuggets and french fries
- Catfish and hushpuppies
- Hot dogs with special toppings, such as cheese, bacon, tomatoes, or chili
- Salad with special toppings, such as shrimp, cranberries, sliced almonds, cheese, avocados, beets, eggs, carrots, and bell peppers
- Tostadas with beans or different shredded meat, cheese, lettuce, and tomatoes
- Macaroni and cheese with hot dogs
- Frozen bagged stir-fry meals

Although you should not rely on fast-food restaurants to do your meal planning, you might also find it necessary sometimes to pick up a quick dinner from one of these establishments. A fast-food dinner might even be a special treat for a Friday or Saturday night. The key to eating food from places such as this is to choose wisely. Most fast-food restaurants now offer healthy, low-fat options on their menus, such as grilled chicken wraps and salads.

O N   T R A C K

You are on track if you can list 1 week's worth of main dinner ideas that would work for your household.

Monday: _____

Tuesday: _____

Wednesday: _____

Thursday: _____

Friday: _____

Saturday: _____

Sunday: _____

Mentor Moment

I always write out my weekly menu and put it on the refrigerator by Saturday morning. That way, I can check out what I have in the cabinets and see what I need to get from the store when I go shopping. I also save time and money when I go shopping because I know exactly what I need to buy, and I don't buy extra items on impulse. Best of all, no one ever asks, "What's for dinner?" because the answer is right there on the fridge!

Neela from Columbus, OH

Shopping

Making the most of your shopping time and money comes down to creating a shopping list. You can save time and money when you shop with a planned menu and grocery list because you know exactly what you need and you will not buy extra items on impulse. Saving even just $5 per week on your groceries can add up over the course of a year ($5 per week $\times$ 52 weeks = $260). Although creating a grocery list takes time, in the end it helps to create stress-free dinner-times and more focused study time later on.

How you go about creating your shopping list will depend on how often you go shopping. Your list should begin with all of the items you use on a regular basis, such as milk, eggs, toilet paper—whatever items your family cannot do without during the month. You might need to walk around your house or apartment to determine what you buy on a regular basis. Once you have a list of these items, you can figure out how often you need to buy them and add them to your shopping list accordingly. You will probably need to purchase some of these items each time you shop, but others might be necessary only every other week or once a month. For example, if you buy toilet paper in bulk, you might need to add it to your shopping list only once a month. Because of this, you might want to plan out your shopping for these basic items on a monthly basis. Planning in this way has several advantages. It can help you to save money by letting you see in advance which items you need to buy. You can also buy items in bulk or stock up when they go on sale.

Once you have your monthly shopping list ready, you can use each week as the basis for your weekly shopping lists. Before you go shopping, look at your meal plan for the next week and add to the shopping list any items that you will need to make the meals you have planned. Be sure to check your shelves or pantry to see what you already have so that you do not buy anything that you do not need. (See Box 2.7 for more money-saving shopping tips.)

> **BOX 2.7** TIPS FOR SAVING MONEY WHILE SHOPPING
>
> - Cut coupons from circulars or weekly papers.
> - Download coupons from the Internet.
> - Buy fruits and vegetables that are in season.
> - Buy generic or store brand items.
> - Buy what is on sale.
> - Cut out items that do not contribute to the well-balanced nutritional value of your meals.

Cooking

There are also ways to save time and money when it comes to cooking meals. For example, you can cook more than one meal at a time and then just reheat them throughout the week. Cooking one-pot meals is also a good idea. In fact, a slow cooker could be your best cooking utensil when you are going to school. All you need to do is place some type of meat, vegetables, and potatoes in the slow cooker and let them cook all day long while you are at work or school. When you get home, you will have a delicious meal waiting to be served. An added benefit is that you have created more time to study after dinner.

Sharing Responsibilities

Coming home to a household full of chores is hard after a long day at work and school. Another way you can create quality study time in your day is to share with others the daily tasks that you must accomplish. Asking family members to share in household responsibilities, such as dusting, vacuuming, feeding pets, washing dishes, taking out the trash, and washing and folding clothes, is a good way to get these routine chores done more quickly, allowing you to have more stress-free study time. It is also a good way to relieve some of the stress you might feel. When your home is in order, you will have an easier time focusing on your reading and homework assignments.

As part of your support team, your family members should be happy to help. In fact, going to school might even give you an opportunity to ask for more help around the house, which you might have needed for a while. Remember that, as a family, everyone should be involved in sharing the household chores. Your significant other could understand that school is now a major priority in your life and should be willing to show his or her support by taking on a few more responsibilities around the home.

If you have children at home, you might tend to do things for them because you think it is faster. But you should remember that including them in household tasks teaches them responsibility and boosts their self-esteem, which helps them to become independent, self-sufficient, responsible adults. Think of it as teaching your children survival techniques. If you have older children, you might already be asking them to undertake certain household chores, such as making beds and cleaning up toys. Do not leave out the little ones, though. Younger children are usually eager to help out, and although you may need to oversee them and they will not always meet your standards at the beginning, as they grow older they will learn how to independently complete tasks in a satisfactory manner. The earlier you can start sharing the responsibility of chores with your children, the more helpful and successful they will be, and the more you can raise the level of responsibility your children have, the more study time you will create for yourself. And throughout that process, you can turn the time you spend with them completing chores into quality time together. (See Box 2.8.)

BOX 2.8   LETTING EVERYONE HELP OUT

Depending on how old your children are, you have probably already begun to teach them some responsibility. Even at an early age, you model good behavior for your children by washing their hands, making meals, and putting away their toys, books, and clothes. Allow them to share in family responsibilities by assigning daily chores. Just make sure that the chores you assign are age appropriate. Here are some ways that children of any age can share in family responsibilities.

Toddlers

- Cleaning up toys
- Helping with laundry (such as matching up socks)

Preschool-age children

- Cleaning up toys
- Getting dressed
- Brushing their teeth
- Feeding pets dry food
- Putting clothes in the hamper
- Dusting
- Stirring food in a bowl when cooking

(box continues on page 78)

BOX 2.8 LETTING EVERYONE HELP OUT (continued)

School-age children

- Picking up toys
- Getting dressed
- Folding clothes
- Setting the table
- Raking leaves
- Emptying wastebaskets

Adolescents

- Cleaning their rooms
- Making their beds
- Doing their own laundry
- Making lunches (for themselves and for their younger siblings)
- Preparing dinner
- Cleaning bathrooms
- Putting away dishes
- Taking out the trash
- Shoveling snow

The best way to ensure that everyone shares responsibility for household tasks is, yes, to create another plan! When you have a plan, you know that as long as everyone sticks to the plan, everything will get done. As a family, you could sit down and develop the plan together. This gives everyone an opportunity to be a part of the planning process, which increases compliance. The first step in planning might be to explain that, as a member of the family, each person needs to help out with household chores. Throughout the planning process, explain that by working together to complete household chores, everyone will be able to have more time for the things they want to do.

As part of the plan, be sure to include the following:

- A list of chores to be completed
- The name of the person who is responsible for each chore
- The time allotted to complete the chore
- The number of times per week the chore must be done
- Standards of achievement (spell out expectations)
- The consequences for not completing the chore (privileges taken away)

O N T R A C K

You are on track if you can begin to list the chores that need to be completed in your household.

1. _____

2. _____

3. _____

4. _____

5. _____

6. _____

7. _____

8. _____

9. _____

10. _____

Once everyone understands and agrees to the plan, you can write the plan on a chart that everyone can see. You can list everyone's name on one side of the chart and then list the chores that need to be completed across the top of the chart. The chart helps everyone to visualize his or her chores and serves as an incentive. Older children will feel proud that they have more responsibilities than younger children, and they might even be able to help younger children complete their chores. You can even use the chart to keep track of whether tasks have been completed by placing stars or checkmarks next to items when they have been accomplished. (See Figure 2.7.)

Motivational Moment

❝ The victory of success is half won when one gains the habit of setting goals and achieving them. Even the most tedious chore will become endurable as you parade through each day convinced that every task, no matter how menial or boring, brings you closer to fulfilling your dreams. ❞

Og Mandino, motivational speaker and author of
The Greatest Salesman in the World

Name	Change Clothes	Make Bed	Clean Room	Household Chores	Do Homework	Good Language	Sharing	Total
Janel	*	*	*	Empty waste baskets *	*	*	*	7
Tyler	X	*	*	Set table for dinner *	X	X	*	4
Jacob	*	*	X	Dust *	*	*	X	5

FIGURE 2.7 Sample chores chart. *Note*: this chart shows the chores for which each person is responsible 1 day of the week. You would create a different chart for each day of the week, although some chores will be daily chores. If the person completes the task on his or her own, the person receives a star. If not, he or she receives a checkmark. If you decide to use a reward system, you might want to base your rewards on the number of stars achieved per week.

You might also want to make rewards a part of your household chore system. Some people feel that the reward is being able to feel good about contributing to the family, whereas others build in a system of monetary or other special rewards. Neither system is right or wrong. The key is to decide what will work best for your family. If you do decide to reward your children for accomplishing their chores, remember to keep rewards age and budget appropriate. Here are some reward suggestions.

● Receiving allowance
● Having an ice cream sundae at the end of the week
● Staying up 30 minutes past bedtime on Friday night
● Getting to play video games for an hour on Saturday
● Going bowling
● Making cookies or cupcakes
● Going to the park
● Getting more cell phone minutes for the month
● Staying overnight at a friend's house
● Renting a movie.

When you reward children for doing a good job, they tend to want to repeat the good performance. You might even choose to involve your children in picking their own rewards. Doing so helps them to feel like more active participants in the process and helps them to know what they are working for as a reward.

No matter what, do not let rewards and chores become a source of stress for you. Ultimately, this system is designed to help you lower stress and create more quality study time. Stay focused on this goal.

Even if you do not have children at home, you can use your schooling as an opportunity to revisit the division of labor in your household, trying to ensure that both you and your partner share responsibilities. Hopefully, your partner will be willing to accept some changes in this area, at least while you are in school. However, for some people, a problematic marriage is the reason they go back to school. Becoming independent enough to get out of a tough situation is one of the main motivators for making it to graduation. If you are in such a situation, your partner might not be one of your cheerleaders and might not be as willing to help out with household chores. You can still use the planning and organization ideas to help you create as much study time as possible for yourself so that you can reach your goals of becoming independent with a new career and a new life.

Mentor Moment

When my girls were 5 and 7, I allowed them to help me make chocolate chip cookies every Sunday afternoon. Then I packed these chocolate chip cookies in their lunches during the week. The first time we made chocolate chip cookies, I had flour and sugar all over the table and floor. I had to clean up quite a mess, but it was a small price to pay. Those cookies were a lifesaver—they not only gave me something to pack with lunches, but they gave us quality time together, taught my girls responsibility, and increased their self-esteem. They were always so proud of their cookies. As they grew older, they continued to bake cookies together—only I didn't have to help them or clean up!

Margaret from Austin, TX

Household responsibilities can also be shared with those outside your home. You can enlist the help of parents, in-laws, and other relatives who live close by. For example, they can help you directly by taking care of household chores or by watching your children so that you can do the chores. If you do not have any family who can help, get creative. Ask friends and classmates to kid-swap so that you can each have more time to get things done. If you can afford to, have someone come in and do the heavy cleaning for you. Treating yourself to maid service every once in a while, even just once or twice a year, helps. This small treat you can give yourself will give you peace of mind that will help you to focus on your studying and, ultimately, your goals.

Enjoying Quality Time

Quality time is something that many people forget to schedule in their daily planner. Most people assume that quality time will just happen when they get their other priorities out of the way. Unfortunately, when that happens, quality time rarely gets to see the light of day. Quality time is important for everyone, but it can be especially difficult to schedule if you have a family. Remember, however, that when you *create* quality time to spend with your family, you create guilt-free study time for yourself after they go to bed. You can create quality time to spend by yourself, with a significant other, or with your family in some very simple ways.

Quality Time for Yourself

Although your commitment to reach your goals will require you to work hard, you might find that you are becoming burned out if you work too hard without taking any time-outs for yourself. Taking quality time for yourself is important to keep your body healthy, your attitude positive, and your mind focused on your goals.

If you have a family, you might be used to not having much quality time to yourself. You probably spend much of your time looking after the other people in your life, with your own concerns being an afterthought. Remembering to schedule some "me time" in your day is even more important for you. Scheduling even 15 minutes per day to yourself can make a major difference in how you feel and how you approach the rest of your day. Make sure that everyone knows when you are having your personal quality time, and make it a rule that no one can bother you during this time. You can spend this uninterrupted time meditating, working out, reading for leisure, checking your personal email, surfing the Internet, or doing anything else that helps you to relax.

If you are lucky, you might even be able to schedule a whole afternoon to yourself some time. If that happens, here are some ways to spend your quality time to yourself without spending a lot of money:

- Look into getting a massage at a massage school for a very low cost.
- Get a pedicure at a beauty school.
- Go to a library or bookstore and read the latest magazines.
- Go to a coffeehouse and slowly drink a cup of gourmet coffee.
- Take a long hot shower or bath. Place scented candles around the tub to enjoy some aromatherapy.
- Slip away for an afternoon at the movies (matinees are cheaper!). Remember to bring snacks with you to save money at the concession stand.

O N   T R A C K

You are on track if you can list three ways that you would like to spend your "me time" and if you can commit to making time in your schedule (at least 15 minutes once per week) for one of these activities.

1. _____

2. _____

3. _____

Quality Time With a Significant Other

Your significant other can play an important role in the journey that you take to graduation. This person will know that, while you are in school, your free time will be limited. Hopefully, this person is supportive and encourages you to pursue and achieve your goals anyway. However, even if your significant other is your biggest cheerleader, that person might begin to resent that fact that you are going to school if you no longer have any time for him or her. Spending quality time with your significant other is just as important as spending quality time by yourself. It not only shows your significant other how important he or she is to you, but it keeps your relationship healthy, which will allow you to maintain your focus on your studies.

Just as you need to schedule quality time for yourself, you also need to schedule quality time with your significant other. Although you might not have as much time to spend together as you did before you started your program, finding some time to spend together is important. One way to work this time into your schedule is to plan a date night. Work together with your partner to find one night a week or every other week where you have a scheduled evening together. You should do this even if you are married and have children; just explain to your children that mommy and daddy need time alone together. If you have met your children's needs by spending quality time with them, then they are more likely to understand and accept your date night (see the next section, Quality Family Time).

Just like "me time," date nights need not involve spending a lot of money. In fact, keeping to a date night budget can help prevent becoming stressed out by the night instead of enjoying it. For example, going out for ice cream or coffee with your significant other alone after dinner, without the noise of the kids, might seem like a mini-vacation. Having one-on-one time with your significant other gives you each an opportunity to catch up with what the other one has been doing and talk about any issues that need to be discussed.

Quality Family Time

If you are a parent, then you will also need to consider how to create quality time to spend with your family. If you have more than one child, it is important that you not only spend time all together as a family but also that you spend quality one-on-one time with each child.

Motivational Moment

66 Other things may change us, but we start and end with family. 99

Anthony Brandt, American author

A great way to create quality time that you can spend as a family is to plan for a "family night" once a week. On this night, the entire family gathers together to participate in a fun activity. (See Box 2.9 for some fun ideas for family night activities). The activity can change each week. You can even let your children take turns deciding what the family will do on family night. Friday is sometimes a good night for family night because everyone can usually sleep in a little later on Saturdays. How much time you spend together will depend on how much time you have and need for the activity. You should aim to spend at least an hour, though. The main goal of family night is for your family to spend some quality time together. You will benefit from having this time away from your studies, and you will also likely find that your family looks forward to spending the time with you.

BOX 2.9 FAMILY NIGHT ACTIVITIES

- Playing a family-friendly game, such as Go Fish, Candy Land, Uno, Yahtzee, or Monopoly (make sure your game is age appropriate)
- Going out for ice cream or a special juice drink
- Renting and watching a movie
- Going swimming in the apartment pool
- Learning a new card game, such as bridge, canasta, or pinochle
- Having a contest with computer games
- Spending time outside together, playing catch or sledding in the snow, depending on the weather
- Going roller-skating or ice skating
- Playing miniature golf
- Going bowling
- Completing a puzzle

To get the most out of your family night quality time, you can follow these simple rules:

1. No interruptions. This means turning off the house phone and all cell phones.
2. No unfinished homework. Before the evening starts, *everyone* must complete their homework—that means you, too!
3. No one is left out. Everyone in the family should participate in the family night activity.
4. No arguing. Family time should be enjoyable for everyone so, unless you are debating who answered a question more quickly or how much Boardwalk is really worth, arguments should be banned from family night.

If family night does not work for your family or if you have trouble agreeing on activities to enjoy together, you might want to focus instead on making sure that your entire family spends quality time together during meals. Everyone needs to eat, thus mealtimes are a good time to come together. Having breakfast together offers an opportunity for everyone to check in with each other about what the plan is for the day and what family tasks need to be accomplished. If breakfast does not work, then try dinner. Family dinnertimes can give everyone in the family a chance to share how their days went and what they did. Make sure that everyone tales a turn. Your children might be proud to tell you and their siblings about how they got an A on a recent test or quiz—and you might do the same. Sharing these little victories with your family will help them to understand how important school is to you and will include them in the important journey you are taking.

Creating one-on-one quality time with each of your children is also important. Doing this can be hard because children tend to compete for their parents' attention. However, taking the time to devote special attention to each child individually will build their confidence in themselves and their relationship with you. One way to create quality time with your children is to block off a portion of your day and turn a room in your house into "one-on-one space." That space might be your kitchen or it might be your living room. The room is not important. What is important is that you allow only one child in the room with you at a time and that you focus your attention solely on that child when you do. You can color, do puzzles, read, go over homework, or just talk. The only rule is that no other child can enter the room during that time. The room belongs to you and that one child. Do this for 15 to 30 minutes for each child if you have the time. Use a timer to help you keep track of time if you need to. After the time is up, you are ready to spend time with the next child. You can do this each day, every other day, or just select one day of the week that works for you. This devoted uninterrupted time alone with you will make your children feel special. Do not be surprised if your other children stand outside the room anxiously waiting for their time alone with you.

Another way to incorporate quality time for your children into your day is "television time." Allow each child to pick one special program that they watch with you. Then turn that time in front of the television into quality cuddle time. Hold your child on your lap or sit with your arm around your child while you watch that program. This simple activity allows you to give 100% of your attention to each child, and you can do it even if you are tired.

Creating quality quiet time before bed can be as simple as sitting on the bed and talking with each child. You can take this time to talk about problems or to review the events of the day. Just be sure that you agree that this is not the time for arguments or yelling—just soft voices, patience, and understanding. This quality time will give your children a good night's sleep and give you some peace of mind to study.

O N   T R A C K

You are on track if you can list three activities for family night that your family might enjoy together.

1. _____

2. _____

3. _____

Success Journal

1. List three problems or issues in your life right now. Then practice your positive thinking skills by adding three new ways of looking at those problems that put a positive spin on them.

   1. _____

   Positive spin: _____

   _____

   2. _____

   Positive spin: _____

   _____

   3. _____

   Positive spin: _____

   _____

2. List three ways in which you will create quality time for you and your family.

   1. _____

   2. _____

   3. _____

(continues on page 88)

Success Journal (continued)

3. Use the chart below to create a monthly grocery list for your household.

Basic Items	Fresh Fruits and Vegetables	Dairy	Meat and Deli Items	Frozen Foods	Toiletries and Medications	Snacks

4. Create a weekly menu for breakfast, lunch, and dinner. Be sure to indicate whether you plan to cook or eat out.

Monday	Tuesday	Wednesday	Thursday	Friday	Saturday	Sunday
BREAKFAST						
LUNCH						
DINNER						

5. Create a household chores chart. List the names of your children along with their ages. Then list the household chores for which they are currently responsible or for which you would like them to take responsibility. Consider indicating whether the child will receive an allowance or other reward for each task or chore.

Making the Adjustment to School

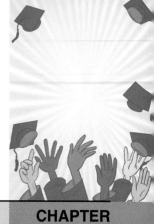

Learning Outcomes

After reading this chapter, the student will be able to:

1. Recognize commonalities that students share.
2. Create a support team that will help to maintain a focus on graduation.
3. Identify cultural beliefs and customs that affect patient care

Fitting in with the Diverse Student Population

Starting something new is always exciting and a little nerve racking at the same time. As mentioned in the previous chapter, school and your future career will require you to become a new *and improved* version of yourself who is ready to take on challenges, learn fresh information, and prepare for a new life ahead. Given all of this, you may be wondering, "How will I fit in at school?"

Fitting in at school might not be as difficult as you are expecting it to be because you will find that you have a lot in common with your classmates. People of all ages and backgrounds who are motivated to change their lives make the decision to pursue their education at health professions educational institutions. In fact, the program in which you are enrolled is designed for such a diverse population. The classes are intended for people like you who want training outside of the usual school setting and take you from your first day of school to your new career without extra classes that are not related to your field of study. Because these educational institutions cater to such a diverse population, the students who attend classes with you might seem different from you in some ways. However, you will soon find that you have a great deal in common with them.

Motivational Moment

66 Strength lies in differences, not in similarities. 99

Steven Covey, author of **The Seven Habits of Highly Effective People**

Age

Some people assume that education in general and vocational schools and colleges specifically are intended for students in the 18 to 20-something age-group. However, educational institutions such as these attract a diverse population of students from all age-groups. Some students have just graduated from high school and want to return to school to continue their education in a career. Other students have been out of school and in the workforce or at home raising children for some time before deciding to return to pursue an education in the health professions field. Health professions educational institutions are designed to provide the education and skills necessary for people of any age to change their lives. Each age-group faces a unique set of challenges in returning to the classroom. However, they also *all* share a common goal of succeeding in a health professions program and beginning a new career.

The 30-something age-group commonly represents the largest group of students in health professions programs. They also sometimes face the most challenges because they have small children at home who make the task of going back to school even more challenging. Children have a way of changing one's perspective and goals. However, if you find yourself in this situation, use it to your advantage. These new goals will help you to stay focused on graduation.

If you fall into the 30-something age-group, you have probably also had certain life experiences that will be advantageous to you in your new program and your new career. For example, you are probably already used the following:

- Getting up early before the rest of your family
- Going to bed after the rest of your family
- Putting other people's needs before your own
- Completing a job when you are tired

Raising your family and managing your home have taught you how to allocate your energy and build your endurance to complete all of the tasks for which you are responsible during the day. Now that you are in school, you are probably finding that you need to continue these routines in order to find time to study and complete assignments. Remember, however, that while you are in school, putting other people's needs before your own requires that you also make quality study time for yourself.

In addition, raising a family and managing a home have taught you many skills.

- The ability to multitask
- Organization of daily activities
- Prioritization of tasks and chores
- Accounting
- Leadership and management
- Decision making and planning
- Problem solving

You can use all of these skills to your advantage during your health professions education and in your new career in the health professions field. For example, your ability to multitask will help you to complete all of your assignments on time. Your ability to prioritize your family's needs and activities will transfer into the ability to prioritize patient needs, which is necessary for triage. Remember to give yourself credit for these skills and capitalize on them by making them a part of your resume and presenting them as strengths during the interview process.

Mentor Moment

When I became a single mom at age 34, I decided it was time for me to go back to school. With two kids in elementary school, I knew I was in for a challenge. My days were full; however, I managed by asking my family to help watch the kids while I took on a part-time job and went to school at night. I won't say it was easy, but I was encouraged to get through those tough times because I knew that after a few months I would have my diploma. Besides, juggling had become second nature to me since my kids were born. School just became one more ball that I had to juggle, and I did!

Louisa, from Santa Fe, NM

If you are one of the many people in the over-40 crowd who is returning to school, you have probably developed the same skills as the 30-something crowd, only you have been using these skills for a longer time. In fact, you might have already used them to help your children complete their educations and get jobs or careers of their own. Your children might no longer live at home, and you are now looking for the opportunity to fulfill your own needs by pursuing a career in the health professions field. You can take the loving, nourishing attitude that raising a family has given you and transfer those skills to the health professions field, where they can benefit patients and their families.

Your life experiences probably also include various jobs that have given you experience and taught you valuable workplace skills and lessons that you can use to your advantage in your new education and career. For example, you probably understand customer service responsibility and the importance of treating customers with respect. Transfer this knowledge to the classroom by being respectful of your instructors and your classmates, even when their opinions differ from your own. Doing so will give you practice for setting a respectful tone for your patients. The more experience you bring to complement your new career skills, the more valuable you will be to your new employer. If you have managerial or supervisory experience, you could create a track to become an office manager. You have the ability to use your life experiences to reach your full potential in your new career.

As a member of the over-40 crowd, one of the biggest challenges you might face is self-doubt. You might be thinking, "It has been so long since I studied. How will I learn?" Do not worry. Each student has his or her own learning style, and although your learning style may change, as you get older, there are successful ways for each student to study within their style. Once you understand those different styles of learning and define yours, you will be able to make the most of the study time that you have. (See Chapter 5, "Learning and Studying Tips.")

Another challenge is allowing yourself to be open to new methods and procedures. As people become older, they generally become more and more set in their ways. Changing your thinking and being willing to entertain and accept new solutions and points of view that are different from your own can be difficult. However, doing so can enhance your education and will help you to be open to new ways of solving patient issues when you are in your new career.

Mentor Moment

When my husband was killed in a car accident, my life changed in an instant at age 46. I had two teenage girls, and although we were all grieving, they were the ones who encouraged me to find a way to move on and do something with my time. Doing so was hard because my heart hurt, but a friend told me that helping other people might help me to heal. I finally called a medical vocational school and enrolled in a medical assisting program. It was the best thing I have ever done. I was always caring for my family, and becoming a medical assistant and caring for patients was just a natural step for me. It helped me to move on with my life and make something wonderful of it.

Tyra from Dover, DE

Even young students who move directly from high school education to vocational education or community college face challenges. Although they might be used to taking notes and tests, which can be an advantage, they also commonly face the hardest challenge, which is being committed to attending classes. If you fall into this age-group, you must remember that your education is a full-time commitment—and it is a commitment that you made to yourself. You cannot attend class only when you feel like it or are in the mood. If you were to go to school only when you felt like it, you might never go! Finding things to do that are more interesting or more fun than going to school is easy; however, you must keep in mind your goal of finding a new career and let that be your motivation to attend class and to make the most of each class by being prepared, paying attention, and taking notes.

Motivational Moment

66 Age is only a number, a cipher for the records. A man can't retire his experience. He must use it. Experience achieves more with less energy and time. 99

Bernard Baruch, financier and political economic consultant

If you just recently graduated high school, another challenge you might face is the class schedule and intensity of classes. The material that you cover in one day of class in a health professions school or college can be a week's worth of material in high school. For example, in high school you probably took different classes on different days. Maybe you only had a given class for 1 hour a day three times per week. Therefore, your learning was spread out. However, learning in a vocational institution or other postsecondary educational institution is commonly much more condensed and requires greater concentration. You are expected to be in one class for 4 to 5 hours per day 4 to 5 days per week. This intense schedule will require you to stay focused on one subject for a longer period, which can be difficult. Even the testing schedule is more condensed in health professions school. Unlike high school, where you probably had two or three major tests throughout the course of the school year, in health professions school you could be given a major test as often as once a week. Although these changes can be challenging, the best way to overcome them is to commit to attending class every day.

On the flip side, the more recently you attended high school, the more likely it is that you are able to maintain a routine of studying and homework. These tasks have been a part of your life, and continuing to allow them to be a part of routine should not pose much of a challenge for you. You might also benefit from less responsibility, a more positive outlook and more enthusiasm for life, a willingness to be open to new ideas, and greater endurance. These skills will make up for the lack of experience you might have.

Mentor Moment

I was just out of high school when I began my health professions education, and I had an "I know it all" attitude of life. High school was easy. I would go, or not go, whenever I felt like it, and I always did well anyway. However, I soon realized that if I missed *one* day at health professions school, it was like missing a week. I ended up being lucky because I sat next to a guy who later turned out to be valedictorian at the age of 57 years young. He helped me learn how to study and kept class interesting.

David from Firth, ID

O N   T R A C K

You are on track if you can list three ways in which your age and life experiences will benefit you in school or in your new career.

1. _____

2. _____

3. _____

Ethnic and Cultural Background

People who attend health professions educational institutions also come from many different ethnic and cultural backgrounds. In fact, the number of minority students in postsecondary education increases each year in the United States and is expected to continue to increase.[1] You might remember learning the term "melting pot" in high school to describe the mix of different cultures that can be found in the United States. These cultures not only reflect the diverse populations you will encounter in health professions school, they also reflect the diverse population of people you will encounter and care for in the health-care field. In fact, health professions educational institutions are now making a commitment to recognize the need to prepare health-care professionals with the knowledge and skills essential for culturally competent care. Most textbooks even have a chapter that deals with cultural diversity and its importance in caring for patients in all settings.

When it comes to diversity, you will find it helpful to know several key terms:

- **Culture:** A set of beliefs, values, traditions, and behaviors that are shared by a racial, religious, or social group and that are usually passed from generation to generation
- **Cultural awareness:** Knowledge of different cultural and ethnic practices and worldviews
- **Cultural sensitivity:** The ability to be aware of and accepting of cultures that are different from your own
- **Cultural competence:** The ability to interact effectively with people of different cultures

Your degree of cultural awareness will depend on the experiences that you have in life. Think now about these questions:

- What other cultures have you encountered in your life experiences?
- Are any of your friends from cultural backgrounds or ethnicities different from yours?
- If so, what customs and beliefs do they have that might be different from your own?

Your ability to answer these questions gives some indication of your degree of cultural awareness.

O N   T R A C K

You are on track if you can list all the cultures you have encountered in your life experiences. Think about all the people with whom you have been friends, been in class, been coworkers, and played sports or engaged in other activities.

_____

_____

_____

_____

_____

_____

Although personal interactions are a good way to learn about other cultures, they are not the only way. You can also learn about other cultures through formal and informal education, such as by reading news stories, watching the news or documentary programs, and even watching popular television programs. An important note to remember about cultural awareness, however, is to make sure that your cultural awareness is free from cultural stereotypes. Such stereotypes can lead you to make assumptions about people before getting to know them.

Motivational Moment

66 We all should know that diversity makes for a rich tapestry, and we must understand that all the threads of the tapestry are equal in value no matter what their color. 99

Maya Angelou, American poet

Understanding the diverse characteristics that make up culture serves as the foundation for cultural sensitivity (see Box 3.1). Cultural sensitivity means that you think about what you say before you say it to make sure that you don't make offensive remarks to someone of a different cultural or ethnic background. Although it is almost always a good idea to think before you speak, cultural sensitivity requires that you take that process one step further by examining your own beliefs and making sure that you do not make assumptions about people based on stereotypes and biases.

BOX 3.1   CULTURAL CHARACTERISTICS

Primary Characteristics of Culture

- Nationality
- Race
- Age
- Generation
- Color
- Gender
- Religion

Secondary Characteristics of Culture

- Education status
- Political beliefs
- Enclave identity
- Socioeconomic status
- Occupation
- Marital status
- Parental status
- Gender issues
- Military status
- Urban versus rural residence
- Physical characteristics
- Sexual orientation
- Reason for immigration (sojourner, immigrant, undocumented status)

Source: Purnell, L. (2009). *A Guide to Culturally Competent Health Care*, 2nd ed. Philadelphia: F.A. Davis, p. 4.

Cultural awareness and cultural sensitivity should combine to give you the cultural competence you need to interact effectively with people of different cultures, both in class and in your new career. Throughout your education in the health professions, you will have the opportunity to encounter diversity all around you. The instructors, administrators, and other students at your educational institution might have cultural backgrounds that are different from your own. This unique situation offers you the opportunity to increase your cultural aware-ness and cultural sensitivity from first-hand experience. In many cases, intoler-ance of a cultural background can be overcome by interacting with and learning more about people from that background. You might find that school is a great opportunity to do this. You and your classmates can help each other learn about and embrace different cultures by talking about your backgrounds, discussing your cultural traditions, and maybe even sharing an international potluck lunch or dinner.

Motivational Moment

> 66 Diversity is the one true thing we all have in common. Celebrate it every day. 99
>
> *Anonymous*

You might even think of your educational institution as a training ground where you can develop the cultural competence that will be required of you in the health-care field. The culturally diverse populations that you encounter in school will help to educate you on the customs, beliefs, and behaviors of the diverse people you will encounter in your new career as well—both your coworkers and the people you care for. Diversity is inevitable in the medical field, and health-care workers must tend to all patients without regard for cultural differences. As a member of the health-care field, you will be expected to treat all of your patients with respect.

If you are a minority, your background might make you feel different or separated from your coworkers in your current job. However, the health-care field embraces employees from all races and nationalities. In fact, bilingual employees are a huge asset to health-care institutions because they help the staff to communicate better with their patients, and better communication results in better health care. So if you are bilingual, you can say "thank you" to your parents or grandparents who made sure you could speak the native language of your ancestors. If you are not bilingual, do not worry. Just take every opportunity you can to learn about the unique nationalities and cultures of the people who live in your area. You can also buy or borrow language books and CDs and take classes to learn a second language. Doing everything you can to increase your cultural competence will increase your ability to provide the best possible care to everyone you encounter.

Mentor Moment

I was in the best program at my school: medical assisting. My class was full of lots of different types of people, but everyone was friendly, and we really worked together to learn our medical terminology. My favorite memory from school was when we shared a potluck dinner. Each student brought in a dish that he or she would cook at home. While we were eating, my instructor asked each student to talk about the dish, explain how it was made, and discuss any traditions related to the dish. Not only was the food delicious, but I learned a lot about different cultures!

Simone from Providence, RI

Because cultural backgrounds affect not only customs and beliefs but also behaviors, rituals, and even diets, health-care workers must be culturally competent in order to help patients and their families do the following:

- Understand their health-related needs
- Understand their risk for certain illnesses (see Box 3.2)
- Make decisions about care that are in line with their cultural beliefs, including decisions about end-of-life care

Cultural differences can even affect to whom you talk regarding health-care decisions. For example, Filipino, Japanese, and Indian cultures have a strong history of allowing only the male head of the household to communicate with health-care workers and make decisions regarding health care for everyone in the family. You might even witness conflict among family members concerning cultural traditions, as traditions that were once important to older generations lose their importance among younger family members. Even if you do not understand or disagree with the way a family approaches its health-care decisions, you must respect the patient's and family's wishes and incorporate their cultural beliefs into the way you handle the patient's care. Although this level of care is most likely to fall on a physician's or registered nurse's shoulders, as an entry-level employee you will need to understand and be supportive of the cultural position and procedures that are part of the office, hospital, or clinic in which you work.

BOX 3.2   CULTURALLY RELATED ILLNESSES

A person's cultural background can play a factor in his or her risk of developing certain diseases. Knowledge of these relationships can help you to understand the important role that cultural background plays in diagnosing a disease and determining appropriate treatments.

Here is a sample of some diseases that are prevalent among certain cultural groups:

- African Americans: sickle cell disease, glaucoma, hemoglobin C disease
- Appalachians: cardiovascular disease, diabetes mellitus, cancer
- Filipinos: coronary artery disease, diabetes mellitus, hypercholesterolemia
- Germans: myotonic muscular dystrophy, cystic fibrosis, hemophilia
- Mexicans: lactase deficiency, cardiovascular disease, diabetes mellitus
- Chinese: lactose intolerance, thalassemia, glucose-6-phosphate dehydrogenase deficiency

Source: Purnell, L. (2009). *A Guide to Culturally Competent Health Care,* 2nd ed. Philadelphia: F.A. Davis.

Cultural competence can also help you stand out during the interview process, increasing your employability for a position in the health-care field. If you take the time to learn about other cultures and develop your cultural competence, you will be able to highlight your experience with and ability to deal with multicultural populations as a strength in your interview.

Mentor Moment

I'll never forget this one family I encountered during my practicum. The father was clearly in charge of making all of the decisions for his family. However, his ability to understand and speak English was limited, and he became frustrated trying to communicate his wishes to the health-care team. Therefore, his oldest daughter had to serve as a translator between her father and the medical staff. It was an interesting cultural clash that taught me to pay attention to my patients' cultural *backgrounds and needs.*

Pamela from Scranton, PA

Religion

In addition to having diverse cultural and ethnic backgrounds, you will find that students in health professions schools have different religious backgrounds (see Box 3.3). For many people, religion involves more than taking time out to say a prayer before eating or going to bed. Religion is a system of values, beliefs, and practices that typically helps to explain the purpose of life and guides behavior. It can affect every decision a person makes in life, including decisions about health care. In fact, when you study the history of medicine, you will learn that it is closely linked to religion. Ancient tribes had elders in their communities (sometimes called "shamans") who served as religious leaders and healed illnesses by removing evil spirits from the soul. Because there were no physicians, hospitals, or clinics, these healers, who used herbal and spiritual remedies, offered the only form of medical care available. They played a big role in the lives of people at that time, both individually and as a community, and many of their treatments are still used today.

Patients commonly receive strength and meaning from their religions, and they undergo their health-care experiences within the context of their religious beliefs. Religion can help patients cope with stress and illness, and it commonly creates hope for a better quality of life. It can also affect medical decisions. As a caregiver in the health profession, you need to be aware of the importance of religion in the health-care experience. For example, a patient might refuse care on a religious holiday or certain day of the week because the day is considered

BOX 3.3   COMMON RELIGIONS IN THE UNITED STATES

- Christianity
  - Catholic
  - Protestant
    - Baptist
    - Methodist
    - Mormon
    - Lutheran
    - Episcopalian
    - Presbyterian
    - Adventist
    - Jehovah's Witnesses
- Judaism
- Muslim
- Hinduism
- Buddhism
- Sikhism
- Rastafarianism
- Shinto
- Scientology
- Atheism

holy. Religion also serves as a foundation for hope when people are seriously ill, and it plays a large role in how people prepare for death physically, mentally, and emotionally. For example, some patients will ask to see a spiritual leader before their passing to give them and their family comfort and support during this difficult transition. By understanding the beliefs and practices of different religions, health-care providers can assist families and individuals in reaching strength and self-fulfillment, even in the face of devastating medical problems.

Like cultural competence, your understanding of diverse religions and religious beliefs will help you to better understand your patients and care for them in the best way possible. You can take the opportunity to develop religious competence by being respectful of and knowledgeable about the religions of the people you encounter. This learning can begin in school with your classmates and instructors and should continue as you grow in your new health professions career. The longer you are in the health-care field, the more you will see how religion and culture play important roles in patients' decision-making process concerning their health care.

Mentor Moment

I learned a lot about other cultures when I was in health professions school, but nothing I learned could have prepared me for my first cultural clash in the real world. I worked in an oncologist's office, and a physician was recommending that a child receive a transfusion of blood platelets. The child's parents refused the blood transfusion due to religious beliefs. At first I didn't understand, but then I had a flashback to school when we talked about the importance of cultural and religious beliefs in patients' lives. I remembered that my role in such a situation was to respect the family's beliefs and do everything I could to help the patient get well.

Charles from Ann Arbor, MI

Some of your own religious practices, such as special prayers or observance of religious holidays, may affect your studies or class attendance while you are in school. Because class attendance is part of your grade, you might be subject to certain consequences, or at least need to complete makeup work, if you need to miss time everyday due to prayer or you need to be absent on a religious holiday. Each educational institution has its own policy and consequences for missing class due to religious observances, within the guidelines of their accreditation agency. However, your institution's attendance policy should be fair and just to all students. If you have any restrictions based on your religion, be sure to discuss them with your instructors, the director of education, or the campus director.

Gender

Although throughout history positions such as doctors and medical researchers have typically been held by men, the gender divides in education and in the workplace have been crumbling since the women's movement in the 1960s. In fact, more women than men now pursue education after high school, many of them, like you, in the health professions field.

The new opportunities to earn an education and have a career in the health professions have made the field attractive to women. Many of those women face unique challenges that place them at risk for not completing their postsecondary education. Some are older women who are returning to their education after raising families or becoming divorced, some are single parents who are responsible for both raising their children and earning enough money to support their families, and some have learned that a well-paying position is their path to independence from an overbearing partner or spouse. However, these situations are also the motivating factors that push many of these women to achieve their goal of having a career in the health-care field. With the help of the faculty and staff at their educational institutions, women from all backgrounds and life circumstances are able to reach graduation.

Women can also go farther in their education than ever before. Women who start out as medical assistants can move on to become registered nurses, medical or physician assistants, or physicians, depending on their interests and motivation to continue their education. The "glass ceiling" no longer prevents women from reaching their highest potential.

Motivational Moment

66 Success is to be measured not so much by the position that one has reached in life as by the obstacles which he has overcome. 99

Booker T. Washington, American political leader and educator

The women's movement opened up new career opportunities for women— and also for men! No longer does society view such professions as teachers, administrative assistants, and nurses as female-only positions. Men are more openly accepted into all levels of the medical field than in the past, from nursing to medical assisting. All professions are open to both sexes; gender is no longer a limiting qualification. Given these advances, your classes will have both male and female students who are all embracing the same dream of graduation and a better life with a new career.

In addition to opening up employment and educational opportunities to both sexes, the women's movement changed gender roles in the United States. In the past, men were customarily the sole head of household, and women's only responsibility was to raise children. An unwillingness of either gender to blindly accept these former roles has changed the makeup of modern families. Today, the role of head of household is usually a shared responsibility among married couples. However, more families are undergoing divorce and more people are becoming "single parents," a term that can apply to either a man or woman who serves as the sole parent in a household. These changing family roles might not only affect your family and play a role in your new educational path, but they will also affect the families of the patients for whom you provide care.

Education

Another area in which your background may differ from that of your classmates is the area of education. Students in health professions schools have varied levels of prior education, ranging from high school diplomas or general equivalency diplomas (GEDs) to some college classes or maybe even a degree in an unrelated field. No matter what his or her educational background is, each student enters the health professions program at the same point: the beginning. In addition, each student has met the same admissions criteria to be accepted to the program. You should feel proud and secure knowing that you qualified for admission just like everyone else—no matter what your education level is at admission. This also gives you something in common with your new classmates; you are all qualified to be here and you have all shown your dedication and desire to gain new knowledge that will lead you to your new career.

Every health professions student also begins his or her education with a clean slate. A person who was a D student in high school can change his or her attitude and learn to become an A student in health professions school. Having a positive attitude, visualizing your future, prioritizing your education, and attending and participating in class will go a long way toward helping you achieve the new goals that you set for yourself.

Building Your New Support Team

Despite the diverse backgrounds and prior experiences of the people with whom you attend school, you will find that you all have some common interests and goals. Each of your classmates is there for the same reason as you—to pursue an exciting new career in the health professions field. Focusing on those commonalities, rather than the differences, when you meet new people will help you to feel more comfortable and form new relationships and friendships. You can use these new relationships as opportunities to build your *new* support team, which will help you make it to graduation.

Classmates

Although you are not attending school to make friends, you will find that sharing the intense experience of school with your classmates creates an undeniable bond upon which new relationships can be built. These relationships can range from close friendships to study and group project partnerships.

When you attend your first day of school, you will find that you are only a stranger in the classroom for a few seconds. Your instructor will welcome you to class, and some of your new classmates will probably greet you as you arrive. If they do not, they may be more shy than you are, so take the initiative to introduce yourself to them. Take advantage of this opportunity to meet as many of your new classmates as you can because it might benefit you later on. Although you might not remember everyone's name, you will have opened a door that will make future communication easier.

If you do not get the opportunity to meet your classmates before class, do not worry. On the first day, some instructors ask students to introduce themselves to the class and say a little bit about their background. Think about this before you go to class and consider what you might want to tell people about who you are. What details of your life define you? You can use this introduction as an icebreaker by telling your classmates interesting information about yourself that might intrigue them enough to want to know more and by learning interesting facts about others. Try to think of the most unique thing about yourself that you would be willing to share with a group of people you just met. Keep it interesting, but keep it truthful. Remember to include information such as your name, educational background, marital and parental status, and age, if you want to share those details. But also remember to include a small bit of information that will help others get a sense of who you are or that will set you off from the crowd. For example, have you ever lived anywhere interesting? Is there something you consider unique about yourself? Have you ever had an unusual experience that others might find funny? Is there something about you that others might be surprised to learn?

O N   T R A C K

You are on track to building new relationships if you can write a brief statement about yourself that you could use to introduce yourself to others on the first day of class.

_____

_____

_____

_____

_____

Once you make it past all of the initial introductions, you will find that the best way to make new friends is to just be yourself. Nobody does it better! You just need to open yourself up to the opportunity, even if you are typically a little more introverted. Remember that this whole experience is an opportunity to reinvent yourself as the person you would like to be!

Making new friends should be easy because each of your classmates has the same goal as you. This shared goal, as well as some of the challenges you will face to reach it, is a bond that you have with your classmates before you even get to class. Each person's determination to make it to graduation should help to inspire and motivate his or her classmates to do the same. You might find that you are giving support to a classmate or that a classmate is helping you. Either way, you will share a special bond with your classmates when you all walk across the stage to receive your diplomas or degrees. You might even be able to help each other overcome some of the daily non-education-related challenges you will face in the months ahead (see the next Chapter 4, "Identifying and Overcoming Personal Challenges").

Making friends can even directly benefit your studies. For example, as you get to know other students in your class, you might find that some will make good partners in a study group. Even if study groups are not for you, you will find it beneficial to have someone to bounce ideas off and share information. For example, if it has been a while since you sat down to read a textbook or do research to gather information, you might find someone in your class who can offer you some helpful hints that will save you time.

Motivational Moment

66 Faith is taking the first step, even when you don't see the whole staircase. 99

Martin Luther King, Jr., American civil rights leader and minister

Keep in mind while you are making new friends that your old friends might feel threatened and begin criticizing you for going back to school. They might make fun of you and laugh about how you are wasting your time and money for tuition. If this happens, just take a few seconds to return to your visualization of yourself in your cap and gown . . . in just a few months you will be at graduation. Go back to your vision board to remind yourself of the reasons you are working so hard. The people in your life who criticize you for those goals are probably unhappy with themselves and are afraid that you will be leaving them behind if you make a better life for yourself. You cannot let that stop you from realizing your dreams. Remember that you must surround yourself with cheerleaders!

Staff and Faculty

In addition to your classmates, you will be traveling this new path with the faculty and staff of your health professions institution. Your instructors, the director of education, the academic dean, student services staff, advisors, and mentors or student ambassadors will all be there to help you succeed and graduate. By talking with your instructors and other staff members, you might find that you have a lot in common. They are likely to share some of the same interests that led you to the health professions. In addition, many of them have taken a path similar to—if not the *same* as—the one you are on right now. They had to learn the same medical terms and vocabulary you are now committing to memory. Their advantage is that they have practiced their skills in the health professions field, some of them for many years. The good news is that they became educators so that they can share with you the knowledge that they have learned. They can show you how to achieve your goals, avoid as many "speed bumps" as possible, and overcome any challenge that you are facing. Remember that the faculty and administrators at your school are there to help you graduate. They want to see you succeed and achieve your full potential.

O N   T R A C K

You are on track if you can write the names or positions of three staff members to whom you could turn if you needed help overcoming a challenge.

1. _____

2. _____

3. _____

Success Journal

1. Get to know the people in your class. List the names of three students you go to school with who:

   a. **Live near you.**

   1. _____

   2. _____

   3. _____

   b. **Have the same number of children as you or children the same age as yours.**

   1. _____

   2. _____

   3. _____

   c. **Are around the same age as you.**

   1. _____

   2. _____

   3. _____

2. Think about your own cultural and religious beliefs. What beliefs do you hold dear that could affect your family's medical care?

   _____

   _____

   _____

   _____

   _____

   _____

_____

_____

_____

3. Now think about other situations in which cultural and religious beliefs can affect health-care decisions. Can you list three beliefs that others might have that could play a role in health-care decisions, including those regarding end-of-life care?

1._____

_____

2._____

_____

3._____

_____

4. How might your cultural and religious awareness influence your decision regarding the type of medical office in which you would like to work?

_____

_____

_____

_____

_____

_____

_____

BIBLIOGRAPHY

1. U.S. Department of Education, National Center for Education Statistics, Integrated Postsecondary Education Data System. "Fall Enrollment Survey" (IPEDS-EF:93–99), Spring 2001 through Spring 2008; and Table 22, Enrollment in Degree-Granting Institutions by Race/Ethnicity Model, 1980–2007. Retrieved from http://nces.ed.gov/programs/projections/projections2018/tables/table_22.asp?referrer=list

Identifying and Overcoming Personal Challenges

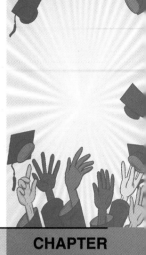

Learning Outcomes

After reading this chapter, the student will be able to:

1. Identify personal challenges that could affect school success.
2. Describe different coping methods for dealing with these personal challenges.
3. Identify outside resources that can provide assistance in coping with personal challenges.
4. Develop and maintain a budget while attending school.

Understanding Common Challenges

As you begin your educational program, you might have already identified some areas in your personal life that could challenge your success in education. Some challenges might threaten your ability to attend class, whereas others might make finding study time seem impossible. Everyone has challenges such as these. You just need to identify what yours are and then overcome them. One way to approach these challenges is to try to look at each as an opportunity for growth and development.

O N   T R A C K

You are on track if you can identify three major challenges you need to overcome before they interrupt your success.

1. _____

2. _____

3. _____

The best way to overcome your challenges is to anticipate them and then put plans in place that will help you to meet them head-on. When you are planning how you are going to overcome your challenges, you should always have a plan A and a backup plan B. Having a backup plan is good because it offers you choices, and it also means that you will not have to scramble for a solution when plan A fails to meet your expectations. You should also plan to continue to monitor the effectiveness of the solutions you choose because the issues you face while you are attending school can resurface again and again and demand your attention.

Motivational Moment

66 Success is not final, failure is not fatal: it is the courage to continue that counts. 99

Sir Winston Churchill, former Prime Minister of the United Kingdom

When developing your plans, you should remember to take advantage of the resources that are available to you. You might want to start by making your challenges known to your faculty and school administrators. As previously mentioned, your faculty and school administrators want you to succeed and will be willing to help you overcome any challenges that you are facing. They also likely possess years of experience helping other students with issues just like yours, and they might be able to offer you the advice and information you need to help you come closer to a solution. You might also find it helpful to talk to your new classmates about the challenges you are facing. Not only may they be attempting to overcome some of the same challenges, but together you may help each other find solutions.

If you start to feel like the challenges you face are too hard to overcome, remember that no obstacle or issue is more important right now than *going to graduation.* Education is the best way to get out of your current situation and to reach the goals you have set for yourself. The key to your success is to put yourself in a box that you have to climb out of to see your dreams on the horizon. Attending health professions school is going to make those dreams a reality. Remember, it is never too late to achieve your dreams, and your new positive attitude will be a key to making them a reality.

Three common personal challenge areas students like you face while attending health professions school are money, transportation, and day care. Although this chapter covers only these three common challenges in detail, you might face other challenges, such as issues with housing, health care, domestic abuse, and substance abuse. No matter what challenges you face, you will notice a common theme among the solutions—that is, you do not need to do it alone. There are many resources available to help you with any issue you may encounter during your education. You just need to know where to go for help.

Managing Money Problems

Because the opportunity to make more money is one reason that many people choose to attend health professions school, it's not uncommon for students like you to face money issues while they are pursing their education. Most likely, lack of money was a challenge that you already knew you would have to face when you decided to return to school. It might even be a reason that you wanted to return to school and why some of the nonsupporters in your life have criticized you for doing it.

A health professions education is not cheap. Your education might cost you anywhere from $10,000 to $65,000, depending on the length of your program and the type of diploma or degree you will attain. In addition to the cost of tuition, you could need to spend money on school supplies, such as books, lab fees, and scrubs. You might also need to adjust your work schedule in order to be able to attend classes. If you are already struggling to support yourself or support a family, these costs are certain to put an even greater financial strain on your situation.

Hopefully, you have already explored and taken advantage of the financial aid that is available to you in the form of federal loans and grants. If you are eligible, financial aid can help to pay for or defer the costs of your education. Even if you have received financial aid, you may still have to cope with money issues while you are completing your program. Although coping with these financial demands will be challenging, you must remind yourself that you are making an investment in your future and that making some sacrifices now will pay off later. In addition, keeping your money organized now will help to ensure that you maintain good credit, which may play a role in your future job search (see Chapter 12).

Motivational Moment

66 An investment in knowledge always pays the best interest. 99

Benjamin Franklin, inventor and statesman

Maintaining a Budget for Your Household

The best way to manage money problems is to look at your finances and plan a household budget. You should do this as soon as possible because once you become stressed over a lack of money, that stress will interfere with your ability to study. The sooner you can overcome the financial issues that you might have, the sooner you can focus all of your energy on making it to graduation!

To make sure that you have an accurate picture of your finances, you should start by gathering all of your financial information, including your bank statements, checkbook, credit card bills, utility bills, loan agreements, and pay stubs, so that you can see how much money you have coming into your household (your income) and the how much money you are spending (your expenses). Remember to collect records of the bills that you pay both online and by check, including those that are directly withdrawn from your bank account. You can look at your finances on a weekly basis or on a monthly basis, whichever works best for you. Many people find that looking at monthly expenses is easier, though, because most bills are due monthly.

The next step is to calculate your total household income. Start by making a list of all of the money that comes into your household. This should include the money that you earn at your job as well as the earnings of anyone else in your household who works. It should also include any child support and alimony payments you might get as well as any other sources of income or financial assistance that help you to pay your bills or contribute to paying your expenses. If you or someone else in your household has a job that does not pay a fixed salary, or if you work a different number of hours each week, then you will have to calculate an average weekly or monthly income. Remember to use your total income after taxes, as this is the actual amount of money that you have available to you for spending.

The next step is to make a list of every expense that you have. If you have a family, you might want to make this a family activity to be sure that you consider each family member's spending. Expenses can be broken down into two categories: fixed and variable. Fixed expenses are those that stay relatively the same each month; these expenses are essential and not likely to change. Common examples include rent or mortgage and utility bills. (Although utility bills usually vary slightly from month to month and more so from season to season, they are generally considered fixed expenses because you must pay them on a regular basis; calculate these using an average cost.) In some cases, fixed expenses occur on a yearly basis (e.g., children's school supplies and sports equipment) or occur regularly but not necessarily monthly (e.g., grooming expenses such as haircuts, waxing, and manicures); remember to account for these in some way as well. For example, you might choose to calculate how much you spend per year on these items and then divide the total by 12 months to get an average monthly cost. Variable expenses change from month to month and are usually the expenses for which savings can be found. (See Box 4.1 for examples

---

BOX 4.1   EXAMPLES OF FIXED AND VARIABLE EXPENSES

Fixed

- Rent or mortgage
- Groceries
- Car loan
- Utilities
  - Water service
  - Electric service
  - Phone service
  - Cable service
  - Internet service
- Insurance
- Allowances

Variable

- Gasoline
- Credit card debt
- Entertainment (e.g., movies, eating out)
- Gifts

of fixed and variable expenses.) As you list your expenses, you should remember to add in the new expenses that you have for school supplies and transportation to and from class. You must also remember to account for the little things that you spend money on each day, such as coffee, bottled water, and snack foods. These items can be considered "luxury items" because they are not absolutely necessary. However, over the course of a month, the cost of those little items can add up.

If you take the time to list all of your expenses in detail, you will have a real picture of where you spend your money daily. The process of sitting down and listing one's household expenses can be quite an eye-opener. Many people do not really know where their money goes each month, and they are surprised to learn how much they spend on certain items. You might find that you are spending more money than you realize on luxury items that you do not really need. And every little purchase you make that is not a necessity can hurt your wallet. Once you have listed all of your expenses, you should add them all up.

O N   T R A C K

You are on track if you can keep track of your flexible daily spending for 1 week using the chart below. Remember to include everything that you spend money on, from coffee and candy bars to school supplies for you and your family. At the end of the week, add up your spending.

Flexible Daily Spending Calendar						
Monday	Tuesday	Wednesday	Thursday	Friday	Saturday	Sunday

TOTAL SPENDING FOR 1 WEEK: $ _____

Once you know where and how you are spending your money, you should compare your total spending to your total income—either on a weekly or monthly basis, whichever is easier for you. Just make sure that you are comparing apples to apples; in other words, if you are looking at your *monthly* income, you should make sure to compare it to your *monthly* spending. Subtract your total amount of expenses from your total income. If your income is higher than your expenses, you are off to a good start. However, if your expenses are higher than your income, then something must change. Either you need to find a way to earn more money or you need to put a plan in place to ensure that your household spending is not greater than your household income. Creating a financial plan, or a budget, is a good idea for every household, even if you find that your current income is sufficient to pay for your expenses. It helps you to keep track of your spending, identify unnecessary spending, and make the most of your money. If you find that you need to cut some of your expenses in order to make your budget work, there are several things that you can do. Sometimes, making small changes or cutting out those little luxury items can help you to find the extra cash that you need to make it through the month. (See Box 4.2 for some suggestions on how to save money.) If you focus on saving money, you can do it. In fact, you will be amazed to see how much you can save when your whole household is committed to the idea of saving.

O N   T R A C K

You are on track if you can go back to the list of daily spending that you created in the previous On Track exercise and cut out unnecessary expenses.

BOX 4.2   MONEY-SAVING TIPS

Groceries and Other Food Expenses

- Create a fixed budget for grocery spending. Although the food you eat each week might differ, you should try to keep your grocery spending at a fixed amount.
- Clip coupons for grocery purchases.
- Buy grocery items that are on sale or buy generic or store brands, which are cheaper.
- Make meals at home instead of ordering take-out. Certain convenience take-out foods, such as pizza, are easy to make at home using premade pizza dough, pizza sauce, and cheese.
- Pack lunches and snacks instead of buying them out.

(box continues on page 120)

BOX 4.2 MONEY-SAVING TIPS (continued)

- Brew your own coffee at home and bring it with you in a thermos instead of paying $3 to $5 per cup at a local coffeehouse. (Just this one expense every day can add up to $15 to $25 a week, or $60 to $100 a month.)
- Bring water in a bottle from home rather than buying bottled water.

Utilities

- Adjust your thermostat to a higher temperature in the summer and a lower temperature in the winter. Just a few degree's difference in each season can offer some savings.
- Turn your thermostat up or down, depending on the season, when you are not home. Alternatively, invest in an electronic thermostat that you can program to automatically adjust the temperature for you when no one is home.
- Turn off lights when you are not in a room.
- Fix leaky faucets.
- Do not leave water running while you wash dishes or brush your teeth.
- Time yourself in the shower to cut down on water.
- Cook more than one meal at a time in the oven.
- Cut your phone service down to only the basic services with no extras (no call waiting, no long distance, no caller ID.). Basic service can cost as little as $10 in some areas.
- Alternatively, if you have a cell phone, disconnect your home phone altogether. Use your cell phone number as your main number. Shop around to find a plan that works for your entire household, and make sure that it has a fixed cost that you can afford.
- Cancel your cable service. Although having hundreds of channels can be nice, it is not a necessity, and your family will find ways to spend their time if watching cable television is not an option.

Credit Cards

- Pay off your credit cards. Credit cards have high interest rates. Once you accumulate a large balance on them, paying off that balance can become very difficult, especially if you make only the minimum payments each month. Your goal should be to create a monthly limit for credit card spending and to pay off the bill when it arrives each month.
- If you cannot pay off your credit card debt, consolidate it. Especially look at retail store credit cards, which typically have higher interest rates than standard credit cards, such as Visa and MasterCard. Select a card that gives you special rewards or bonuses, such as points that you can use on gift certificates for travel or for eating out.

BOX 4.2 (continued)

Other

- Cancel your daily newspaper subscription. Instead, find the news on television or on the Internet.
- If you have an older car that is paid off, talk to your insurance agent about the best and lowest possible insurance for the make and age of your car. You might be paying for more coverage than you need.
- Conserve gas by completing grocery shopping and other errands during one trip, carpooling to and from school, and carpooling your children to school and other events.
- Go to a local beauty school to have your hair cut.
- Swap household items, outgrown children's clothing, and other items you do not need with friends for items that you do need.

If you have money left over after you have covered the costs of all of the items that are necessities, you might want to budget some amount for each family member for a luxury item of their choosing. Your luxury item might be having a manicure done once a month or having a gourmet coffee once a week at a local coffee shop. Your son's luxury item might be joining a soccer league over the summer. Although luxury items are nice to have, they are not necessary, and if your family has no money left over, these items should be cut from the budget. And even if you cannot afford to plan for luxury items, you might still be able to afford them occasionally. For example, try saving up your loose change in a jar. This money can add up faster than you think, and when you have saved enough money, you can splurge on a luxury item for yourself or for the family. Saving in this way for a luxury item will make you appreciate it even more when you can afford it.

You should also try to save money to create an emergency fund for unexpected expenses that might occur, such as car and home repairs. Forgo luxury items until you have saved up enough money for the emergency fund—for example, $200. You might also want to save money to create funds for other occasional expenses, such as a car, Christmas, and birthdays. Last, you might want to consider using any extra money you have to pay down your credit card debt so that you can get rid of your debt faster. The faster that debt is paid off, the sooner you will have more financial freedom to spend your money in the way that you want.

Although saving money might seem impossible right now, you can find ways to save that you will not even notice. For example, when you use cash for purchases, you can save your leftover change in a special place. The small amount that you collect each day by doing this can add up over time. Saving money can be difficult, especially when you are already faced with financial burdens, but it is necessary and you need to start somewhere. So start small and make saving a little money each month part of your household budget and monthly goals.

Motivational Moment

66 Optimism is the faith that leads to achievement. Nothing can be done without hope and confidence. 99

Helen Keller, American author and political activist

Sticking to a budget might require a commitment from each member of your family. Most likely, everyone will need to make sacrifices in order for your new budget to work. However, these sacrifices are necessary for you to improve your life for you and your family members. Approaching the situation as a family and working together to create a budget will increase the chances of success. You might be surprised at the cooperation you receive when your family comes together to create the budget and determine which items are luxury items instead of you dictating or asking your family to live without certain things.

Mentor Moment

I was never a big coffee drinker, but when I started school I found that I would drink a café latte each afternoon to stay awake for my night class. Later, during our class break, I would go across the street for another café latte. I was not simply surprised—I was shocked—when I added up how much this routine was costing me. In order to save money, I started to bring a thermos from home instead. So I didn't feel like I was missing out, I splurged a little and bought my favorite flavored creamer to go with it.

Jennifer from New Smyrna, FL

If you determine after planning your budget that you need more money and are unable to cut your expenses down enough to manage them on your current income, you will need to find a way to increase your income. Start by looking for opportunities within your current job.

- Are there more responsibilities you could take on that would increase your pay?
- Are there opportunities for promotion?
- Can you take on extra shifts or work extra hours?

Consider discussing these possibilities with your boss. If you find that the opportunities at your current job are limited, you may need to look elsewhere for part-time work. If you are just a little short on cash each month, you might find that doing simple chores for your friends and neighbors, such as mowing their lawns, babysitting, or cleaning their houses, can provide you with just that little bit of extra cash you need. If these opportunities are not available to you or will not work for you, then you might need to look for a more formal part-time job.

Finding a Part-Time Job

If your current income is not sufficient to meet your needs while you are in school and if your current job lacks the opportunities for you to make more money, then you will probably need to get a part-time job. Facing up to this fact is not an easy thing to do, and trying to fit this one additional responsibility into your schedule will be challenging. However, you must remember that you are in a position to make a change in your life. If you have a family, making this change will require everyone in your family to make some temporary adjustments and sacrifices until you have graduated and started your new career. You will need to think of your part-time job as another brick wall that you will need to overcome. Just remember that overcoming that brick wall will reveal how determined you are to reach your goal.

O N   T R A C K

You are on track if you have determined whether your current income will be sufficient for you to meet your needs while you are in school. If you have determined that you need more money, you are on track if you can commit to finding a part-time job by completing the following statement:

I, _____(name)_____, promise to myself (and to my family) that I will find a part-time job within ___ week(s)

One tool that you will need when looking for a part-time job is an information sheet about yourself, known as a resume (see Box 4.3). Although the resume you will need to find a part-time job will not be as formal as the one you will need when you look for your career, it should contain certain information that will help prospective employers understand who you are and what your goals are (see Chapter 8 for more information on how to create a professional resume). Many people overlook this important component when looking for a part-time job. Therefore, coming prepared to each employment opportunity with your resume in hand will help you to stand out from other job seekers. If you need help understanding how to write a resume, talk to the staff in your school's career services department. They will give you the direction you need and will most likely have someone available to proofread your current resume for you and offer suggestions.

You should also be sure to come to each employment opportunity neat, clean, and professionally dressed. If you need help understanding how to dress professionally, talk to the staff in your school's career services department. (Also see Chapter 10 for more information on dressing professionally.)

Types of Part-Time Jobs

If you determine that you need to get a part-time job, remember that any job that generates enough money will do for now. Although taking on such a job might seem like a step backward, remember that you will only need to work this job until you have accomplished the goal of a new career. Think of it as a stepping-stone to that new career, a means to an end. You must do whatever you need to in order to make the money that you need to stay in school. This is no time to let your ego or pride get in the way of doing what you need to do in order to achieve your dreams. Any job that provides the money you need to pay your bills, put

---

BOX 4.3   CREATING A QUICK RESUME

Although the resume you need when looking for a part-time job will be more in-formal than the one you need when looking for your career, you should be sure to include certain information, such as the following:

- Name
- Address
- Phone number, including cell phone number
- E-mail address
- Work experience (listed in chronological order, starting with your most recent job and working backward no more than 5 years), including this information:
  - company name
  - dates of employment
  - your position or title
  - your job responsibilities
- References page (people who can speak highly to your character, integrity, and punctuality, such as former employers)

You should also hold on to this resume after you find a part-time job because it will form the basis of your more formal resume later on.

BOX 4.3 (continued)

Example

STUDENT GENIUS
1234 Career Path
Future, USA 12345
H: (123) 456-7890, C: (098) 765-4321
Email address: studentgenius@email.com

Objective
I am looking for an opportunity to transfer my skills from my work experience to a part-time position.

Transferable skills
• Excellent customer service experience answering phones
• Retail register experience
• Attention to detail in data entry
• Team player with large and small staff

Work Experience
Dollar Store   2009-present
Sales and register experience.

Video Store   2008-2009
Sales and data entry of video returns

ABC Pizzeria 2006-2008
Front desk, customer service, and phones

Reference
Susan Smith
ABC Pizzeria supervisor
(123) 555-1234

food on your table, and pay for school supplies is a good job. Companies that operate 24/7 (i.e., are open 24 hours per day, 7 days per week) are ideal workplaces for students because they commonly offer various shifts and flexible schedules.

Mentor Moment

I knew before I even started my program that I was going to need a part-time job as soon as possible to help pay for school supplies and other expenses. But I didn't know how to find a job. Luckily, a spokesperson from the United Parcel Service (UPS) came to my campus and presented students with information about various job opportunities, including their salary and benefits. UPS was willing to work around the class schedules of students like me, and it was great because I ended up working with UPS during my entire program.

Brian from New York City, NY

You need to remember that everyone must start somewhere, and success generally takes hard work and compromise. Few successful people began their careers doing just what they hoped to do. Just think about all of the stories you have heard about people who are now rich and famous who started out working low-paying jobs before they got their big breaks in Hollywood. For example, Beyonce Knowles worked in her mother's salon sweeping up hair; Gwen Stefani worked at a Dairy Queen; Bill Cosby sold produce, shined shoes, and stocked shelves at a supermarket; and Brad Pitt wore a giant chicken suit to promote a restaurant. These people did not find such jobs below their dignity. In fact, some people consider these types of jobs as opportunities, opportunities that serve as stepping-stones to new goals and careers.

The part-time job that you will take on while you are in school is an opportunity for you in more ways than one. It will be the opportunity that you need to create your very own success story. Without that opportunity, you would be stuck in your current situation, hoping for something better to come along in your life. The flexibility offered by such a job is also a major opportunity for you because you will need a good amount of flexibility in order to be able to fit the job into your already hectic schedule. In fact, flipping hamburgers, delivering pizzas, and bagging groceries are perfect opportunities for you in your current scenario because they are relatively stress free, can be found almost anywhere, and are sometimes open 24 hours a day, 7 days a week.

In fact, you are likely to find several fast food and pizza restaurants near your campus. These types of establishments are generally open early in the morning for breakfast and close late at night, allowing you to find a job that works around your school program. However, these are not the only types of part-time jobs that are available to you (see Box 4.4 for other opportunities you might want to consider).

O N   T R A C K

You are on track if you can list three possible jobs that you would be willing to do that you could work into your schedule.

1. _____

2. _____

3. _____

Looking for a part-time job will also be an opportunity for you to practice your career search strategies. Although the process will probably not be as formal or professional, you will need to use the same strategies and skills in searching for a part-time job as you will for your new career position.

Ways to Find a Job

Although opportunities for part-time jobs are everywhere, you might not know where to begin your job search. You can approach your search in several different ways, depending on your needs and preferences. No matter which method you choose, however, you should remember to keep yourself open to any opportunities that arise. Also, keep your mind filled with positive thoughts that you will find the right part-time job for you.

BOX 4.4   PART-TIME JOB OPPORTUNITIES

- **Restaurants:** Waiter or waitress, waiting assistant, cook, host or hostess, cashier, delivery driver
- **Retail and grocery stores:** Stocker, cashier, inventory clerk, customer service clerk
- **Hotels or motels:** Front desk clerk, housekeeping attendant, porter, valet
- **Transportation companies:** Driver, dispatcher
- **Convalescent or assisted-living homes:** Receptionist, food service
- **Temporary agencies:** Various short-term placement positions

The Classified Approach

A common way to find a job is to look at classified ads in local newspapers, free employment papers, or online. Printed papers are generally available at convenience stores and supermarkets, if you do not have one delivered. You might even find copies of these papers around your school, such as in the career services department. Free employment papers are sometimes found in boxes near public transportation sites, such as bus stops and train stations.

The classified sections of newspapers and free employment papers usually come out on certain days of the week. They generally list jobs in alphabetical order, sometimes grouped into certain markets. Scan these listings with an open mind and consider your skills and previous work experience to see the jobs listed as opportunities. Look for certain details that might help you to determine whether the job will be a match for you.

- **Location:** You should not waste your time looking for jobs that are too far away from your local area; a job that is either near your home or school would be best.
- **Hours:** If the job requires someone to fill a specific shift and those hours conflict with your school schedule, you should not waste your time inquiring.
- **Experience:** Although some companies advertise that they are looking for a certain level of experience and are willing to consider candidates with less experience, you should use your judgment about pursuing jobs that specify a type of experience that you do not have.

When you find an opportunity that might work for you, write down any information that is provided in the ad, such as the company name, phone number, contact person, and pay rate, if available. Leave some space below this information so that you can write notes when you contact the company later on to find out more information. Be prepared when you call to ask about the job responsibilities, the hours, and any other concerns that will help you to determine if the job is right for you.

Searching online classifieds works in a similar manner. Most large newspapers list their classified ads online in addition to printing them. Another online option is job search websites, such as CareerBuilder.com and Monster.com. These sites allow you to type in key words and search for jobs based on your zip code. In the advance search options, you will often find an option to choose part-time positions. Alternatively, you could include the words "part time" in your key word search. If you have some idea of what type of work you might like to do (e.g., food service, housekeeping, hostess), you can type in that key word or phrase to find jobs that might interest you or you can go directly to the web sites of local businesses with such positions. For some people, an online search is the fastest and most effective way to find a local part-time position. Some companies even allow you to apply online, speeding up the process even more.

The Career Services Approach

Another place to find job opportunities is at the career services department on your campus. The people who work in this department might be aware of currently available part-time opportunities and may have a list of employers who are willing to hire students and work with their school schedules. In fact, many employers contact local colleges and vocational institutions looking for student employees to hire on a part-time basis. Explain your needs to the career services staff, along with your commitment to school and a part-time job. Make sure you leave your name and phone number with the career services department before you leave. Plan to visit the department daily or at least weekly until you are hired. Your persistence will show the staff that you are determined and serious about getting a part-time job.

The career services department might also be able to provide you with information on local job fairs. A job fair is an event, usually sponsored by a local community, at which representatives from multiple employers gather to meet prospective employees and explain the opportunities available in their companies. Job fairs are wonderful opportunities for employment because you can meet as many as 150 employers at one time.

When you visit a job fair, you will see booths identified with company names. Most booths provide information sheets about the company and its employment opportunities. At each booth, you will also find people you can talk to about the company; sometimes they will even interview you on the spot. The most important part of visiting a job fair is to avoid getting caught up talking with companies that are not offering part-time jobs. You know how valuable your time is, and so you must spend it wisely every chance you get. Remember: You must work the job fair; do not let the job fair work you.

You should come to the job fair prepared to talk to employers about yourself and prepared to ask questions about the employment opportunities available. Also come prepared to hand out your resume to as many companies as interest you. You might need to have as many as 30 copies with you; it is better to come prepared with too many than not enough. Remember that coming prepared with a resume will help you to stand out from other job seekers.

The Walk-and-Talk Method

Another good way to find job opportunities is to use the walk-and-talk method. This method involves simply walking to the local fast food restaurants, supermarkets, hotels, motels, and any other small business around your campus and asking if they are looking for part-time help. When you arrive, ask to speak to the manager or supervisor. If you get to speak to someone in this position, be sure to ask the following:

- What part-time positions are available
- What shifts are available

- What is the salary range
- Whether the uniform is provided
- Whether you can interview for the position
- When you can start

Even if a manager or supervisor is not available to speak with you, ask whomever you do speak with whether you can complete an application for employment. Note that some stores, such as Target, Wal-Mart, and some supermarkets, have computers available in their customer services department where you can complete application forms electronically. Others might direct you to apply directly on their websites. In fact, some large retail stores and restaurants *require* you to apply online, even when you show up in person.

If you use walk-and-talk method, be sure to dress properly and be ready to present your resume in case you have an instant interview. Do not begin using the walk-and-talk method until you are ready to answer some basic interview questions, such as the following:

- What can you tell me about yourself?
- Why do you think you will do well here?
- What can you tell me about your work experience?
- What are your strengths?
- What are your weaknesses?

Although you will need to be honest with your prospective employer about your current situation, you might want to hold off on telling the person who interviews you that you are in school. The fact that you are in school is something of which you should be extremely proud; however, a prospective employer might not be willing to go through the trouble to train you for a job if they know you are only going to be working for a few months, which will require them to train another employee. If you wait until you are working out a work schedule to tell your employer that you are in school, you will have already given yourself the opportunity to make a good first impression.

The walk-and-talk method has several advantages:

- You will know that you are limiting your search to convenient jobs that are located walking distance from your campus, which will save time and gas if you are hired.
- You have the opportunity to make a real impression, becoming something more than just a name on a resume. The employer will see you and hear how you present yourself in your introduction.
- Small businesses usually have a small staff and need people to help during the evening and on weekends.

The best part about the walk-and-talk method is that you can make immediate progress. In just a couple of hours in one afternoon, you can apply for employment to several businesses. If you get to speak directly to a hiring manager when you arrive, you might even be hired on the spot after a short interview.

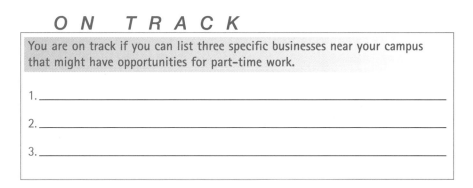

O N   T R A C K

You are on track if you can list three specific businesses near your campus that might have opportunities for part-time work.

1. _____

2. _____

3. _____

If you are a little nervous about using this approach, make the first place you go be a "tester" location, where you just try out the approach and practice the interview process by answering some questions for a manager or someone else at the store. If your interview does not go well for some reason, make note of what you might have said that affected the outcome. That way, you can learn from the experience before you approach your next opportunity. Keep in mind that some businesses simply will not be looking to hire anyone. Do not take this personally; just move on to the next opportunity and be confident that you will find a part-time job that works for you.

Motivational Moment

66 Failure is simply the opportunity to begin again, this time more intelligently. 99

Henry Ford, founder of Ford Motor Company

The Ask-Everyone Approach

As the final step in your part-time job search, you need to reach out to your inner circle of family, friends, and classmates. Do not let the fact that you are looking for a job be a well-kept secret. Talk to everyone about your job search. Other students, especially those who are further along in their programs, can be an excellent resource for employment opportunities, as they have likely gone through the process themselves. They might be able to help you save time by telling you which businesses to avoid. You might even find a student who is preparing to leave a part-time position during his or her practicum or after graduation, creating an employment opening for you.

When contacting your family and friends about your job search, take advantage of all that modern technology has to offer you. Use your e-mail contact lists, cell phone lists, and even social networking sites, such as Facebook and MySpace, to send out the message that you are looking for a part-time job. You never know who will be able to help.

Mentor Moment

When I was looking for a part-time job, I sent out an e-mail to all of my friends and contacts and asked them to send it out to everyone that they knew. I listed my goals and qualifications and I attached my resume. Within days, I received three job offers! Once I sent out that e-mail, the only hard part about finding a job for me was deciding which job to take.

Elizabeth from Colorado Springs, CO

Remember throughout your part-time job search that your ego is not looking for a job. Although you will want to pick the job that will best fit your preferences, schedule, and needs, you should consider all opportunities that come your way. Your determination to go to graduation plus your financial needs should be your guidelines when looking for part-time employment.

Motivational Moment

66 Don't let what you cannot do interfere with what you can do. 99

John Wooden, former basketball player and UCLA coach

Finding Transportation

Along with money issues often come issues with transportation. If you are attending classes at a campus rather than online, transportation issues could be a real problem for you. Depending on your current situation, you might not have a car or you might have to share your car with other members of your household. Even if you have a car, you might be worried about its reliability. Fixing your car might not be possible right now, especially with your other current financial commitments. If this is the case, online classes are not an option, and your school is not within walking distance, you might find yourself in need of transportation to and from class.

If you are worried about how you are going to get yourself to and from school, develop a plan to solve this transportation issue now. Although transportation problems, such as having car trouble, are not something you can control, you cannot let them become an excuse for you to miss class. As previously mentioned, attending class is essential to your success. Like most good solutions, your transportation plan should include a plan A and a plan B. That way, you will know that you will not have to worry about missing class, which could damage your chances of making it to graduation.

If getting a car or fixing your car is not possible right now, consider these other transportation options.

Public Transportation

Public transportation is a great option for people who do not have access to their own vehicle. Most areas have some sort of public transportation available for commuters. Examples of public transportation include buses, trains, and subways. Check with your school's admissions or student services offices to find out which types of public transportation are accessible near the campus. They might even keep bus schedules on hand to help students solve their transportation needs. If not, you can check for local public transportation schedules online at the provider's website. If you know you will need to take public transportation on a regular basis, look into getting a weekly or monthly pass to save money on this expense. Your school might even sell passes or tell you where you can obtain one.

Although taking public transportation might seem like a challenge in itself, it does have some advantages. For example, it provides you with quiet, quality time that you can put to good use by studying, putting your notes in order, and reading assigned chapters. You might even want to use that time as your own personal "down time," if it is the only opportunity you have to find time for yourself when you are not in class or at work. In addition, depending on your personal transportation situation and the age of the vehicle you are using, public transportation might be more reliable than personal transportation. The reality is that public transportation is merely a means and a stepping-stone to your graduation. If taking public transportation bothers you, just remember that it is a temporary situation that you will have to endure until you have achieved your goals. Remember that you can do anything if it will help you enter your new career field.

Carpooling

Carpooling, or ride sharing, is another option for people who do not have access to their own vehicle or for people who share a vehicle with someone else and might only have access on certain days of the week. If you have a car available to you some of the time, carpooling is a great way to save money on gas, find rides on the days you need them, and even make new friends. If you do not have a car, consider offering other trades, such as bringing someone lunch in exchange for a ride. If you can find people who live near you to carpool with, then you can work out a schedule where you drive to school on certain days of the week (e.g., Monday, Wednesday, and Friday) and then they drive on the other days (e.g., Tuesday and Thursday). The more people you bring into your carpool, the fewer days you will need access to your own transportation. Just make sure the carpool schedule you develop works for everyone in the carpool. Also make sure that you carpool with people who are reliable and have reliable vehicles.

Finding someone to carpool with does not have to be difficult. You are certainly not the only student in your school who is facing the challenge of finding a way to get to and from school. First check to see if any of your family members or friends drive near your school when they go to work. Maybe they could drop you off in the morning or pick you up after school. If you cannot find someone at school to carpool with, look on student bulletin boards, ask your instructors, and check with your student services department to find other students who are looking to carpool. Also ask the new friends you have made in class if they would be willing to share rides to school. To make carpooling work for you, you might need to arrive at school earlier than necessary; however, just use this extra time to study.

Mentor Moment

When I was in school, I took one bus to drop off my two children at the day-care center and then I took a second bus to get to my campus. Most of my classmates took one bus and complained about it. I was up by 5:30 a.m. every day to make it to school. I wanted a new career and nothing was going to stop me from achieving my goal.

Angela from Montgomery, AL

Finding Child Care

If you have children at home, especially children who are younger than school age, you might have to face the challenge of finding appropriate and reliable child care. You might need someone to watch your children during the day, while you are in class; at night, while you are at work; or both. Although this challenge might seem daunting, you must look at it as just another brick wall that needs to be overcome. Your children are probably a part of your motivation to go back to school and create a better life for yourself. You want to make sure that they are in good hands at all times, especially when you cannot be there to care for them yourself. As a parent, you will be better able to focus on your studies if you know that your children are safe and supervised.

If you already have child care arranged and are happy with the care being provided, then you are ahead of the game. If not, you will need to explore your child-care options and determine which one best accommodates your situation.

Day Care

Day care is a common and popular choice for child care. Although there are different types of day care, most follow certain standards for child care, such as child-to-teacher ratios and requirements for teacher certification and education. The rules and regulations that each day care must follow vary by city, county, and state.

You will probably need to consider many factors when choosing a day care. Not the least of these considerations will be price. *Private day cares* are for-profit businesses that care for children. They tend to be more expensive than some other day-care options because they have a curriculum based on preschool and enrichment. However, if price is not an issue for you, you might find that overcoming the challenge of child care is as simple as finding a reliable and affordable private day-care facility in your area. Another, sometimes more-affordable option for child care is a *community day care.* Schools, churches, and synagogues commonly provide such day-care services. Even if you think you cannot afford day-care services, you might want to look into your options because most communities have state or federally funded agencies that offer discounted day-care rates to qualified applicants.

To help determine which day-care facility is best, many people visit several different day cares to talk with the caregivers, check out the environment, and observe class activities. Consider looking at facilities that are close to your home or your school to make transportation easier. When "shopping around" for a day care, you should come prepared to ask certain questions about their policies and procedures. For example, you will want to ask about the day care's hours and policies. You must be aware of all of the facility's policies and procedures so that you will know what to expect when something does not go as planned, which is bound to happen at some point. Many have scheduled times for dropping off and picking up children. They also have rules regarding extra fees that you must pay if you are not on time for pick up. Another policy that you will want to ask about is their sick-child policy. Some day cares take sick children, whereas others do not. Although many private day cares are more likely to allow parents to drop off their children when they are sick, they might also charge an additional fee for this service. (See Box 4.5 for a list of questions you will want to ask when you interview day cares.)

BOX 4.5 QUESTIONS TO ASK AT DAY CARE

- What are the fees and what do they include?
- What are your hours of operation? In other words, what time can I drop off and pick up my children?
- What are your rules regarding picking children up late or dropping them off early? Is there a charge?
- Are you closed on any specific days or holidays?
- How many children do you care for each day?
- What are some of the major rules you have the children follow?
- What is the daily routine like?
- How do you discipline?
- How do you disinfect the areas where children play?
- Do you have an outside yard for the children?
- How much television do you allow the children to watch? Which programs are they allowed to watch?
- Are meals provided?
- Do you offer discounts for two or more children?
- Do you have provisions for sick children? What do you consider "sick"?
- Are you licensed and bonded?
- Do you have references?

You can use several strategies to find out about the day-care options that are available in your area. You might want to start by asking people you know in the community or at class whether they know of reliable and affordable day cares. You can also check the telephone book for private day cares as well as schools, churches, and synagogues in your area that might offer day care. Make a list of the possibilities, including their phone numbers, and then call each facility to ask if they provide day care. If the school or church does not offer day care themselves, they might have the name of local providers they could give you. Be sure to explain to the day-care facilities that you contact that you are a student on a career path. They may need information from you about your income or from your school, such as your admissions paperwork or an enrollment agreement, to verify your situation and be able to offer you a discounted rate.

Informal Child-Care Options

If you cannot afford to pay for day care, overcoming this challenge can be much more difficult. You might need to enroll your parents, other relatives, and friends in your plan. Asking for this type of help can be difficult, but your friends and family will be supportive of your efforts to go back to school and better your life. You will probably be surprised to learn that they will be willing to help in any way that they can. Even if someone cannot help by offering to provide full-time day care, they might be willing to fill in during emergencies or to help out on a part-time basis, in which case you can divide your day care up among more than one trusted care provider.

Mentor Moment

I was on my last choice on my list of possible sitters when I asked my sister-in-law if she would babysit. I convinced myself that she would never want to do it. I was so surprised when she said "yes." I found out we could trade the days for some weekend time. You never know until you ask. Ask *everyone* is my advice.

Twylah from Louisville, KY

If family and friends are not able to provide day care for you, you might want to take advantage of the new friendships you have made in class by asking classmates if they know of a good day care or babysitter. If these classmates are facing a similar challenge, they might even be willing to share a sitter with you or trade child-care responsibilities with you, which could save you both money.

O N   T R A C K

You are on track if you can take the time to stop and list all of the people who might be able to provide day care for you. Be sure to include all friends, family members, classmates, and coworkers who you might trust with this important responsibility.

1. _____

2. _____

3. _____

4. _____

5. _____

Backup Child-Care Options

Unfortunately, when it comes to child care, sometimes even the best-laid plans go wrong; therefore, you will need to have a backup child-care plan ready at all times. Doing so might seem impossible, especially if you have trouble lining up child care in the first place. However, having this plan in place will reduce your stress, leaving you prepared and focused to face each day, even when it does not go as planned. If your first choice for day care cannot provide care on a regular basis, find out if he or she would be willing to occasionally substitute for your regular day-care provider. Having to deal with this situation can be frustrating, but you must remember that your friend or family member is doing you a favor by providing child care. Remember not to take that fact for granted and to be grateful for the times that work out without problems. Of course, if someone becomes completely unreliable, you should seek out another alternative.

Finding Resources for Assistance

No matter what challenges you face while you are in school, the one important fact to remember is that you are not alone. In addition to the new people you will meet in school who will be there to offer their assistance to you, such as administrators, instructors, and classmates, many outside resources are available to help you overcome your challenges. You just have to know where to find them and not be afraid or ashamed to ask for help. Remember, everybody needs help from time to time.

Box 4.6 lists some national organizations that offer assistance to people in need. You can also ask your student services office whether there are local organizations in your community that offer similar assistance, such as community food banks, shelters, community health centers, and legal assistance. In addition, you can find a list of state, county, and city agencies that provide various types of assistance in the front of your local phone book. Most counties have social services offices that provide assistance such as food stamps, heating assistance, children's health services, and child-care assistance. You can find your local social services office in the front of your local phone book or by searching the Internet for the term "social services office" and the name of the county in which you live. Each social services office provides different services, so be sure to contact your local office to find out what assistance may be available to you.

BOX 4.6   NATIONAL ASSISTANCE ORGANIZATIONS

General Assistance

Catholic Charities USA

Through its more than 1,700 local Catholic Charities agencies, Catholic Charities USA offers services to help reduce poverty, support families, and empower communities.

Contact information:
Sixty-Six Canal Center Plaza
Suite 600
Alexandria, VA 22314
Phone: (703) 549-1390
Fax: (703) 549-1656
Website: http://www.catholiccharitiesusa.org/
Services:
Housing assistance
Emergency services
Health care
Child care

Salvation Army

The Salvation Army helps people throughout the United States receive the basic necessities of life, such as food, shelter, and warmth.

Contact information:
615 Slaters Lane
P.O. Box 269
Alexandria, VA 22313
Website: www.salvationarmyusa.org
Services:
Food programs
Youth camps
Disaster relief
Missing persons assistance
Recreation
Elderly services

Society of St. Vincent de Paul

The Society of St. Vincent de Paul assists people in need on a person-to-person basis.

(box continues on page 140)

BOX 4.6 NATIONAL ASSISTANCE ORGANIZATIONS (continued)

Contact information:
58 Progress Parkway
St. Louis, MO 63043-3706
Phone: (314) 576-3993
Fax: (314) 576-6755
E-mail: usacouncil@svdpusa.org
Website: http://svdpusa.org
Services:
Food programs
Emergency financial assistance and transportation
Rent and mortgage assistance
Low-cost housing
Shelters for people who are homeless or abused
Thrift stores
Free pharmacy services
Education programs
Youth programs
Camp programs

United Way
Through its nearly 1,300 local organizations in the United States, the United Way creates opportunities for a better life by providing assistance with education, income, and health.

Contact information:
Phone: (703) 836-7112
Website: http://www.national.unitedway.org/
Services:
Education assistance
Financial assistance
Health care

Young Men's Christian Association (YMCA)
The YMCA is a nonprofit community service organization that is committed to helping children, families, and individuals.
Contact information:
YMCA of the USA
101 North Wacker Drive
Chicago, IL 60606
Phone: (800) 872-9622
Website: http://www.ymca.net/

BOX 4.6 (continued)

Services:
Child care
Financial assistance
Health and well-being programs

Young Women's Christian Association (YWCA)

The oldest and largest multicultural women's organization in the world, the YWCA provides assistance to women that aims to eliminate racism, empower women, and promote peace, justice, freedom, and dignity for all.

Contact information:
YWCA USA
1015 18th Street, NW Suite 1100
Washington, DC 20036
Phone: (202) 467-0801
Fax: (202) 467-0802
E-mail: info@ywca.org
Website: http://www.ywca.org/
Services:
Child care
Financial assistance
Health and well-being programs

Child Care Assistance

ChildCare.gov
ChildCare.gov is a comprehensive online resource that can be used to help parents find child care information and assistance.

Contact information:
ChildCare.gov
U.S. Department of Health and Human Services
Administration for Children and Families
370 L'Enfant Promenade, SW
Washington, DC 20447
Website: http://www.childcare.gov/index.html
Services:
Resources for child-care information

Domestic Violence Assistance

Safe Nest
Safe Nest provides confidential assistance and services to individuals who are experiencing domestic violence, including physical, sexual, emotional, and verbal abuse; destruction of property; pet abuse; and social isolation and economic dependency.

(box continues on page 142)

BOX 4.6 NATIONAL ASSISTANCE ORGANIZATIONS (continued)

Contact information:
2915 W. Charleston Blvd., Ste. 3A
Las Vegas, NV 89102
Hotline: (800) 486-7282
Phone: 702-646-4981; TDD: 702-647-8584
Website: http://www.safenest.org/
Services:
Shelter
Food
Clothing
Counseling and education

Food and Nutrition Assistance

National School Lunch Program (NSLP)

The NSLP is a government-assisted meal program that provides nutritionally balanced, low-cost or free lunches to children in public and nonprofit private schools and residential child care institutions.

Contact information:
U.S. Department of Agriculture, Food and Nutrition Service
3101 Park Center Drive, Room 914
Alexandria, VA 22302
Phone: 703-305-2286
Website: http://www.fns.usda.gov/cnd/Lunch/default.htm
Services:
Food assistance
Nutritional education
*Ask an administrator at your child's school whether they participate in the National School Lunch Program and how you can apply for your child to receive this assistance.

Supplemental Nutrition Assistance Program (SNAP)

SNAP is a federal nutrition program administered by state and local agencies that helps low-income people and families buy the food they need for good health.

Contact information:
U.S. Department of Agriculture, Food and Nutrition Service
3101 Park Center Drive, Room 914
Alexandria, VA 22302
Phone: (800) 221-5689
Website: http://www.fns.usda.gov/snap/

BOX 4.6 (continued)

*Apply for benefits by finding your state's application form at the above website.
Services:
Food assistance
Nutritional education

Woman, Infants, and Children (WIC) Program

WIC provides temporary nutritional education and assistance to low-income pregnant, breastfeeding, and non-breastfeeding postpartum women and to infants and children up to age 5.

Contact information:
U.S. Department of Agriculture, Food and Nutrition Service
Women, Infants, and Children Program
3101 Park Center Drive, Room 914
Alexandria, VA 22302
Phone: (703) 305-2286
E-mail: wichq-sfpd@fns.usda.gov
Website: http://www.fns.usda.gov/wic/
Services:
Supplemental food assistance
Nutritional education
Breastfeeding education and support
*Visit the WIC website to find the toll-free number for the WIC office in your state.

Housing Assistance

U.S. Department of Housing and Urban Development (HUD)

HUD is a government agency that provides subsidies to make housing more affordable.

Contact information:
451 7th Street S.W.
Washington, DC 20410
Phone: (202) 708-1112; TTY: (202) 708-1455
Website: http://portal.hud.gov/portal/page/portal/HUD
Services:
Low-income housing
Rental assistance
Public housing

(box continues on page 144)

BOX 4.6 NATIONAL ASSISTANCE
ORGANIZATIONS (continued)

Substance Abuse Assistance

Alcoholics Anonymous

Alcoholics Anonymous is a worldwide fellowship of more than 2 million men and women are recovering from alcoholism.

Contact information:
11th Floor
475 Riverside Drive at West 120th St.
New York, NY 10115
Phone: (212) 870-3400
Website: http://www.aa.org/

Narcotics Anonymous

Narcotics Anonymous is a community-based association of recovering drug addicts that helps people who want to overcome substance addiction.
Contact information:
PO Box 9999
Van Nuys, CA 91409
Phone: (818) 773-9999
Fax: (818) 700-0700
Website: http://www.na.org/index.php

Success Journal

1. Take one of the challenges that you need to overcome and turn it into an opportunity by developing plan A and plan B solutions. Plan A should be the most obvious and realistic answer to your challenge. Plan B should be your "thinking out of the box" idea or backup solution.

Plan A:

_____

_____

_____

_____

_____

Plan B:

_____

_____

_____

_____

_____

(continues on page 146)

Success Journal (continued)

2. List some jobs that you would be willing to do on a part-time basis in order to make it through your education.

_____

_____

_____

_____

_____

_____

_____

_____

3. List five ways that you can cut down your household spending.

1. _____

   _____

2. _____

   _____

3. _____

   _____

4. _____

   _____

5. _____

   _____

4. Complete the chart below to get a true picture of your total monthly spending.

EXPENSES	
Expenses	**Amount**
Fixed Expenses	
Rent or mortgage	
Groceries	
Car loan	
Utilities	
Phone	
Cell phone	
Cable	
Electric (may vary by season, but use an average)	
Water	
Sewage	
Insurance	
Car	
Homeowner's	
Life	
Alimony	
Child support	

(continues on page 148)

Success Journal (continued)

EXPENSES	
Expenses	**Amount**
Long-term fixed expenses (e.g., haircuts, school supplies, sports equipment)	
Variable Expenses	
Gas and other travel expenses	
Credit card debt	
Credit card 1	
Credit card 2	
Credit card 3	
Entertainment (e.g., eating out, movies)	
Luxury spending	
Gifts	

5 List one to three issues with which you might need assistance. Then, for each, list the name and contact information for one specific organization that might be able to assist you with this issue.

1. _____

Organization name: _____

Contact information: _____

_____

2. _____

Organization name: _____

Contact information: _____

_____

3. _____

Organization name: _____

Contact information: _____

_____

Learning and Studying Tips

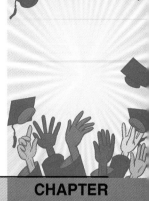

Learning Outcomes

After reading this chapter, the student will be able to:

1. Differentiate between the three major learning styles.
2. Identify techniques to enhance personal study skills.
3. Understand how to create and manage a productive study group.

Learning to Learn

To make the most of the little time you have to study, you should first learn to become an effective learner. The first step in this process is for you to understand that there are different learning styles. Figuring out your learning style and using it to your advantage to make the most of your study time is just one more skill that you can learn and use along your new path to graduation.

You must also recognize that learning as an adult is different from learning as a child. (See Box 5.1.) As an adult, you have more personal responsibilities than you did when you were a child, and you are also more likely to take personal responsibility for your education. Postsecondary educational institutions capitalize on these learning differences to assist the adult learner to be successful:

- *An adult learns best when he or she can see the outcomes of success.* Starting right from your admission process, your school has been fostering this vision. The admissions representative explained to you that your program will take months instead of years, enabling you to envision your success as a reality in the near future. Someone probably gave you a tour of the campus, where you might have seen some sort of "wall of fame." Perhaps the wall displayed pictures of graduates now working in the field or a list of where some of the school's graduates are now working and how much they are making. Each campus has a special way of showing pride in its graduates. As you walked by this information, you probably imagined how your picture or your name would look up on that wall. The admission representative might even have shown you a binder with letters from graduates. Your ability to visualize your success is why you will be successful in entering your new career in the health-care field. Your motivation to learn is high, and your performance on exams and quizzes will exceed your past performance because you can see the success that awaits you and how it relates to your learning.
- *An adult learns by questioning and might reject information that does not follow his or her belief system.* Postsecondary educational institutions present information in a way that does not challenge the student's own personal belief system but instead expands on and enhances existing beliefs and fosters the development of new beliefs based on the health-care field. These new beliefs are presented in such a way that they are embraced by the adult learner and incorporated into the existing personal belief system. Because patients are from various nationalities and have differing cultural beliefs, the health-care field needs employees with cultural awareness, sensitivity, and competence (see Chapter 3). A health professions education bonds adult learners with new beliefs that enable them to assist anyone in need of medical care, despite differences in the major cultural belief systems of the health-care provider and patient.

● *An adult learner is more internally motivated.* Your initial motivation gave you the courage to call a postsecondary educational institution for an appointment. Later, your motivation moved you to make a commitment to sign up for a health professions program. Now you are motivated by your deep desire to achieve certain goals, such as graduation and a new career.

Being an adult learner brings more responsibility to your commitment to learn and reach your goal of graduation.

Motivational Moment

66 Get over the idea that only children should spend their time in study. Be a student so long as you still have something to learn, and this will mean all your life. 99

Henry L. Doherty, American businessman

Understanding Learning Styles

You might be wondering, "What is a learning style?" Simply put, different people learn in different ways. A learning style describes how you learn—in other words, how you process and retain new information. Some people learn best by simply reading and memorizing written information, whereas others engage more of their senses in the learning process to increase their retention

BOX 5.1 ADULT LEARNER VERSUS CHILDHOOD LEARNER

Adult Learner	Child Learner
Is more self-directed in obtaining material	Depends on others for material
Has a role as a doer, using previous learning to reach success	Has a primary role in life as a learner
Learns best when he or she can see the outcomes of success	Learns what he or she is told to learn
Will question and even reject information if it does not follow his or her belief system	Is usually more open to new information
Is more internally motivated	Is more externally motivated

of information. How you process information, along with your life experiences, helps to formulate and change your point of view, actions, and goals.

Types of Learning Styles

There are many different types of learning styles, and many different terms have been used to describe them. The three most common styles are as follows:

- **Auditory learners:** Auditory learners learn best by listening and discussing. Verbal lectures and discussion or study groups are a foundation for learning for these types of learners because they tend to absorb information that they hear. They are able to pick up on and interpret the importance of information based on changes in a speaker's pitch, voice tone, and volume. Hearing information verbally helps them to remember it; they are less likely to benefit from written information, as they might have more trouble discerning what is important. Thanks to such modern technologies as voice recorders, cell phones, MP3 players, portable listening and reading devices, and portable computers, auditory learners have more tools to use for learning than ever before.
- **Visual learners:** Seeing and visualizing information is the foundation of learning for visual learners. They are able to ascertain meaning and recall information from visual aids such as charts, diagrams, flip charts, and, especially, PowerPoint presentations. They also tend to sit in the front of a classroom so they can see the teacher's body language, gestures, and facial expressions without other visual distractions. This helps them to fully understand the important concepts of a lecture. Some visual learners also have photographic memories. They might take detailed notes as a visual way to process and retain information.
- **Kinesthetic learners:** Kinesthetic learners reach a strong level of understanding by becoming actively involved. They benefit greatly from such activities as labs, which allow them to touch, do, and move as they practice new techniques and skills. This hands-on approach to learning helps kinesthetic learners to better absorb information, understand how things work, and retain meaning from the world around them. They could have a hard time sitting in class for a long period of time unless the teacher uses class activities to engage them.

These definitions are important to understand because they can help you to realize that there are different ways of learning. In reality, each person has a unique learning style that probably incorporates some aspects of all three of these learning methods. However, most people tend to favor one style as their dominant learning style. Being able to identify and capitalize on one's dominant learning style gives a person the upper hand when it comes to making the most of his or her study time.

Mentor Moment

I always loved school, but I never got great grades. I was pretty much a C student, and I had to work very hard for the few B's and A's I did get. I wear glasses, and I never really got into music, even as a teenager. But I never thought those things would have anything to do with my grades—at least, not until health professions school. Participating in labs taught me that I learn best when I can work with my hands and be involved with my learning. Once I learned that, I was able to reach for and achieve more A's.

Angela from Kansas City, MO

Defining Your Own Learning Style

Now that you understand what a learning style is, what some of the different types of learning styles are, and how learning styles can affect your studying, it is time to discover what learning style, or combination of learning styles, best suits you. You can make the most of your study time by defining your own learning style and then tailoring your studying to techniques that work with that style.

Defining your learning style can be difficult. To begin, answer the questions in Box 5.2. Remember, though, that you could have a combination of these traits and learning styles.

BOX 5.2   LEARNING STYLE-RELATED BEHAVIORS

People who share similar learning styles also tend to share certain behavior characteristics. Place a checkmark by each of the descriptions below that you feel applies to you. Your checkmarks will help to indicate which type of learner you are (if most of your checkmarks are under one heading, that's probably the type of learner you are). Remember that not all of the behavior characteristics for a given learning style will apply to you and you might find that you have behavior characteristics for all of the learning styles.

Auditory Learner

❏ I am a "talker."
❏ I am not physically coordinated.
❏ I like telling jokes and long stories.
❏ I remember spoken material.
❏ I have poor handwriting or an inability to draw.
❏ I love music.

(box continues on page 156)

BOX 5.2 LEARNING STYLE-RELATED BEHAVIORS (continued)

❑ I do not have a good sense of direction.
❑ I enjoy study groups.
❑ I enjoy small gatherings.
❑ I enjoy long walks with friends.

Visual Learner

❑ I enjoy reading books.
❑ I learn best when someone shows me how to do something.
❑ I do not enjoy learning a foreign language.
❑ I tend to be a good "detail person."
❑ I am not very talkative in class.
❑ I find it hard to sit still.
❑ I like organization.
❑ I like written directions.
❑ I like using websites to find information.
❑ I like texting.

Kinesthetic Learner

❑ I love building things and taking things apart.
❑ I love sports and group activities.
❑ I find it hard to sit still.
❑ I have great physical coordination.
❑ I love to touch things and hug people.
❑ I am a good note taker.
❑ I learn best by doing things myself and working with my hands.
❑ I enjoy puzzles.
❑ I like creating ceramics, pottery, or picture albums.
❑ I like to play card games.

In addition to personal behavior characteristics, societal norms and other environmental factors also have an influence on learning styles. Although this topic has been debated among researchers, there is some evidence that environment influences learning. For example, in the early part of the 20th century, the invention of radio led families to gather together in the evening to listen to news and be entertained by stories such as the *Shadow Mystery Series*. Generations that grew up listening to the radio in this way might have a better ability to gather information as auditory learners. With the invention of television, media became more visual, and many people who grew up during that generation could be visual learners. Today, the multifunctional use of MP3 players and other auditory technology might lead some people to return to a tendency toward auditory learning. Others who continue to be drawn in by television and other visual media, such as computers and video games, might favor visual and kinesthetic learning. In addition, the modern educational system has always tried to incorporate kinesthetic learning by involving students in making, doing, and creating at all levels of education.

Motivational Moment

66 When you change the way you look at things, the things you look at change. 99

Dr. Wayne Dyer, author and self-development speaker

As a student in the health professions field, you will be exposed to all styles of learning, which will allow you to be successful. The hours you spend in the classroom listening to lectures and asking questions will engage your auditory learning; you will learn data-entry skills and how to present projects, which will expose you to visual learning; and your clinical lab and computer lab classes will be a rewarding experience as part of your kinesthetic learning process. Finding ways to capitalize on your primary learning style and to involve all of your senses in your learning process will increase your retention of information and increase your chances of being successful. (See Box 5.3.)

BOX 5.3   TIPS FOR EACH LEARNING STYLE

Now that you understand the different types of learning styles, you can use these tips to incorporate all different types of learning into your educational experience or to focus your learning on how you learn best.

Auditory Learner

- Read your textbook aloud when you are studying to help retain information. Also consider taping yourself so that you can listen to the chapter instead of rereading it when you need to review.
- Ask your instructor if you may tape the lectures so that you can listen to them again later.
- Form a study group so you can talk with and listen to others.
- Sit toward the front of the class to distinguish your instructor's tone and pitch and to help determine the meaning of the lecture.
- Ask questions during the lecture to make sure you understand the concepts being presented and can hear an explanation of the information in another way.

(box continues on page 158)

BOX 5.3 TIPS FOR EACH LEARNING STYLE (continued)

Visual Learner

- Sit toward the front of the class to see your instructor's body language and facial expressions to help determine the meaning of the information.
- Focus your attention on visual presentations of information in your textbooks, such as medical charts and diagrams. Also, ask your instructor where you can go to see additional charts and diagrams that will help you understand the information.
- Take complete and detailed notes to help you process and retain information and to have for review later on.
- Use visual aids, such as flash cards, to help you review and remember important information.
- Retype your handwritten notes from class into a word-processing program on the computer so that you can see the ideas on the screen.

Kinesthetic Learner

- When taking notes in class, leave space so you can go back later and add in real-life examples.
- Join a study group to learn through active participation.
- Plan to take a leadership role in the lab to ensure that you stay with a subject or procedure until you have fully learned the details and feel confident.
- During lab, bring your instructor to your group to answer questions.
- Perform more lab skills than are required to really learn the techniques.
- Help someone else to learn his or her lab skills.

O N   T R A C K

You are on track if you have identified your primary learning style or styles. Rank them here from 1 to 3 in order of how you think you learn and retain knowledge, with 1 being your primary style.

_____ Auditory

_____ Visual

_____ Kinesthetic

Improving Your Study Skills

Now that you understand learning styles and have identified some ways to use them to your advantage, you can focus on improving some other important study skills that will help you to be successful. You are preparing to enter one of the fastest growing professional employment fields. The number of positions in the medical field are increasing faster than those in any other career path. However, you will be competing for those positions with other students like yourself. To get ahead, you will need to master the health-care field's special medical vocabulary, laboratory procedures, computer schedules, and computer billing. That means you will want to achieve a grade of no lower than a B on your clinical and computer lab assignments. As previously mentioned, this begins with your attendance because you cannot learn if you do not attend class. This important rule applies whether you are taking classes in a classroom, online, or both. But what you do outside the classroom is important as well. You must make the most of your study time, and the best way to do this is by sharpening your study skills. Improving your study skills begins with managing your time effectively so that you can have uninterrupted study time.

Managing Your Time

The term "time management" is misleading; it gives the impression that you can manage time (for example, by finding a way to create more hours in the day); however, each day has only 24 hours for you to decide how to spend. If time were a resource, it would be an equal opportunity resource. Everyone, no matter his or her race, creed, or nationality, has exactly the same number of hours to spend each day (24 hours) and each week (168 hours)—no more, no less, no matter what you do. You cannot change or control time; you can do your best to make sure that you are making the most productive use of the time you have each day. While you are in school, you will find this task to be particularly challenging because you will probably be trying to manage and balance family, work, class, and study time and maybe even try to squeeze in some exercise time. Creating quality study time is difficult, even for people who do not have a family. Faced with this challenge, you will find that organization now has a priority in your life.

Because each person has only 24 hours to spend, or waste, each day, the management of those 24 hours is the responsibility of each individual. In terms of both long-range planning and daily scheduling, each day requires you to make decisions about how you are going to spend your time. So, when you think about the term "time management," instead think about it as prioritizing your time.

Now is the time for you to take control of your time. When you say that you do not have enough time to do something, you might really be saying that you are not spending the time you *do* have in the way you want to complete all the chores, projects, and tasks you need to complete.

Good time management gives you a chance to spend your most valuable resource—time—the way you want to on your priorities. One of your main priorities during the time you are in school is studying, which includes reading chapters, reviewing lecture notes, completing homework and projects, and reviewing for tests and quizzes. However, you will also need to find time for other necessary tasks, such as sleeping, eating, commuting, and possibly working and caring for your family.

The best way to ensure that you have plenty of time in your schedule for studying is to develop a plan. Although planning out how each day will go can sometimes be difficult because unexpected tasks pop up, planning how you need (and want) to spend your day beforehand will help to keep you on track and will remind you of what you still need to accomplish when each day is done. If you have not done so already, you can combine your daily time management plan with your daily to-do list (see Chapter 2) by using a daily planner that is divided into hours. A daily planner such as this makes the concept of the finite 24-hour day a reality, and it will help you to see that you can realistically accomplish only so much in one day. Even if you cannot commit now to keeping a daily planner, take the time to plot out your daily tasks for 1 day over a 24-hour period. Do not forget to include time for necessities, such as sleeping and eating. In fact, begin with those tasks because you will need to complete them no matter what else you accomplish in a day. Then account for the time that you must spend each day at work and in class. The time left over after you have completed all of those tasks will be the time that you have left to allocate to your family and to studying.

O N   T R A C K

You are on track if you can look carefully at how you need to spend the 24 hours you have in each day and can determine how much study time you have. Use the list below as a starting point to calculate the amount of time you need for routine activities. Note that not all of these items may apply to your personal situation. Add to the list as necessary to make sure you have included all of your personal tasks.

ITEM	TIME
1. Sleep	_____
2. Morning preparation: Self	_____

3. Morning preparation: Family   _____

4. Breakfast   _____

5. Morning commute (include dropping children at school or daycare)   _____

6. Work   _____

7. Class   _____

8. Afternoon commute (include picking up children at school or day care)   _____

9. Dinner and family time   _____

10. Preparation for bed: Family   _____

11. Preparation for next day   _____

12. Preparation for bed: Self   _____

13. _____   _____

14. _____   _____

15. _____   _____

Total   _____

Once you have completed your list, total the number of hours that these tasks will take and then subtract that total from 24 hours. This remainder of time is your potential study time.

Once you see how much time you have left in each day, you need to focus on your priorities and create quality study time. Your schedule should be guided by your short-term goals (e.g., reading a chapter or reviewing for your next test) and long-term goals (e.g., passing your national exam and being hired for your new career position). Again, the key here is to make sure that the hours you do have for studying are spent as *quality* study time. The fewer hours you have, the more important it is for you to focus on your studies both in class and out of class.

In addition to study time, relaxation time will be competing for those left-over hours that you have in the day. This is where your time management skills will more importantly come into play. Although you might be tempted to unwind in front of the television after a long, hard day, you will need to choose to show your commitment to graduation by studying instead. Remember that scheduling quality time during the week—for yourself and your family—will help you to stay on schedule and focus on your studies when necessary.

Motivational Moment

66 The price of greatness is responsibility. 99

Winston Churchill, former Prime Minister of England

Building Your Study Skills Set

To ensure that you are making the most of the study time you have, you need to develop good study habits. You will be working very hard to create the study time that you have, so you want to be sure to make the most of it. Although you may have been told when you were growing up that you had to study and that studying is important, most people have never really been taught *how* to study. It is not too late. Now is the time for you to learn about good study habits and incorporate them into your study skill set. Doing so will serve you well not only now as you reach to meet your new career goal but also in the future as you embark on other journeys.

Good study habits start with the following:

- **Having a strong motive and interest in your subject:** You have selected a health professions career for your future.
- **Having a strong mental attitude:** You are feeding your mind with positive thoughts that will help you to reach graduation.
- **Avoiding stress:** You are reducing your stress by being organized.

By following the advice in the previous chapters, you should be well on your way to achieving these three objectives that will serve as the building blocks for building your new study skills set.

To build your study skills set, you will need to learn new study habits for both inside and outside the classroom. Following these suggestions will help you to make the most of your study time, no matter what style of learner you are.

In Class

Whether you attend class in person or online, you can make the most of your time there by following certain suggestions. Here are some ways to get the most of each classroom session (obviously, some of these suggestions do not apply to online courses):

- **Sit toward the front of the classroom:** When you sit toward the front of the room, you help to minimize the distractions that can keep your mind from focusing on the information being presented. Remember, class is not a social event; it is a learning situation. Although you will want to build new relationships with your classmates, do so during breaks and not during class time.

- **Pay attention:** As you have already discovered, your study time is precious and you must make the most of every minute. That includes your time in class. You will get the most out of each class and can minimize the time you need to spend studying at home by simply paying attention. Paying attention means listening carefully to the instructor as well as to your classmates and, if you are taking online courses, shutting out the world around you. Your listening in the classroom should be at a different level than when you are in a casual conversation with a friend or family member. Focused listening will allow you to connect ideas in ways that will help you to better understand them and better grasp their relevance to the functions, standards, and policies you will encounter in your new health professions career.

- **Ask questions:** You are making an investment in your education. Be sure to get your money's worth by not being afraid to clarify information that you do not understand. You should raise your hand to ask a question the minute you do not understand what the instructor is presenting. Lessons can build on themselves; therefore, not understanding a key piece of information early on might cause you to miss the entire point of the lecture. Asking for clarification about a topic also forces the instructor to present the information in a different way, which reinforces the concept in your mind. Questions can also spark discussions, which may afford you with a deeper meaning of the information. Never leave class until you understand the ideas and concepts presented that day.

Mentor Moment

Like most other people I attended health professions school with small children, my study time was limited. This made me realize that I needed to become a more efficient learner. In other words, I needed to understand as much new information as I could the first time around. So I really learned to listen in class. If I did not understand something, I raised my hand and asked a question. I did not want to leave class not understanding something because I was working hard to pay for my education, and I wanted to make sure I got every penny's worth!

Donna from Chicago, IL

- **Take notes:** Note taking involves your ears, mind, and hand in the learning process. The more senses you involve in learning, the better. Taking notes reinforces the information presented in class and also gives you documentation to which you can refer later on. (For more information, see "Note Taking" later in this chapter.)
- **Record your lectures:** Taping the audio from your lectures gives you a record of the lesson to which you can refer later. You can use these recordings to make sure that the notes that you have taken are accurate and also to enhance your review of your notes. Having information available to you in this portable form also gives you an opportunity to reinforce your learning at times that you might not otherwise be able to study. For example, you can listen to your recorded lectures during your commute or even while you are grocery shopping. However, be sure to get approval from your instructor before taping any lectures.
- **Come prepared:** Being prepared for each class by completing your assignments in advance is the best way to make the most of each session. Review the chapters before each lecture so that you can be ready with questions to ask the instructor about the meanings of words and concepts.

Motivational Moment

66 There are no secrets to success. It is the result of preparation, hard work, and learning from failure. 99

Colin L. Powell, statesman and former U.S. Army general

While Studying

Building your study skills set will also require you to learn good habits for studying outside the classroom. Sometimes making the most of your study time means simply selecting the right place to study (see Box 5.4). Studying at the same time and in the same place each day helps to establish it as a habit. Be sure to plan your time appropriately. If you think an assignment will take 1 hour to complete, plan on 2 or 3 hours. Projects usually take much more time than you estimate.

Making the most of your study time also means making sure that you are up to the task by being physically prepared. One way to do this is to be sure that you get enough sleep at night. For most people, 6 to 8 hours is sufficient. Although you cannot always help what time of day you study, you should make sure that you are alert as possible so that you can focus on, understand, and retain the information. Study difficult or boring subjects first, when you are most alert. You should also make sure that your eyes are up to the task of studying.

BOX 5.4   SELECTING THE RIGHT STUDY ENVIRONMENT

Here are some ways to make sure that you have the proper study environment:

- **Noise:** Select a quiet space away from ordinary noise. Although you will want to reduce your exposure to household noises, such as a blaring television and children yelling, you might want some background noise to help you focus. For example, some people like to study with headphones on or very low music on in the background. This "noise" filters out outside noises that can creep in and disrupt your concentration.
- **Light:** Study in a place with good lighting. You do not want to have to squint to see the type on a page. You will find that you will be able to study longer with the correct lighting.
- **Temperature:** Keep your environment at an even temperature to make the most of your study time. A warm room will make you sleepy, whereas a temperate room will help you to study longer and concentrate better.
- **Seating:** Choose a place to sit that is comfortable, but not too comfortable. Avoid reading in bed or in a cozy chair, such as a recliner, because you will tend to fall asleep. A straight-backed chair is best. A kitchen table or a desk is a good choice, as long as you are in a room away from household noises.
- **Interruptions:** Commit to your study time by not allowing yourself to get interrupted. For example, take your phone off the hook or turn your cell phone to vibrate. You might even want to consider telling your friends to call only during certain hours.

Use reading glasses if necessary to help you better read the type on a page. If you get headaches or your eyes burn after reading, you may need an eye examination. Such conditions as illness, hunger, and thirst can also keep you from doing a good job of studying. Take care of all of these conditions in advance so that you are at your best when it comes to study.

When Reviewing Chapters

Another important study skill is to learn how to review a chapter. As you read, your intent should be to understand the information being presented, not just to look over the words quickly on each page. Reviewing chapters again after an exam can also help you to learn because you can go back and focus on what is important and pick up information from the exam questions that you missed.

To learn to read a chapter for understanding, you should first learn how a chapter is written. Under each topic heading, which is usually in boldface or colored type in your text, you will find several paragraphs that define the subject and present information and examples. Each paragraph typically begins with a topic sentence, which identifies what the paragraph is about. Although the topic sentence may be just a general sentence that clearly states the topic, in many cases it is phrased in the form of a question or even a teaser to get your attention. Paragraphs generally have only one main topic sentence; however, they could have more. The paragraph should then go on to present details, evidence, examples, and opinions to support or illustrate the concept. Last, the paragraph should end with a summary or concluding statement that ties the ideas of the paragraph together. All of the paragraphs under a given heading should build on each other to explain and illustrate the main topic of the heading. Understanding this general format will help you to quickly identify the main points of a chapter. (See Figure 5.1.)

Here are some suggestions for making the most of your review of a chapter on your first pass.

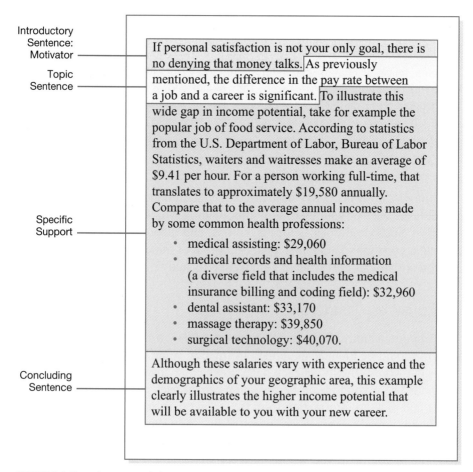

FIGURE 5.1 Sample paragraph format.

Before You Read

- **Get the assignment right:** All learning styles require that you *listen* to the assignment when it is stated by the instructor, visually *see* the assignment on the board, and finally *write* the assignment down with every detail. Make sure to ask the instructor for clarification if you are not sure of the homework assignment.

- **Check the chapter table of contents:** The table of contents is a preview that shows you the development of topic information from the first heading to the last. It should help you to understand the focus, direction, and point of view of the author. Some learners benefit from getting this view of the whole picture before getting into the details.

- **Scan the chapter:** Quickly reviewing the chapter before you read also gives you a preview of what is to come. As you visually scan the chapter, read the main section headings and look for topic sentences and summary statements. Think of this process as a warm-up exercise, where you engage in some "mental gymnastics" to try to test yourself and figure out the point of the chapter before you start to read it. In many cases, this preview will pique your interest in the topic and motivate you to read.

- **Go to the back of the chapter:** Read the chapter summary and questions at the back of the chapter so that you know what you will be expected to learn by the time you finish reading. This technique helps you to read with more purpose and an intention of answering the questions in the back of the chapter. It gives you a hint as to what you should be focusing on as you read.

As You Read the Chapter

- **Read for understanding:** As previously mentioned, when you read, your goal should be to understand the information that is being presented. This will require you to read carefully, not just skim through the paragraphs quickly. Completing one focused read of the chapter will make it easier for you to complete your assignments and labs and will help you to understand more fully the information that your instructor presents in class. In addition, reviewing the chapter correctly the first time will save you time when you study for exams later on.

- **Highlight key ideas:** Highlighting is a way to make key ideas stand out. Begin by highlighting topic sentences and summary statements. Also highlight details that the instructor references in lecture. But remember, highlighting should be used sparingly. If you highlight an entire page, you are coloring, not highlighting. Highlighting the key points and words as you read will trigger you to remember the important information later, when you review. (See Figure 5.2.)

Careers, on the other hand, lead you down a path that is created by you, your dreams, and your goals. They usually require special training and allow you to build your skills and experience over time. The payoff for this is generally a higher salary and benefits. In some cases, careers are also accompanied by greater security, flexibility, and responsibility. People who enjoy their careers find a sense of personal satisfaction in what they do. Careers offer people the opportunity to challenge themselves, nurture their personal growth, and feel they have made a difference in the world.

FIGURE 5.2 Sample of highlighted paragraph. *Note:* This illustration shows how to properly highlight key words and phrases in a paragraph. Notice that by reading only the highlighted areas, you can still understand the message of the paragraph.

- **Look up unfamiliar words:** As you read, write down any new words that you encounter in the chapter, look them up, and write down their definitions before you proceed. When you do not understand the vocabulary, the meaning of a sentence or paragraph can be lost. Take the time to learn the words that are unfamiliar to you, as they may appear again in assignments, in lectures, on handouts, and on tests and quizzes. If you still do not understand the meaning of a word after looking it up, ask your instructor. Keep the list of definitions you created, so that you can use it to study later on.
- **Write down questions:** As you read, you are bound to come across information you do not understand, is not fully covered in your text, or seems irrelevant. If you have a question about any specific information, write it down so that you can ask your instructor when you cover the material in class.

As You Review the Chapter
- **Focus on the highlights:** As you review the chapter, focus your attention on what you decided the key points were during your first read. Remember that you need not, and should not, have to read the chapter again in its entirety.
- **Remember your lectures:** As you review the chapter, also try to tie the text material into the instructor's lecture. The instructor should be pulling important information from the text during the lecture. The phrases, "This is important," "Did you understand . . .?", and "Do you have any questions about . . .?" will usually precede important information. Try also to remember examples that your instructor presented in class to help clarify information, as they will not appear in your text.

- **Rephrase the main ideas:** Take each main idea and turn it into a question (see Box 5.5). Write these questions in your notebook and then provide answers. Try to create answers in your own words. You might even use these questions later when reviewing with your study group.
- **Create flash cards:** Write all definitions, important details, and technical terms on flash cards, making sure to spell each word correctly. This will help you to master the language and vocabulary of the health-care field. You can carry your flash cards with you so that you have them to review whenever you have a few extra minutes, such as before class or during breaks. The creation of flash cards is a learning experience for all types of learners. Visual learners benefit by seeing the cards, kinesthetic learners benefit by making the cards, and auditory learners benefit by hearing the sounds of the words as they review the flash cards out loud. (See Figure 5.3.)

Note Taking

Note taking is the process of writing down the important topics covered in class. Notes tie previous, current, and future lessons together. Think of note taking as the thread that connects the information you are learning and makes it relevant for you. You are more likely to remember this information if it is relevant to your goals.

BOX 5.5   HOW TO REPHRASE MAIN IDEAS AS QUESTIONS

Main Idea	Question
Butterfly blood draw	Under what conditions should I select a butterfly needle?
	What are the steps in a butterfly blood draw?
Data entry of an insurance form	What patient information is most important on the insurance form?
	What is the most common error on the insurance form?
Deep tissue massage	Under what conditions should I not attempt a deep tissue massage?
	Does a deep tissue massage have any danger signs of which I should be aware?

Front	**Back**
Cardiologist	*Heart physician*
Oncologist	*Cancer specialist*
Orthopedist	*Bone physician*

FIGURE 5.3 Sample flash cards.

To get the most of out your note-taking experience, follow these suggestions:

- Be prepared to take notes each day by coming to class with the proper equipment. A binder or spiral notebook is useful for keeping all of your notes together in a safe and orderly manner. You can also takes notes on your computer, if permitted by your facility and the instructor. If you cannot use your computer in class, you might find it helpful to retype your notes on your computer later.
- Focus on the lecture. As you listen, think about how you will apply the information being presented in your new career.
- Listen for repetition of ideas and emphasis of key words. Also listen for key words, such as "therefore," "but," "also," and "besides," which indicate a change in the ideas and thoughts being presented.

- Keep your notes brief and clear.
- Copy what is written on the board. If an idea is important enough for the instructor to take time to write it on the board, you should write it down in your notes.
- Use shorthand if necessary to keep up with your note taking during the lecture. Use a system of shorthand that makes sense to you. For example, use symbols instead of spelling out whole words every time (e.g., the symbol "w/" can be substituted for the word "with"). In addition to the shorthand you create for yourself, as a medical professional you will be learning medical symbols to use for particular words. If your instructor used a symbol you do not understand, be sure to ask.
- Date and label all of your notes.
- Use key words as headings in your notes.
- Take notes in an outline, bullet, or paragraph format.
- Make sure to write quotations, definitions, formulas, and dates correctly.
- Mark any information that you did not understand with a question mark, and if you do not get a chance to ask the instructor during class, ask afterward.
- As appropriate, use diagrams to help you understand the topic.
- To get the most out of your notes, review them within 24 hours and again weekly. You might even find it helpful upon your first review to edit or rewrite your notes. Doing so gives you a chance to fill in missing information and organize your notes.
- Highlight important information. Just as when you review a chapter, you can save time by highlighting important information in your notes during your first review and then focusing only on the highlights at subsequent reviews. If you decide to rewrite your notes and cut out extraneous information during that process, you might not need this step.
- If you miss any notes, be sure to get them from a classmate or study group member.

O N   T R A C K

You are on track if you can improve your note taking by using two of the suggestions listed above. Write down which suggestions you plan to try.

1. _____

2. _____

Creating and Working with Study Groups

Another great way for you to learn is to form a study group so you can talk with and listen to others. A study group will assist your learning because it requires your active participation. Study groups have been a mainstay for students in many fields, including law, business, and medicine.

The people you include in your study group play an important role in how successful the group will be and how much you will get out of the group. Unfortunately, although everyone in your class should have the same goal of making it to graduation, not everyone will show the same commitment to that goal as you do. Therefore, picking the right study partners might not be easy. Start by talking to the students you sit next to in class or by talking to people during breaks. You can ask them a simple question about the lecture or reading assignment to help gauge who is keeping up. Also, listen during class to see which students pay attention and ask questions. Try to determine who has done well on class assignments and quizzes and ask those people to join your study group. Although choosing focused and intelligent classmates is important, you should also be sure to choose classmates you like and respect. Your group should generate energy and active participation from each member to take your learning to a higher level. If you are too shy to ask or are having trouble finding study group partners, you can ask your instructor to help you organize a study group.

Here are some other tips for creating a study group that works:

- *Keep it small.* Select only two or three other students to be a part of your study group. You might find that the smaller the group, the better. (See Box 5.6.)
- *Set a day and time that will work for everyone in the group.* Picking a consistent day and time will help everyone to remember to attend. And remember to mark it on your calendar for the entire length of the course. How often and how long the group meets each time is up to you. Remember that just 30 minutes before each class could make all the difference in your learning potential.

BOX 5.6   ALL YOU NEED IS ONE

Even if a big study group is not your thing, you might benefit from finding just one other person with whom you can study. This person can become your "study buddy." A two-person study group has lots of advantages, including that you only have to work with one other person's schedule, which can make finding study dates and times much more manageable. In addition, the fewer people you have in your group, the less the chances are of someone taking the group off the topic.

- *Meet on a regular basis.* The most productive study groups meet regularly, not just before a major test. The more often you meet, the more productive you will be. However, you need to remember to balance your group study time with your personal study time and make sure that you have enough time in your schedule for both.
- *Decide on a place that works for everyone.* The library or another location at the school might be an ideal spot. Transportation usually is not an issue and everyone knows where to go if you meet at school. Although the school is a good choice, some groups prefer to meet in local coffee shops or bookstores. The key is to agree on a place that works for everyone.
- *Decide on some study group rules that will help you to be productive.* A study group will die a slow death if it is not productive when the members meet. Members will slowly stop attending if they feel it is a waste of their time. Here are some recommended rules:
  - Everyone should make a commitment to arrive on time. Showing up late for study group is not only disrespectful, but it is a waste of your time and others' time. Make it clear that the group waits for no one! Even if one person is late, the study group will go on as planned. Remember, though, that attendance in the study group does not replace class attendance.
  - Everyone should try to be as focused and productive as possible. Remember that your study time is precious and you need to spend it studying.
  - Everyone should respect one another. No opinion is wrong, and no questions are stupid. A study group is no place to be judgmental or conceited. Hostile study groups are not productive. The purpose of the study group is for you to take away a better and deeper understanding of the information by sharing ideas. You cannot do this without respecting one another.

Motivational Moment

66 I am defeated, and know it, if I meet any human being from whom I find myself unable to learn anything. 99

George Herbert Palmer, American scholar, educator, and author

- *Choose a group leader.* The leader will help to keep the discussion on track. He or she should be strong enough to bring the group back to the subject at hand when members start talking about nonessential topics and should also make sure to encourage participation from all members. Everyone in the group should agree on who serves as group leader.
- *Create a discussion format.* Decide as a group what you will discuss each week and how the discussion will progress. Some groups like to compare lecture notes, whereas others benefit more from reviewing the homework

assignments. You might even want to put together a mini-lecture by having each person summarize one of the main concepts from class that week. (See Box 5.7 for a sample discussion format.)

● *Make sure everyone in your group is happy with the decisions you make as a group.* If someone is not happy, he or she might stop coming to the study group, making it less productive.

● *Make sure all members of the group know that they have a responsibility to the group and that they can be voted out if they do not contribute.* This agreement, which can be verbal or written, might help to keep members productive.

If you join a group and then find that it is not working for you, you are in the wrong group. Search for another group or, better yet, consider finding just one other person with whom you can study (i.e., a study buddy).

O N   T R A C K

You are on track if you can list the name of one person who could be your study buddy or if you can list the names of people with whom you could form a study group.

_____

_____

_____

_____

_____

BOX 5.7   SAMPLE DISCUSSION FORMAT

• Take one subject from the text at a time and compare the material with everyone's lecture notes.
• Ask each member to give his or her viewpoint to make sure that the group covers all of the material.
• Try to relate your new material to the material you learned in the past.
• Make sure everyone in the group understands the concept, vocabulary, and main ideas of the topic.

BOX 5.7 (continued)

- Go around again and ask each member to think of a question on the topic. Questions should be current and relate to how the material is useful, applied, compared and contrasted, and how it applies to your program in the health professions field. The question style could be true or false, fill-in-the-blank, matching, or essay, depending on which question styles your instructor uses.
- Each member asks the group the question he or she created.
- Do this with each main topic that you want to review. Your group may decide to eliminate *easy* topics as a way to maximize your group study time. Focus on the subjects, concepts, vocabulary, and procedures you *do not know.*

Success Journal

1. Describe what your study habits were like before your read this chapter.

_____

_____

_____

_____

_____

_____

2. List three ways in which you can improve your study habits.

   1. _____

   2. _____

   3. _____

3. Write down your primary learning style and then list three study habits that you can use to capitalize on your primary learning style.

   LEARNING STYLE: _____

   1. _____

   2. _____

   3. _____

4. List three rules that you think could be useful to a study group.

   1. _____

   2. _____

   3. _____

Test-Taking Skills

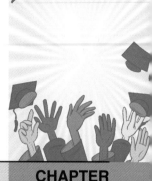

Learning Outcomes

After reading this chapter, the student will be able to:

1. List symptoms of test anxiety.
2. Understand how to study and prepare for taking a test.
3. Understand how to study for and answer different styles of test questions.
4. Identify the resources needed to prepare for a certification or national examination.

Becoming a Confident Test Taker

At this point in your journey to graduation, you have probably made some changes in your life. You might have started by working to create a positive attitude. That positive attitude allows you to focus on your goals and gives you the motivation to keep moving forward, even through the tough times. You have probably also incorporated into your life some new skills that are helping you to achieve your goals. For example, you have used time management techniques to analyze and organize your schedule to create quality study time. You have been breaking down "brick walls" to create new stepping-stones for your path to becoming a health professional. You will continue to make changes such as these in your life as you continue on your journey toward graduation.

One brick wall you may still have in front of you could be taking your first test. In your experience, you have probably heard—and maybe have even said—the phrase "I am just not good at taking tests" or "I am a poor test taker." Everyone responds to test taking differently. For some, simply hearing the word *test* provokes emotions such as anxiety and even fear. If you are young and just out of high school, your testing experience is recent, and so your emotions about it are fresh in your mind. If you are "age experienced," you might not remember much about your testing experience, except the residue of emotion that still lingers with you. However, you need to look at testing with your new positive outlook. Think of testing as a new level of experience.

Mentor Moment

When I was in high school, I made mainly C's and had more D's than I care to count. When I qualified for my vocational college, I was more surprised than anyone. I decided that I would earn good grades. I wanted to make something of myself and also have my kids feel proud of me. I did just that: I made all A's! It was not easy; however, it started with my determination to do my best for the first time in my life.

James from Anchorage, AK

While you are in school, you could experience one test per week for approximately 8 months, excluding your practicum. This totals 32 tests during your program, not including quizzes and other required projects. (If your program is longer than 8 months, then just add 4 additional tests for each month you are in school.) Clearly, you will not be able to avoid test taking while you are in health professions school, so the best way to approach it is to learn some new skills that will improve your confidence, reduce your fear and anxiety, and allow you to focus on conveying the information that you have learned.

O N   T R A C K

You are on track if you can remember the last test you took and how you felt when you were taking it. Write down the experience:

_____

_____

_____

_____

_____

If taking that test was a good experience, keep it as a good memory. If it was not a good experience, leave it here on this page and prepare yourself to create a new experience from your next test in your health professions program.

Believing in Yourself

The first step toward becoming a successful test taker is to believe in yourself. If you have been told by others or your past experience has shown you that you are a poor test taker, then of course you will believe that you are. But this is another one of those moments that you must learn to control. You must learn to *believe* that you can successfully take a test. Think of it this way, life is a journey on which you encounter decision making and problem solving every day. A test is merely an opportunity on your way to graduation for you to decide that you will be successful and for you to use problem solving to figure out how to do it.

Motivational Moment

66 Life is either a daring adventure or nothing. 99

Helen Keller, American author and educator

Creating a new attitude toward testing requires that you accept responsibility for your learning and studying habits. When you do not accept responsibility, you allow yourself to be a victim of fear. Your fear feeds on the negative thoughts and negative images you create in your mind. It grows and can become overwhelming when you try to ignore it. Instead of letting this happen, you must control your mind and create alternative thoughts. Take control of your mind so that you can control your fears. Ask yourself this question, "What would I do if I did not feel afraid?" Maybe your response is one of these outcomes:

- I would accept responsibility for studying.
- I would learn this material.
- I would show myself and others that I can do it.
- I would do well on the test.
- I would prove that I am not a poor test taker.

Now say these outcomes out loud several times until they feel real to you. Imagine these results coming true. Use this image to create the positive attitude you want. It may sound simple, but practicing this exercise will make it easier for you to believe in yourself. Now is the time to take charge, drown out that little voice in your head, and control your test-taking fears.

O N   T R A C K

You are on track if you are able to identify where your current level of confidence is and what steps you need to take to improve it. Answer these questions:

What grade do I think I can earn on my next test? _____

What grade do I *want* to earn on my next test? _____

What steps do I need to take to achieve that grade? _____

_____

_____

_____

_____

Overcoming Test Anxiety

Many people score poorly on tests simply because they suffer from test anxiety. Feeling a little fear, nervousness, and stress before a test is normal. However, test anxiety occurs when those feelings are so intense that they interfere with how a person performs on the test. The person might report having difficulty concentrating or feeling like his or her mind has gone completely blank. Test anxiety can also cause a person to experience headaches, nausea, sweating, light-headedness, rapid breathing and heartbeat, and other physical symptoms.

Becoming a confident test taker requires not only believing in yourself but also being able to overcome test anxiety. Your first level of defense is to discuss this issue with your instructor and follow the suggestions offered here. However, if your anxiety is extremely severe or the suggestions below do not work for you, you may need to turn to a professional for help.

Creating the Right Attitude

Like many other obstacles, learning to control your test anxiety begins with a positive attitude. Start by telling your mind, "I am a skillful test taker." Giving that little voice in your head something different to say will strengthen your test performance. Acknowledge your test-taking fear and nervousness and take control of them. In fact, use them to your advantage by drawing on the energy they generate. Create a new position of strength with your mind. Now is the time to use words such as "I can" and "I will," which create the positive pattern that you need in your mind.

Another way to control your test anxiety is to be prepared. The most obvious way to do this is to study. Studying to the point that you feel *overprepared* for the test will help to build your confidence. Make sure that you have studied the material that the test will cover. Review your class notes as well as the highlights of your readings and any flashcards that you might have created. The more confident you feel, the less likely you are to experience test anxiety. (See the section "Preparing for a Test" later in this chapter for more information on the most effective ways to prepare for a test.)

Another way to feel prepared for your test is to gather together all of the materials you need the night before. Lower your stress by bringing extra pens, pencils, erasers, and other supplies. Also decide what you are going to wear when you take the test. Be sure to choose clothes and shoes that are comfortable. Before the test, get a good night's sleep and take time to eat something so that you are not hungry and can focus during the test. Preparing in advance in this way frees up your mind so that you can focus on correctly answering test questions.

Controlling Your Body's Response

The next step in overcoming test anxiety is to control your body's physical response to it. Test anxiety might cause you to experience fast or heavy breathing. Just experiencing this type of breathing can make you more nervous. You can try to take control of your breathing and calm your test anxiety by following these simple steps[1]:

1. Be aware if you experience fast or heavy breathing before a test.
2. Take a deep breath very slowly through your nose.
3. Hold the breath to a count of 5.
4. Exhale very slowly from your mouth to a count of 5.
5. If fast breathing and anxiety continue, repeat the breathing exercise, holding your lower ribs and abdomen with your hands to make sure you have fully exhaled.

Be sure to perform this exercise slowly to prevent hyperventilation, which can cause dizziness and lightheadedness. If these symptoms occur, use your hands to cup your nose and mouth and rebreathe your exhaled air. When properly performed, this exercise can give you back control of your body by returning your breathing to normal. If you are unable to regain your normal breathing or experience a more severe response, immediately notify your instructor and seek professional attention, if appropriate.

Exercising the rest of your body can also help you to overcome and prevent test anxiety. Exercise helps the muscles to release tension that can make you feel tight and on edge. This physical tension can translate into mental tension that surfaces in the form of test anxiety. Walking briskly to class, stretching, and doing some jumping jacks before you enter your classroom are some easy ways to release body tension before a test.

Mentor Moment

I never did well on tests in high school. For some reason, I would always get really nervous before I took a test because I never felt prepared. To make sure that this did not happen in health professions school, I joined a study group. Studying with other people who were also committed to doing well helped me to feel more prepared to take my tests. I also found that I enjoyed studying more because I was working toward my goal of becoming a surgical technologist.

Paulina from Louisville, KY

Learning from Mistakes

The last step in overcoming test anxiety is to ensure that you learn from your mistakes. Remember that a test is a product of your *performance,* not your *potential.* If you perform poorly on a test, you must go back and review your performance to understand what went wrong:

● If you did not know the answers, ask yourself why. Did you study the wrong material? Did you focus on the wrong points? Did you not pay attention in class? Did you forget to review your notes?

- If you studied and knew the material but still answered the questions incorrectly, ask yourself why. Did you misread the questions because you read them too quickly? Did you not understand all of the parts to a question?
- If you became overwhelmed by test anxiety and your mind went blank or you ran out of time, ask yourself why. Did you try to use the breathing exercise previously discussed? Did you go into the test thinking that you were going to fail?

If you are able to analyze what went wrong and identify the cause of your poor performance, then you are on the path to correcting that problem so it does not happen the next time you have a test. Be sure that you find a way to make your performance a true measure of the knowledge that you have.

If you are unable to figure out the reason for your poor performance, you can enroll your instructor in assisting you to find a solution. Remember, your instructor has encountered many students, and he or she wants to see each student do his or her best and graduate.

Motivational Moment

66 Achievement seems to be connected with action. Successful men and women keep moving. They make mistakes, but they don't quit. 99

Conrad Hilton, founder of Hilton Hotels chain

Preparing for a Test

Although having a positive attitude can take you a long way when it comes to overcoming test anxiety and taking a test, to really do well on a test you also need to prepare. This means taking the time to learn and review the material that will be covered on your test, which will require a significant commitment on your part. Simply attending class is not enough. Your ability to be successful on a test—whether it is a quiz, weekly test, midterm, or final—depends on your commitment to study and prepare.

When it comes time to take a test, do not just "wing it." You have a responsibility to prepare for tests and exams by studying. You owe this responsibility to your family (think about all of the changes you have asked them to make for the benefit of your education) and to yourself (think of all of the changes and sacrifices you have made yourself for the benefit of your education). No one can study for you, and you cannot assume that you will just absorb the information by attending class. As previously mentioned, you must dedicate time in your schedule to study—and the time that you dedicate must be significant, especially when it comes time to prepare for tests. You cannot count on being successful if you allot 90% of your time to other people and events and study only 10% of your time. Remember that you may need to reorganize and reprioritize in order to create quality study time. If you have not done so already, now is the time to make those changes in your schedule that will create quality study time for you. To be successful, you need to think like a winner and study like a winner.

Motivational Moment

66 Winning is not everything—but making the effort to win is. 99

Vince Lombardi, American football coach

Knowing What to Study

Before a test, your instructor will probably spend time reviewing what the test will cover. The instructor will make reference to certain chapters, theories, vocabulary, and concepts from the lectures and handouts. Pay attention to this material and make note of the topics that your instructor mentions so that you can focus on them as you prepare for the test. Also focus your studying on concepts that the instructor emphasized several times in lectures or repeated in different ways, as these concepts are generally the most important.

You need to be aware that your instructor wants you to understand the material. Most instructors will go out of their way to mention important concepts in different ways until they feel you understand the information. They do not intentionally try to mislead you about what concepts are important or what information will be on the test. Some instructors even hold a formal test review day to go over what will be covered on the test. This review usually occurs the day before the test. Because this review will guide your studies and help you to conserve your time by focusing on important information, your attendance on test review day is even more important than it is on most other days. Test review day requires not only your attendance but also your questions. If you do not understand any of the material that will be on the test, you should come prepared to ask questions on test review day. You have an investment in your future, and your investment is reflected in your tuition. Your instructor respects your investment in yourself, and you need to have that same respect and show it by asking questions.

Even if your instructor does not hold a formal test review day, do not be afraid to ask questions about the test. Ask your instructor what material the test will cover, and also ask to review any material that is giving you trouble. Some specific questions you might want to ask include the following:

- Will the test include vocabulary terms? If so, will they be matching or true-or-false questions?
- Will the test include any essay questions? If so, how many essay questions will be on the test?

Asking questions before a test is a good way to increase your confidence and reduce test anxiety. The more information you have about the test, the less anxiety you will feel on the day of the test.

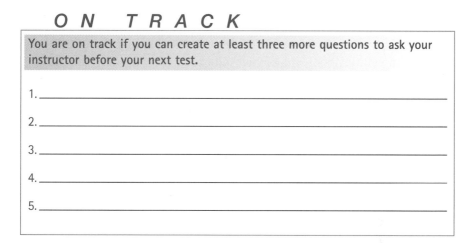

O N T R A C K

You are on track if you can create at least three more questions to ask your instructor before your next test.

1. _____

2. _____

3. _____

4. _____

5. _____

In addition, although it might feel good to answer questions on information you have already learned, you should not waste time studying what you already know. Your study time will be precious, and so you should focus it on studying what *you do not know* when the instructor indicates this information will be on the test. Challenging yourself in this way will increase the knowledge that you have, leaving you better prepared when it is time to take the test.

Understanding How to Study

Just as important as knowing what to study is knowing how to study. You can use one, several, or all of the following techniques to help you prepare for a test.

- **Read your class notes:** If you have taken good notes, they should reflect what the instructor covered in class and in the clinical lab for each chapter. The instructor usually discusses major concepts and important vocabulary terms. The instructor should also describe the reason behind the concepts and policies in your program field. Therefore, reviewing your class notes will not only tell you which concepts the instructor felt were important but also how to apply those concepts. For this reason, reading your notes should help you to answer essay and fill-in-the-blank questions, which are usually based on concepts.

- **Review the material you highlighted in your textbook:** Reviewing the information in your textbook will be important, but you will not have time to review everything. If you took the time to highlight important concepts during your first review of the chapter, then you will save yourself time and agony when it comes time for you to prepare for the test. Your textbook is likely to present information in a very factual manner. For this reason, reviewing the material you highlighted in your textbook should help you to answer fill-in-the-blank, matching, multiple-choice, and true-or-false questions, which are based on facts.

- **Review the questions at the end of each textbook chapter:** The end-of-chapter questions in your textbook are another indication of which concepts are important. Reviewing these questions can help you to judge whether you have grasped the essential information from the chapter. Reviewing the textbook questions is also helpful because instructors commonly use questions from the textbook or from an instructor's guide for their tests. Sometimes these questions are multiple-choice, fill-in-the-blank, or matching format, but instructors might also take or modify essay and short-answer questions from your textbook summary questions.

- **Study your flash cards:** Although you will benefit most from reviewing your flash cards for a short amount of time each day, reviewing your cards before a test is a good way to ensure that you remember all of the important technical terms and concepts that might appear on the test. You might be asked on a test to directly define vocabulary terms, but even if you are not, those terms might appear within the context of other questions and you will need to remember their meanings in order to correctly answer those questions.

- **Review with a classmate (study buddy) or study group:** Studying with others is a good way to increase your confidence about the test material you know. When you are able to explain a concept to someone else, you reinforce it in your own mind and can gauge your true understanding of it. You will also be able to recognize what you do not know. After a study group session, you can take time to focus your studying on what you do not know, rather than reviewing what you already know.

- **Review your lab procedures:** This task might require the least effort when it comes to studying, as you will have practiced these procedures over and over again each day in class. Although you will want to review your lab procedures before a test, do not wait until right before the test to master these procedures. If you are not efficient at an "A" level when you review the procedures in class, you should buddy with a lab partner who is at an "A" level or ask your instructor to help you reach that "A" level. Your ability to understand each lab procedure and execute it will be impressed upon your mind. When you take a test, you should then be able to use visualization to recall these procedures and come up with the right answers.

You should also make the most of your preparation by knowing when to study. This time will be different for each person, as some people are morning people and others are night owls. For example, a morning person might not benefit from pulling an all-nighter studying, whereas a night owl might. If possible, you should choose to study during the time of day that you are most focused and alert. Do not be afraid to accept your strengths and weakness when it comes to studying. Instead, use them to your advantage to make the most of your tudy time.

Motivational Moment

66 First say to yourself what you would be; and then do what you have to do. 99

Epictetus, Greek philosopher

One study approach that it not successful is cramming. Cramming for a test by trying to review a lot of information all at once in a short amount of time creates confusion and fear when test time arrives. Instead, arrange your schedule so that you can study a couple chapters and concepts for a few hours each night. Do not overwhelm yourself by trying to cover too many topics per night, and do not move on to new information until you understand and can remember the first couple of concepts you are reviewing. Covering sections of material each night through repetition in this way is the most beneficial approach for your mind to master the information. Reading your notes before going to bed and allowing your brain to process the information while you sleep is a stronger impact than cramming.

Mentor Moment

When I first started health professions school, I found that I was doing poorly on tests because I did not understand the words in the test questions. I talked with the director of education because I really wanted to pass and go to graduation. By offering to meet with me and go over the test I had just taken that week, the director of education helped me better understand the test questions so that I could do better on my next test. I realized I knew the answers when she read the test questions to me. I was so glad I asked for help. She helped me gain confidence in my testing-taking ability.

Maxine from La Habra, CA

Taking the Test

Preparing for a test is only half the battle. Once you have the information you need to know in your head, you must become effective at actually taking tests and showing your instructor what you have learned. After all, the test-taking experience is the culmination of your education. Your test grades will be a major factor in your overall grade in your class and will determine your ability to go to graduation.

When the test paper lands on your desk, you can experience two major emotions. You might feel confident because you have studied and your brain is full of information. However, you might also feel scared and worry that your past test-taking experiences will "flare up." Understanding how to take a test and trusting the knowledge you have learned and stored in your brain are keys to becoming a successful test taker.

Understanding Test-Taking Thought Processes

How does your brain help you to answer test questions? All of your experiences go into your subconscious. Think of it as your brain's "filing cabinet." The other part of your brain is the conscious part, which is the thinking part. These two parts work together when you are taking a test. Your subconscious provides an answer to your brain once you have read a question. Then the conscious side of your brain lets you know if the answer submitted by the subconscious is correct and tries to prove that the answer is right or wrong. So when you feel like you have a battle going on in your stomach as you take a test, that battle is really in your head.

So, how does understanding how your brain works help you to take a test? Well, have you ever heard the saying that the first answer that pops into your head is usually the correct answer? That is because this answer is the one that your subconscious is providing based on the facts you have stored in your file cabinet. As long as you have taken the time to file away enough facts by studying and as long as you read the question correctly, this answer will usually be correct. Once you have answered a question, you can forget it and move on to the next question. Once you have answered all the questions to the best of your ability, you should turn in the test to your instructor. You can quickly review it to make sure that you have answered all the questions and return to any that you left blank, but do not second-guess the answers that you have completed. Trust that you came up with the correct answer the first time and feel confident as you turn your test over to your instructor. This method works best on tests and exams with objective question types, such as true-or-false, fill-in-the-blank, and multiple-choice questions. By allowing the subconscious side of your brain to do the work, you can improve your test-taking ability and score higher on your next test.

One obstacle to overcome is that your conscious might attempt to place doubt about your abilities. Low self-confidence will probably make you feel like you do not have the right answer, and even worse, that you cannot be right. Have you ever written down an answer and then erased it, only to find out later on that you erased the correct answer? Once again, having a positive attitude is the answer to coping with this problem and being successful. You must be confident in the fact that you have learned the information by preparing for the test and asking questions about topics that you did not understand. Once you increase your self-confidence, you will be able to trust the answers that your subconscious provides. If you have not yet created a positive attitude, now is the time.

O N T R A C K

You are on track if you can write down a positive affirmation that you can verbalize to yourself before you take a test. For example, "I know this information because I studied this information, and I can do well on this test." Write your positive affirmation here:

_____

_____

_____

_____

Understanding Question Types

Understanding the different types of questions you will encounter on a test can help you to not only better prepare for the test but also to better answer questions using the knowledge you have studied and stored in your brain. The types of questions you are likely to encounter are discussed next.

● **Multiple-choice:** Multiple-choice questions generally present you with a question and three or more possible answers. Sometimes the question is preceded by a scenario that you must reference in order to answer correctly. A traditional multiple-choice question has only one correct answer; however, these types of questions can be made more challenging by having more than one correct response that you must identify. Because the answer options are sometimes similarly worded, multiple-choice questions will test your ability to distinguish between definitions and concepts that have slight distinctions.

Which type of specialist would a patient be referred to if he or she has cancer?
a. Cardiologist
b. Oncologist
c. Orthopedist

(The answer is b.)

- **True-or-false:** True-or-false questions generally present you with a statement that you must identify as being true or false. These questions are usually designed to test your understanding of the differences between two concepts. You must understand those concepts in order to make the right choice.

True or False: An orthopedist is a doctor who studies cancer cells in the body.

(The answer is False. An orthopedist is a doctor who deals with disorders and injuries of the skeletal system; oncology is the study of cancer cells.)

- **Fill-in-the-blank:** Fill-in-the-blank, or fill-in, questions generally present you with a statement that is missing one or more key words or terms. You must be able to recognize and insert the term that correctly completes the statement. This type of question will draw on your recollection of vocabulary terms and their meanings.

When my son was born with a hole between the two chambers of his heart, the heart specialist, or _____, said it was a ventricular septal defect.

(The answer is "cardiologist.")

- **Matching:** Matching questions usually present you with two columns and ask you to match an item on the left side with an item on the right side. This type of question format is commonly used for matching vocabulary terms with their definitions.

Match the physician titles to the study of their practice:
1. Cardiologist   _____ Study of cancer
2. Oncologist   _____ Study of the skeleton
3. Orthopedist   _____ Study of the heart

(The correct order is 2, 3, 1.)

- **Short answer:** Short-answer questions require you to draw on your knowledge to write out short answers to a question. In health professions school, short-answer questions commonly ask you to state equipment needed for or the steps of a procedure. To receive full credit for a short-answer question, you will need to remember to include all pertinent steps in the procedure, including those related to patient observation and safety.

Example

List and define at least 10 instruments a surgical technologist would need to perform or prepare for open heart surgery.

(The correct answer would be something like this:

- Cardiopulmonary bypass machine, or "heart-lung machine": functions as the heart and lungs while the surgeon works on the heart
- Hypothermia and temperature units: bring down body temperature to slow the heart's metabolism
- Cell saver: recycles blood that is lost during the procedure back into the body
- Electrosurgical unit or "pencil": necessary for coagulating and cutting purposes
- Suction system: used for disposal of blood and other body fluids
- Ice (slush) machine: used as an adjunct to lower body temperature
- Heart pack
- Drapes (nonfenestrated heart sheet)
- Basin sets, including other sterile supplies such as medication cups and a pitcher for irrigation
- Drains: chest tubes for reestablishing negative pressure in the pleural cavity
- Dressings: according to surgeon's preference
- Scalpel blades, needles, and syringes of various sizes
- Sternal or oscillating saw to open up the chest
- Sternal retractor
- Delicate instruments for the heart for optimal visualization.

One way to ensure that you will be ready to answer any of these question types when you encounter them on a test is to study as if all of the test questions will be in short-answer form. Do not study for true-or-false and matching questions; those question types tend to be easier to answer because they test your knowledge at more basic levels of understanding. They generally require you to simply *recall* information, whereas essay questions require you to *apply* the information you have learned. For example, an essay question might ask you to show that you understand how the concepts, ideas, vocabulary terms, and processes you have learned relate to patient care, safety, and regulations. In addition, you not only need to recall this information so that you can pass your test, but you will also need to retain this information to complete your national and certification exams.

By approaching your studies in this way, you will ensure that you truly grasp each of the important concepts. Of course, understanding the important concepts begins with understanding the building blocks for those concepts, which include your vocabulary terms. Reviewing your flash cards to make sure that you know all of the vocabulary terms and can define them is important, but when you are preparing for a test, you should think about those terms in a broader context, making sure that you understand their importance to the concepts that you must know. For example, it might be important to know that a cardiologist by definition is a physician who studies the heart and its diseases. However, in preparing for the test, you should think about broader concepts, such as what steps would a cardiologist use to repair a ventricular septal defect, what anatomy and physiology concepts are important to understanding this procedure, and what equipment is needed to keep the patient breathing while the defect is being repaired.

Answering Test Questions

Sometimes, even people who study hard and go into a test feeling confident do not perform as well as they would like to. However, learning certain skills can help you to approach test taking in a way that is more likely to have your performance match your potential.

One of the easiest ways to lose points on a test is to not answer one or more of the questions. To avoid doing this, you should review the test when you receive it. Begin by reading the test instructions and then quickly review the questions. Ask your instructor any questions you have about the test and make sure to check the board for any extra questions. If you see a question format that you are not familiar with, ask about it before you start the test. And, as simple as it sounds, make sure you turn the page over to see if there are any questions on the backs of the pages. If you do not understand what a question is asking, ask your instructor to explain it. Although the instructor will not give you the answer, he or she might present the question in a way that you better understand it and can answer it on your own.

Even if you do not know the answer to a question, you should try to provide an educated guess to give yourself a chance of getting the answer right. Although you should avoid blind guessing, you can use the information you do know, the process of elimination, and the information you get from other questions you read in the test to provide an educated guess. For true-or-false questions, you have a 50% chance of getting a question correct just by giving an educated guess. For standard four-option multiple-choice questions, you have a 25% chance. For essay questions, you may be awarded partial credit for answering whatever part of the question you can. No matter what the question type, if you leave a question blank, you will receive no credit for that question, so you are better off putting down some sort of answer.

In addition to losing points, not answering all of the items on a test can also cause other problems. For example, if you are using a computerized test form for your answers, skipping questions could cause you to get your answers out of order. In this case, even questions you answered correctly may be marked wrong. You should take the time to carefully check that you are putting your answers in the corresponding spaces on the computerized test form.

You also need to make sure that you take the time to carefully read each question and read it in its entirety. In fact, you should read each question twice before answering. Doing so gives your brain a chance to process the question. It might even help you to feel a little calmer and lower your test anxiety. Your speed of reading is likely to increase as your test anxiety increases, which in turn will cause you to read faster and miss or misread words in the question.

If you find yourself caught up in this vicious cycle of read fast-feel anxious-read faster, you should practice your breathing exercises to reduce your anxiety.

Reading too quickly can cause you to make the following mistakes:

- **Misunderstand the instructions:** Start with the basics by making sure that you take the time to carefully read and understand the test's instructions. When you misunderstand the instructions, you are more likely to make mistakes on the rest of the test.
- **Misunderstand what the question is asking:** Misreading a question can cause you to quickly decide on an incorrect answer. If you do not give your brain enough time to process the question, you will have moved on without realizing that your answer is incorrect. Again, make sure that you read each question twice, slowly, to ensure that you understand what the question is asking. Do not try to guess what the question is asking or wants as an answer.
- **Miss parts of what the question is asking:** Not answering all parts of a question could result in the entire question being considered wrong or you receiving less than full credit for the test question. One way to reduce confusion and keep track of question parts is to add a letter, such as (a), (b), and (c), by each section of the question that you need to answer. Making sure that you answer all the subquestions in a main question increases your chances of getting full credit.
- **Miss important words in the question:** Key words, such as "not," "except," and "opposite," could be the keys to answering questions correctly.

Once you know that you have read the question carefully, understood it, and provided an educated response, you should keep moving! Another mistake many students make is spending too much time on a question. If you find yourself reading a question several times and you still do not know the answer, then you should move on to the next question. You need to remember that you are in a timed test situation. You do not want to waste time on any one question that is difficult for you because you might be forced to rush through questions later on or you might not get a chance to answer all of the questions due to lack of time. Be sure to mark the question in some way or to write down the question number at the end of your test, which will remind you to return to it when you have answered the other questions on the test. Doing so releases your mind to answer the questions ahead of you. You might even find the answer to the question you are having trouble with tucked in one of the other questions as you move through the test.

Many students lose points because the instructor cannot read their answers. Believe it or not, this problem can occur on all test question types, not just essay questions. Writing clearly is the best way to communicate the knowledge that you have and is the only way to ensure that you will receive credit for the questions you answer correctly. If your instructor cannot read your answer, it will be marked wrong. You cannot expect your instructor to guess whether you knew the correct answer. If you know that your handwriting is bad, then write slowly and print to make your writing as clear as possible. (See Box 6.1.)

Preparing for Your Certification or National Exam

The tests that you take during your health professions program are preparing you for the most important exam, which is the certification or national exam that you

---

BOX 6.1 AVOIDING COMMON MISTAKES

Knowing the 10 most common test-taking mistakes will help you to avoid them, making it possible for you to achieve the highest possible test scores.

1. Not believing in yourself
2. Studying what you already know
3. Studying to memorize rather than learn
4. Cramming
5. Not answering all of the test questions
6. Misreading test questions
7. Spending too much time on a question
8. Misreading key words
9. Blindly guessing
10. Writing illegibly

will probably take at the end of your program. Most health professions programs offer a certification (e.g., medical assisting, billing and coding) or national examination (e.g., massage therapy) that gauges your competency to work in the health-care field. These exams commonly have a test bank of approximately 2,500 questions, and you will be asked to answer as many as 250 on your exam.

Mentor Moment

It takes a great deal of studying to pass the national certification. Really, it is like you are studying for the exam during your entire program. Each time you take a test, you need to keep your lecture notes and study guides so you can keep going over the material. I learned that the hard way. I thought I would just remember everything when it came time for the national exam, but I failed the first time I took it. The hardest part about that was that I had to pay for the test the second time—but I made sure that time that I studied *and passed!*

Sonny from Baton Rouge, LA

Understanding Certification

At this point, you might be wondering, "Why would I want to take another test after I have finished my program?" One reason is that passing a certification or national exam increases your earning potential and helps you to realize your professional goals. Your school might even require that you take a certification exam as a condition of graduation.

Even if certification is not a requirement for your graduation, you should explore the options for certification in your field by doing some research. Find out the following:

- *Is your program specifically accredited?* If you are attending an accredited program, your educational institution will need to follow guidelines that hold your curriculum to a higher standard. Having such a strong curriculum will ensure that you are learning the information needed to pass a certification exam.
- *Is your school a test site?* If your school is a test site, the major advantage is that you will not need to travel on test day.
- *Are your instructors certified, and if so, when did they take the exam?* If your instructors are certified, they might be better able to help you prepare for your exam by emphasizing concepts and subject areas that are important for you to know and understand.
- *What do you need to become certified?* Each organization that issues certifications has specific requirements. They also have certain applications and processes that you will have to follow to schedule your national exam.

- *Who pays for certification?* Sometimes the fee for your first exam is part of your tuition, and sometimes you need to save for this cost on your own.
- *What is the cost of the exam?* The cost for each exam varies. Some exams are more expensive than others.
- *Who is in charge of administering the exam?* Each specialty exam is offered by a different organization, and some specialties have multiple certifications offered by multiple organizations. You can find out which organizations or agencies offer certification in your field by searching the internet.
- *What study aids are available for the test?* By visiting the websites of the organizations or agencies offering certification in your field, you can also find out which books are recommend for studying and may also be given access to sample testing.

Finding out the answers to each of these questions for your specific school and program will lead you to more information about certification. Your department administrators and career services department should be able to provide you with some basic information to get you started.

Knowing What and How to Study

The comprehensive nature of a certification or national exam could be overwhelming to you. You might be wondering how you will know what to study for your exam. The information that will be covered on your certification or national exam depends in large part on your program of study. Some national certification organizations offer study guides that provide a review of the content. Many also offer sample questions on their websites. Your educational institution may also have study materials and online tests to assist you during your preparation time. Check with your instructor to see what type of study aides are available at your campus.

The best way to prepare for your certification or national exam is to focus while you are in school. The exam will test your knowledge and application of the important concepts you are learning throughout your program. If you truly learn those concepts, not just memorize facts that help you to pass a test, then you are already on your way to being prepared to pass the exam.

When it comes time to take the exam, you will still want to review. Studying the exam guide will be essential. Remember to answer any questions included and to check your answers in the back of the guide.

You might find it useful to study for the exam with your study group or study buddy. If you like studying alone, however, then you should inquire whether your campus offers test review questions in a computerized version or on a website. Reviewing sample questions such as these will give you an idea of the types of questions and concepts that will be covered on the exam. You might also ask a student who has passed the exam the following questions:

- How did you study for the exam?
- What areas did you find most difficult?
- What questions surprised you?
- What lab procedures were covered as questions?
- What do you think is the best way to study now that you have taken the exam?

Approaching the exam in this way will give you the one key you need to be successful: you will be overprepared, and that alone will boost your self-confidence.

O N   T R A C K

You are on track if you can list the following information:

1. The name of the person who handles the national exams at your campus _____

2. The steps that you need to take to schedule your national exam

_____

3. The fee for the exam_____

4. The person responsible for paying for the exam

_____

If you do decide to take the certification test or need to as a condition of your graduation, you should make sure that you know exactly when and where the test will be given and have followed the instructions for test registration. As the test day approaches, be sure to double-check the date and time of the test and make sure that you know exactly where you are going. You might even want to drive to the test site in advance to make sure you do not get lost on test day. Arrive early for your test because you will not be permitted to take the test once the doors are closed and the testing begins.

Success Journal

1. Remember a time when you experienced some test anxiety, no matter how slight. Then describe what you could do now to calm yourself down if you experience that test anxiety again.

_____

_____

_____

_____

_____

_____

2. Review the techniques that you can use to prepare for a test and select two approaches that you could incorporate into your new study habits.

1._____

_____

2._____

_____

3. Think about your past test-taking experiences. Write down three mistakes that you have made when taking a test and then explain what you could do to avoid each of these mistakes in the future.

1._____

_____

_____

_____

2. _____

_____

_____

_____

3. _____

_____

_____

_____

4. Do some research to find out what resources are available at your campus to help you study for your certification or national exam and then list three of those resources here. *Hint:* Check with the placement and the education departments at your school.

1. _____

2. _____

3. _____

BIBLIOGRAPHY

1. Nugent, P.M., & Vitale, B.A. (2008). *Test Success: Test-Taking Techniques for Beginning Nursing Students,* 5th edition. F.A. Davis: Philadelphia.

Preparing to Be Successful in Your New Career

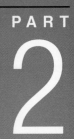

Marketing and Networking to Succeed

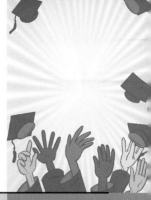

Learning Outcomes

After reading this chapter, the student will be able to:

1. Understand and discuss the importance of marketing oneself early in one's program.
2. List effective networking techniques.
3. Demonstrate the ability to develop a marketing and networking plan.
4. Understand the importance of selecting the right mentor.

Marketing Yourself From Beginning to End

When you think about the term "marketing," you probably associate it with the business concept of advertising that you encounter every day on television, in stores, on billboards, on the radio, and on the internet. In fact, marketing is *big* business. You almost cannot avoid it in life, even if you try. Marketing is all around you.

By definition, marketing is the process that a company uses to promote and sell a product or service. It is commonly used to advertise such products as soft drinks, cars, cell phones, and even medications. It is also used for services such as tax preparation, insurance coverage, and phone and internet service. The goal of marketing is to spread the word about a product or service and present the qualities of that product or service in such a way that it is uniquely differentiated from the other products on the market.

In much the same way that businesses advertise and market their products, to be successful in your new career, you will need to learn to market your product . . . *you!* The goal will be the same: to spread the word about yourself and the services (skills) you offer in a way that makes you stand out.

Motivational Moment

66 When you believe in a thing, believe in it all the way, implicitly and unquestionably. 99

Walt Disney, American animator, entertainer, and philanthropist

Networking is one way in which you will get your marketing message out to other people. Think of networking as a major component of your personal "advertising campaign." Although networking occurs on a more personal level than typical advertising, it is a way for you to promote yourself to other people and make connections by letting them know about your interests, goals, and ideas.

Throughout your health professions program, you will encounter opportunities for marketing and networking that will help you to succeed later on in your career. The more people you can inform of your goals, the wider your opportunity for success will be.

Importance of Marketing Yourself

Depending on your personality, values, self-confidence, and personal history, you might find marketing yourself difficult, uncomfortable, or challenging. You are not alone. Many people are uncomfortable with the concept of marketing themselves because it means that they must talk about themselves to others. However, you must understand that marketing yourself will be a key component of your future success. Unless you are lucky enough to have a career position fall into your lap (but do not count on that), you will need to put significant time and effort into advertising yourself and finding your new career. You cannot let all of your hard work go to waste by being too shy or too afraid to tell people about yourself and your goals.

Motivational Moment

66 Self-esteem isn't everything; it's just that there's nothing without it. 99

Gloria Steinem, American feminist and cofounder of New York *magazine*

Effective marketing begins with believing in your product. In the same way that you might know the reasons why you prefer to buy one cola brand over another, you need to know and be able to communicate the reasons why an organization should invest in you by hiring you for its position. That means you need to be able to recognize and "sell" your best qualities and talents to prospective employers through marketing.

Whether you are just starting out on a career path for the first time or starting over on a new career path, the confidence that you have in yourself will become the foundation for your marketing strategy. Your health professions program should be helping you reach a higher level of self-confidence and self-esteem by preparing you with the new knowledge and skills you will need to enter your new career. Continue to build on that confidence by reminding yourself of all of the strong personal skills and qualities you have as well, including your organizational skills, your ability to work in a team environment, and your ability to learn quickly. You need to think of all of these skills as a marketable product and find a way to effectively communicate those skills to a future employer or to someone who might be able to connect you with a future employer.

O N   T R A C K

You are on track if you can list three things about yourself that make you stand out from the other people in your field.

1. _____

2. _____

3. _____

Steps for Marketing Yourself

To maximize your marketing potential, you should develop a marketing plan and follow it. Although doing so will not always be easy, now is the right time for you to start. You need to begin planning now so that you can be prepared to advertise that you will be ready to be employed in a new career in several months. The sooner you can start spreading the word about yourself, the more opportunities you will create for your future. You can use the steps that follow as guidelines for developing your marketing plan.

Step 1: Learn the Field

The first step is to learn as much as you can about your field of interest. Doing so will help you to start conversations about health-care topics with people you do not know. In other words, this knowledge can be a good "icebreaker" for when you begin to network. Learning about the field will also help to increase your self-confidence and make you sound well-versed and educated in your field, which will assist you to land a position and reach the highest possible salary.

Here are some important points of interest that you will need to know about:

- **What is happening in the field?** To keep up with current events in the health-care field, you should read professional journals, magazines, and newspaper articles. Some of these articles are available online for free. You might also find it informative to watch the news and health-related television programs, such as *The Doctors* and *The Dr. Oz Show*, to see how medical procedures, patient care, drugs, and other health-care issues are changing. Knowing what is happening in the field will come in handy during your career search because it will enable you to show that you are in touch with current issues when you are networking and interviewing. However, you will need to continue to stay on top of what is happening in the field even after you have a position. Medicine moves fast, and employers want to know that their employees are keeping up with current events and advancements.
- **What are some of the current "buzz terms"?** As you learn more about what is happening in the health-care field, you are certain to be exposed to and pick up some new terminology along the way. If you stop to think about it, you have probably already learned some important "buzz" terms from your textbooks and your instructors' lectures. (See Box 7.1.) Keeping up with the latest developments in your field will help you to put those key terms into contexts that can help you better understand their meanings and their application to your new career. Having a knowledge of key medical terms will also give you an edge when you are marketing yourself. Being able to "talk the talk" gives

people confidence that you can also "walk the walk." This initial confidence builder can be key when it comes to marketing. If you sound like you know what you are talking about, people are more likely to want to talk with you and find out more about you.

O N   T R A C K

You are on track if you can list five medical buzz terms that you have heard in practice or learned from your classes.

1. _____

2. _____

3. _____

4. _____

5. _____

- **Who are the current leaders?** The more you learn about what is happening in the health-care industry, the more likely you are to hear about who the leaders are in the field. For example, did someone recently invent a new surgical procedure or medication? Listen carefully to new information and make mental notes of people who are making a difference in your field. You might even begin to notice that the people you are hearing about are the same people who are writing the articles you read or are speaking on television.
- **What new medical products are available?** Knowing when a new medical product or cure has hit the market is important, especially when it comes to new drugs. Drug development is a billion dollar industry that is constantly

BOX 7.1 EXAMPLES OF CURRENT BUZZ WORDS

Buzz Term	Meaning
Cardio	Short for "cardiology"
A good stick	Someone who can do a good blood draw
Medisoft	Medical software program
Record	Patient file
Triage	Front desk and scheduling of patients
ECG or EKG	Electrocardiogram

changing. Drug manufacturers are developing, testing, and marketing new drugs all the time. Once approved by the U.S. Food and Drug Administration, you might see these drugs being advertised on television or in magazines or being prescribed where you work.

- **What medical products have been recalled?** Just as important as knowing when a new drug hits the market is knowing when a drug or other medical product has been recalled. Recalls can affect both prescription and over-the-counter drugs. Some drugs are recalled permanently due to potentially dangerous side effects or for other reasons, whereas others are recalled on a small-scale basis due to manufacturing, production, or distribution errors, such as incorrect dosages or bacterial contamination of the product.

- **What are the new, cutting-edge ideas?** The cutting edge ideas of today could become standard practice tomorrow. Therefore, you should keep abreast of what the latest technology is and how it is being used. For example, current trends in surgery include minimally invasive laparoscopic approaches to some commonly performed procedures and robotic surgery. Such new approaches and technologies can have a huge impact on the health of our nation by decreasing surgery time, improving success rates, decreasing infection, and decreasing recovery time—all concepts you should be aware of in your new career.

- **What issues are currently being debated?** As you learn more about what is happening in the health-care field, you are also likely to learn that many health-care-related issues are up for debate. Currently, and probably for some time to come, the concept of health-care reform is a foremost concern among health-care providers and patients alike. However, controversies surrounding certain medical practices and research practices also exist. For example, debates ensue about stem cell research, the use of certain medications for preventative purposes, and physician-assisted suicide.

Step 2: Create Your Marketing Materials

Once you have "done your homework" by preparing yourself to be able to talk about your new field using appropriate terminology, you will be ready to turn the focus of your marketing plan development on yourself. That means that you will be ready to begin developing your marketing materials, which should include the following:

- Resume
- References page
- Business cards
- Portfolio

Your resume, and sometimes the accompanying cover letter and references page, will be your primary tool when you are marketing and networking yourself throughout your educational program and your new career. Chapter 8 provides detailed information on how to develop and design a professional entry-level resume, cover letter, and references page.

Business Cards

Another important component of your marketing materials is your business card. As discussed in Chapter 1, making a business card is easy. Many common software programs, such as Microsoft Word and Publisher, offer templates that can help you create and print business cards on a personal or school computer. You can also find lots of websites on the internet where you can design a business card and then order copies at a relatively low cost, even as low as $1.99 for 100 business cards, depending on the style you choose and text you want to include. (See Fig. 1.1 for a sample business card.)

Portfolio

The last major component of your marketing materials is your portfolio. A portfolio is a marketing tool that contains a selected showcase of one's work and achievements over time. Unlike an artist's portfolio, which might include drawings or paintings, or an entertainer's portfolio, which might include head shot photos, your portfolio will include a distinctive collection of documents from your education that highlight your performance and progress.

You can think of your portfolio as your own personal "brag book." If you are one of those people who finds it difficult or uncomfortable to "toot your own horn," you can let your portfolio do it for you. Include information that tells people who you are, what your credentials are, and what experience you have. Your portfolio should be unique to you and should help you stand out from other people.

During an interview, your portfolio will help you to show a prospective employer that you have the experience and skills the organization is looking for. Using a binder with plastic pages and organizing your portfolio into sections will allow you to speak about the high points of your past performance and experience in a structured manner. It will also help the prospective employer to experience first-hand your organization skills, professionalism, and dedication. Here are some recommended sections to include in your portfolio:

- **Current resume:** Your resume is an official introduction to an employer listing your experience, skills, and accomplishments for a position.
- **References:** A reference is someone you list on your application. Your potential employer will be allowed to call them to verify your work ethics and integrity.
- **Tutoring assignments or awards:** Your ability to tutor shows leadership and training responsibility and above-average ability in course knowledge in the health professions field.

- **Transcript of your grades:** Your transcript shows your ability to excel in your course of study and reveals your motivation and commitment as a student. You should generally include your transcript if you have a grade point average of 3.0 or better.
- **Letters of recommendation:** Including letters of recommendation from instructors, coworkers, and previous supervisors and managers speaks to our work ethic, good attitude, outstanding customer service, and punctuality. (See Box 7.2.)
- **Attendance awards:** Attendance is key in any organization. Your attendance awards will reassure employers of your dedication and commitment to your career. They will help an employer see that the time spent hiring and training you will be worth the effort because you are the type of employee they want and need in their organization, hospital, office, or clinic.

BOX 7.2 OBTAINING LETTERS OF RECOMMENDATION

A letter of recommendation should provide a prospective employer with personal knowledge of your personality, attitude, work ethics, ability to follow policies and procedures, attendance, customer service skills, ability to get along with others and work on a team, ability to work independently, and other applicable skills and traits that a prospective employer will value. Because your letters of recommendation will become permanent parts of your portfolio, it is important to get the best recommendations that you can.

Finding good people to write you letters of recommendation will be worth the effort. Start with past supervisor or managers because these people understand what other employers are looking for and can honestly say that you have these skills and traits. If possible, you should contact all of your employers over the past 5 years to ask for letters of recommendation. You might even want to ask coworkers with whom you worked closely to write you letters of recommendation.

Here are some other people you can turn to for letters of recommendation:

- Instructors (note that some schools do not allow instructors to give recommendations)
- Clergy member, such as a rabbi, minister, priest, or nun
- High school and grade school teachers
- High school principal
- Colleague at or director of a volunteer organization
- Attorney
- Insurance agent
- Bank manager
- Day care director
- Social worker
- Friends and family

- **Evaluations:** Evaluations indicate your past employment performance, commonly addressing your strengths as well as important traits such as work ethic.
- **Medical vocabulary:** Including a list of the medical vocabulary with which you are familiar illustrates your specific level of knowledge and shows that you are capable of filling out and understanding a patient medical record.
- **Lab skills chart:** You can keep track of your lab skills on a chart so that prospective employers can see what skills your training included and what your skill level is. For example, the chart might show how many blood draws you performed in your program.
- **Test and quiz scores:** You can include outstanding examples of your work, such as class papers, tests, and quizzes, which will give you an opportunity to show off your medical understanding and skills.

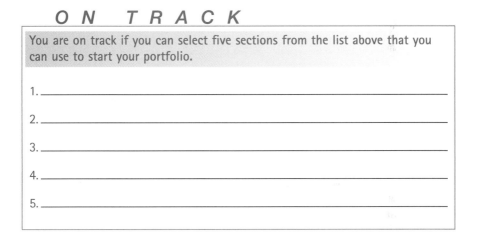

O N   T R A C K

You are on track if you can select five sections from the list above that you can use to start your portfolio.

1. _____

2. _____

3. _____

4. _____

5. _____

Although your portfolio will serve an important role in getting you your first job in the health professions field, it will also continue to be useful throughout your health professions career as you learn new information and advance to new positions. Therefore, you should continue to collect items to add to your portfolio throughout your career. An easy way to do this is to keep a folder called a "Wonderful File," in which you place items that you need to add to your portfolio. For example, you can add your employment evaluations as well as thank you letters and cards from patients who especially enjoyed your caring attitude and great customer service, awards you receive, and certificates for seminars you attend. You can also keep an electronic spreadsheet file that lists by date projects you completed, deadlines you met, and goals you accomplished. These two methods create an easy way to keep track of your accomplishments at work and will make it simple for you to update your resume and portfolio when you are ready to look for a new position.

Without the proper marketing materials, you will not be able to run an effective advertising campaign for yourself. If you need help developing any of the marketing materials previously discussed, talk with one of your instructors or someone in your school's career services department.

Step 3: Make Yourself as Marketable as Possible

The next step in self-marketing is to make sure that you are prepared to present the best possible version of yourself. That begins with making sure that people see the confident *new* you. You must have faith in yourself and believe in your abilities in order to make others believe in you, too. Your new confidence will increase your level of communication so that you can speak up about yourself when you meet people in the health-care field. Remember that you have learned many new skills and have much to offer employers in the health-care field. You just need to have the confidence to be able to advertise these new talents when you are networking, interviewing, and marketing yourself.

Mentor Moment

I had a hard time with the concept of marketing myself. I was uncomfortable talking about myself because it seemed like boasting, and I didn't like to "toot my own horn," so to speak. I was making good grades and was really good at my skills, but I had trouble expressing to others what I had learned. I really wanted a good position, though, so I could support my family, and I let that become my focus. By remembering my goals and keeping them in mind as I met new people, marketing myself became easier.

Sam from Sioux Falls, SD

Another way to increase your marketability is to brush up on and improve your computer skills. Every position you apply for will likely require some hands-on computer skills. Employers will expect you to be familiar with how to use a computer and use certain software programs, such as Microsoft Word, Excel, and possibly PowerPoint. If you feel that your computer skills need some improvement, you could take some classes or ask a friend for help. Just having these basic skills will help to keep you competitive in the market. It might also offer you the opportunity to meet other people in your field and build new relationships with people who have the same interests as you.

Step 4: Finding Advertising Opportunities

The next step in your marketing plan is to attend seminars, trade shows, career fairs, and other career-related functions where you can meet people, make use of your new knowledge, and disseminate your marketing materials. Whether they are speakers, panelists, or other attendees, the people you meet at career-related functions could be connections that lead to possible interviews later on in your career. Your goal at these functions should be to meet as many people in your field as possible. Have you ever heard the phrase: "It is not what you know but who you know"? If so, you might have some idea of the importance that knowing the right person has for your future career search. In some cases, knowing someone who can personally recommend you for a position or deliver your cover letter and resume to a hiring manager can make all the difference in whether you are able to get your foot in the door for an interview.

When it comes to distributing your marketing materials, you should make use of every available opportunity. Although attending career fairs and other functions related to your specific field of interest makes sense, you should not be afraid to broaden your scope to see whether crossover opportunities are available through other health professions. You should be open to and try to attend *all* career fairs because you never know where you will find the right opportunity for you. (See the section below on "Networking" for more information on how you can distribute your marketing materials.)

Motivational Moment

66 Perhaps the most valuable result of all education is the ability to make yourself do the thing you have to do, when it ought to be done, whether you like it or not. 99

Thomas Huxley, English biologist

Step 5: Rehearse

Even with the right attitude and the right marketing materials, you might still be nervous when it comes time to market yourself. One way to calm your nerves is to rehearse. Ask your mentor or one of your "cheerleaders" to role play some questions with you. Practicing how you will answer some basic questions, such as "What are your interests?" and "How did you first become interested in the health-care field?" can prepare you to discuss these topics when you meet new people in the real world. Practicing with another person gives you the benefit of having someone else who can point out where you need improvement. For example, the other person might notice that you pause too long before answering or say "um" too many times while you speak. Knowing what your weaknesses are before you go out to market yourself can help you to address them and prepare to put your best foot forward even if you feel nervous.

Even if you do not have someone to rehearse with, you can practice by rehearsing your introduction and answering some questions about yourself in a mirror. The mirror will show you how you look by revealing your facial expressions, gestures, and posture, all of which convey information about your self-confidence. Analyze these details and make improvements so that you are ready to market yourself when the opportunity presents itself.

These exercises might sound silly, but they are ways to create opportunities to practice how you will introduce yourself to people, inform them of your interests and, when the timing is right, announce to them that you will soon be looking for a position in the health-care field. The more you rehearse and the more experience you have meeting people, the more natural you will feel and the more relaxed you will appear when a marketing opportunity arises.

Mentor Moment

I never liked to speak in front of people, so I never really answered many questions in class and I never volunteered to present anything. The thought of networking and talking to people had my stomach in knots. My instructor kept telling me to practice by looking in a mirror, so I could see how others saw me. Finally, I locked myself in my bathroom and started introducing myself to the person in the mirror. I was really surprised when I noticed how serious and even how scared I looked. The more I practiced, though, the more I began to smile. Networking was never really easy for me, but I think I became kind of good at it!

Robin from Jacksonville, NC

Networking

Networking is a way in which people make new connections with others who share common interests or goals and exchange ideas and information. For you, networking will be another means by which you find opportunities to market yourself. One of the most important concepts to understand about networking is that it does not start when you graduate—rather, it starts when you first put on your scrubs. As you approach graduation, you will be searching for your career position and looking to all of the contacts that you have made through networking for help. That is why *now* is the time to create your foundation for networking.

As a health professions student, you are now searching for the right place to start your new career. Within the first 6 months of your program, you will probably be able to narrow down your search to a specific area of interest or type of office that interests you. This area of interest might be based on the new medical knowledge and lab skills you have obtained or it might be based on the fact that certain information in a test or chapter just clicked with you. In any case, having a focused field of interest can help you make the most of your networking efforts.

Motivational Moment

66 Remember that it is not where you come from, or not even where you are; it is where you are going that matters most. 99

Bo Bennett, author of Year to Success

The disadvantage of networking is that it takes time to cultivate professional relationships. That is why it is important for you to start networking as soon as possible. You should be sure to include in all conversations with new people you meet that you are studying a health profession and will soon be focusing on a career search.

Importance of Networking

Building professional relationships and friendships can benefit you throughout your career. Thanks to technology, position postings generate hundreds of applicants. This is why networking now is important. Networking can give you the professional edge that you will need when you are competing for a position and is a major part of marketing yourself. For example, networking might provide the following advantages:

- Having the right connections might help you to learn about a position posting before others do.
- One of your professional contacts might be willing to vouch for you by giving your resume to a hiring or office manager. The better you know a person, the more willing that person will be to go out on a limb for you when it comes to recommending you for a position or helping you get your foot in the door.
- Knowing the right person might give you an advantage when it comes time for a prospective employer to choose interview candidates.
- Having the right contact might help you to find out more information about the organization, department, position, or hiring manager before you interview. For example, you might benefit by knowing the size of the organization, the hours, the benefits, or the salary range of the position.

Not only are you more likely to learn about available positions through your network, you are also more likely to learn about good positions. Stop and think about it. Wouldn't you rather be hired by an office or organization that you have heard good things about from someone you know? Many people are so focused on finding a position when they graduate that they forget to look for or do not think they have the luxury of finding a *good* position at an organization where they will be happy. You should remember that not all offices are the same.

Certain details about a position or organization might determine whether the position is right for you. For example, consider these questions:

- Is the office small or large?
- How many physicians are in the office?
- What are the physicians' personalities?
- How many other employees work in the office?
- What are those employees like?
- What is the personality of the office manager?
- What kind of standards does the office manager expect?
- What are the office's policies on weekend hours and overtime?
- When do employees begin receiving benefits and paid time off?
- What is the procedure for annual reviews?

In a similar way, networking can help you to learn about positions to stay away from as well. For example, you might decide that a particular organization is not the right match for you if you learn that it has some negative characteristics:

- It does not have a pleasant working atmosphere.
- The physician has a quick temper.
- Most externs quit after 2 days.
- The employees in the office tend to gossip.
- Employees are required to work on weekends or at night.
- The organization offers no benefits.

Knowing certain information about an organization ahead of time can help you to find a position in which you will be happy right from the start.

When it comes to networking, you should also remember that it goes both ways. You could help your classmates by telling them about an opening in an office that fits their interests or you might want to recommend a classmate for a position in your organization. Be sure to offer your help and advice to other people when you have a chance because you never know who will be able to help you in the future. In addition, sharing "inside information" with the people in your network to give them an upper hand provides you the chance to give back and share in that wonderful feeling of helping someone else.

Mentor Moment

I started my networking by making a list of all my friends and former classmates who had graduated from the school. When I thought about it, I realized that I now knew lots of people who were working as medical assistants and billers and coders. I added the names of the places where they were working and their phone numbers. This became the networking list I used 2 months later when I graduated and was ready to send out my resume.

Marion from Alexandria, VA

Networking Strategies

The most important networking strategy for you to employ is to network with everyone you know. Your networking plan should include visiting the career services department at your campus as well as using online social networks, business networks, and websites.

Visiting Your Campus's Career Services Department

The career services department on your campus is a good resource for many different aspects of your marketing and networking strategies. For example, as previously mentioned, the staff there will be able to help you develop professional-looking marketing materials that you can use in your search. In addition, the career services department is a good place to find out about marketing and networking opportunities such as career fairs, as well as position openings, when you are ready to look for your new career.

Because the information at the career services department will be constantly changing, you should plan to visit the department once a week to make sure that you are learning about all new opportunities that become available. You might even want to select a particular day of the week and add your visit to the career services department to your schedule.

Networking Online

In today's job market, another important networking strategy is networking online. Social networks, such as Facebook and Twitter, are fast becoming the way to reconnect with old friends, make new ones, and keep in touch with all of the people you know. These connections could come in very handy when you are ready to let others know that you are beginning your career search. With just one posting on your social network page, you can alert everyone you know that you are going to be graduating soon and looking for a new position.

The online social networks are also fast becoming popular connections for business. Many companies are now using these types of sites to reach customers and connect with potential employees. Other sites, such as www.LinkedIn.com, were designed specifically for the purpose of business networking.

You can also network online by finding the websites of professional health professions organizations and other medical websites and making connections on those sites. (See Box 7.3.)

O N   T R A C K

You are on track if you can list two professional health care–related websites that might offer you networking opportunities.

1. _____

2. _____

BOX 7.3 PROFESSIONAL HEALTH PROFESSIONS ORGANIZATIONS

Most health professions and other health care–related organizations have websites that offer opportunities for you to connect with other people in your field. For example, most of these organizations hold annual or semiannual meetings or conventions. Some also hold seminars and have local chapters that also hold meetings. Joining one of these associations or attending one of their events is a good way to find marketing and networking opportunities. Visit the following websites to find out more information or do an internet search to find other organizations related to your specific field.

General Health-Related Organizations

- **American Health Care Association (AHCA):** The AHCA is a nonprofit alliance of assisted living, sub acute care, and other providers. http://www.ahca.org
- **American Medical Association (AMA):** The AMA's goal is to "promote the art and science of medicine and the betterment of public health."[1] Its site offers valuable resources to health professions students, including a *Health Care Careers Directory* that lists information about more than 80 careers in the health-care field. http://www.ama-assn.org/
- **American Public Health Association (APHA):** APHA, the oldest public health organization in the world, is a nonprofit association dedicated to improving pubic health. http://www.apha.org/
- **Association of Schools of Allied Health Professionals (ASAHP):** This nonprofit professional association serves administrators, educators, and others who are concerned with critical issues affecting the health-care field. http://www.asahp.org/index.htm
- **Health Professions Network (HPN):** The HPN is a nonprofit group of professionals working to increase the quality of health-care. http://www.healthpronet.org/

Billing and Coding

- **American Academy of Professional Coders (AAPC):** The AAPC is dedicated to elevating the standards of medical coding through training, certification, networking, and job opportunities. www.aapc.com/

BOX 7.3 (continued)

- **American Medical Billing Association (AMBA):** The AMBA provides education and networking opportunities. www.ambanet.net/AMBA.htm
- **Medical Association of Billers:** The Medical Association of Billers offers billing and coding specialists reliable information about the field as well as opportunities for certification. http://www.e-medbill.com/

Dental Hygiene

- **American Dental Association (ADA):** The ADA is a national dental society that provides oral health–related information to dentists and patients. www.ada.org
- **American Dental Hygienists' Association (ADHA):** The ADHA is a nonprofit organization that offers professional support and educational opportunities to its members while enhancing the profession. www.adha.org

Health Information Management

- **American Health Information Management Association (AHIMA):** AHIMA promotes quality health care through quality information and offers various certifications to health information management professionals. www.ahima.org

Massage Therapy

- **American Massage Therapy Association (AMTA):** The AMTA works to enhance the practice of massage therapy through training, education, and legislative efforts. /www.amtamassage.org/
- **Massage Therapy Foundation:** The Massage Therapy Foundation is a group of therapists, educators, and other professionals dedicated to promoting the knowledge and understanding of massage. www.massagetherapyfoundation.org

Medical Assisting

- **American Association of Medical Assistants (AAMA):** The AAMA is a certification organization that promotes professional medical assisting practice through education and credentialing. www.aama-ntl.org

Pharmacy Technology

- **American Association of Pharmacy Technicians (AAPT):** The AAPT is an international nonprofit organization that offers education opportunities to technicians practicing in hospitals, extended care facilities, and other settings and to those working as educators. www.pharmacytechnician.com
- **National Pharmacy Technician Association (NPTA):** The NPTA is dedicated to advancing pharmacy technician practice. www.pharmacytechnician.org

(box continues on page 220)

BOX 7.3 PROFESSIONAL HEALTH PROFESSIONS ORGANIZATIONS (continued)

Surgical Technology

- **Association of Surgical Technologists (AST):** The AST helps to ensure that surgical technologists and assistants offer top-quality care. www.ast.org
- **National Board of Surgical Technology and Surgical Assisting (NBSTSA):** The NBSTSA benefits the medical community and its patients by offering certification for surgical technologists and surgical assistants. www.nbstsa.org

Miscellaneous

- **American Medical Technologists (AMT):** The AMT is a nonprofit agency that offers certification to medical technologists, medical laboratory technicians and assistants, medical assistants, phlebotomy technicians, dental assistants, and certain other health professionals. http://www.amt1.com/

Tips for Networking

The more networking you do, the more you will find out that you should not just "wing it." You cannot meet someone and go right away from "hello" to "I will be looking for a new position in a few months." So, what should you say when you meet someone? How should you bring up in conversation that you will be looking for a health profession? Here are some tips to help you make the most of networking and to make networking work for you:

- **Create a networking action plan (NAP):** During or before your third month in your program, you will need to create a plan for networking. Your NAP must be more than words on paper; it must translate into steps that you will take. These steps will help you focus when you meet new contacts and will include creating a Verbal Career Card that you can use to help you to break the ice. (See Boxes 7.4 and 7.5.)
- **Plan time to network:** When you plan your week, add networking time to your calendar. For example, you might want to schedule 30 minutes per week to visit the career services department at your campus or do online searches to find information or networking opportunities. You might also want to consider making it a goal to attend one career-related function per month. The more time you can devote to networking, the more opportunities you will create for yourself.

BOX 7.4 STEPS IN A NETWORKING ACTION PLAN

As mentioned in previous chapters, the more organized you are, the more successful you will be in everything you do. Therefore, having a plan for networking is important. Here are just a few ideas for steps you should include in your networking action plan:

- ❏ Make a list of your classmates, friends, colleagues, and other contacts with whom you can share your goal of searching for new employment in the health-care field.
- ❏ Make a list of the medical offices in your area.
- ❏ Make a list of organizations in your field that might be holding local meetings.
- ❏ Make a list of upcoming career fairs in your area.
- ❏ Make a list of websites where you can network.
- ❏ Collect business cards.
- ❏ Schedule time in your routine for networking research and actual networking time.

BOX 7.5 VERBAL CAREER CARD

A Verbal Career Card is a three- or four-sentence statement that you can use to introduce yourself to people in a professional manner. It should list your current interests, personal strengths, qualifications, and medical skills.

The further along you are in your health professions program, the more you can expand your Verbal Career Card. When you are first beginning your educational program, your Verbal Career Card might simply relate to your transferable skills. However, as you continue in your health professions program, you will be able to add lab skills and other skills that relate specifically to the health care field.

Example Verbal Career Card for a Student in Months 1 to 3 of a Health Professions Program

Hello, my name is Sally Rogers. I have extensive experience in customer support, and I am known for my communication skills. After an extensive hospital stay, I became interested in the health-care industry. I am now studying to be a medical assistant at ABC Health Professions School and will be looking for opportunities as a medical assistant in a pediatric office or clinic.

(box continues on page 222)

BOX 7.5 VERBAL CAREER CARD (continued)

Example Verbal Career Card for a Student in Months 4 to 9 of a Health Professions Program

Hello, my name is Sally Rogers. I am currently a medical student at ABC Health Professions School, where my attendance during my program has been stellar, as my attendance awards in my portfolio reveal. I excel in blood draws and injections as part of my lab skills. I also have outstanding communication skills and a firm grasp of medical vocabulary. I will be graduating as a medical assistant in May and will be looking for opportunities in a pediatric office or clinic.

- **Always be prepared to network:** Networking is a full-time opportunity because chances to network can present themselves anywhere you go. Do not try to judge which opportunity is the "right" opportunity for you. Network at every opportunity. Make yourself comfortable with networking by always being prepared. Have your Verbal Career Card committed to memory, and always keep some of your student business cards and copies of your resume with you. You can keep these items in a folder in your car so that they are always on hand and always look nice and neat.

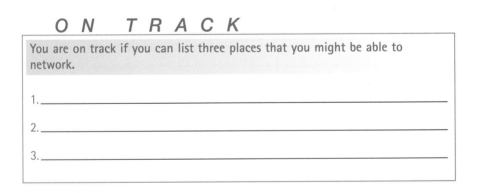

O N T R A C K

You are on track if you can list three places that you might be able to network.

1. _____

2. _____

3. _____

- **Bring a positive attitude to all networking opportunities:** Because any event can turn into a networking opportunity, you must bring a positive attitude with you wherever you go. People like meeting people who have energy and a positive attitude. Social gatherings are a time for you to sparkle and shine. The more positive, upbeat, and outgoing you are, the more likely you are to meet new people and strike up conversations about your interests, which can become a perfect time to network. Never bring troubles to a social gathering, including family gatherings. Instead, use these opportunities to share your goals and practice your new professionalism. Whether you like it or not, others will judge you based on their first impressions of you. Make sure to always put your best foot forward by having a positive attitude.

● **Make the most of every networking opportunity:** Whether you are networking in person or online, you should take advantage of the opportunity to network with everyone you know, including family, friends, casual contacts, friends of friends, physicians, and teachers. Think outside the box when it comes to the people who might be useful contacts and do not leave anyone out. For example, you should even network with waiters, travel agents, insurance brokers, retail clerks, clergy, and so on. Tell everyone you meet and use all the technology available to you (e.g., Facebook and Twitter) to announce that you will be looking for a position in the health-care field when you graduate. Your search should not be a secret. Also, when you meet someone new, you should ask for a business card and offer him or her one of your own.

● **Network forward and backward:** Network forward with all of the new friends you make at school. Some of these contacts will be entering the field before you and might help you learn of available opportunities in the field when you are ready to graduate. Network backward by contacting old friends as well as former colleagues, coworkers, and bosses. Let them see how professional you have become in your training for your health professions career.

● **Create a networking notebook:** You can use a notebook to keep your networking contacts and events organized. Start your notebook by making a list of all of the professional people you know. Keep in mind that it is not necessary for these people to work in the health-care field. Professional people visit doctor offices and know other professional people who know doctors and other potential contacts who could be helpful to you. This is just a possible contact list. Do not make any judgments at this time; just write down the names of all of the professional people you know.

O N   T R A C K

You are on track if you can make a list of professional people you know. Start your list here and write the names of at least three professional people you know.

1._____

2._____

3._____

- **Be yourself:** Be true to yourself in your interactions with others. When you pretend to be someone you are not, you can come across as being fake or a schmoozer. This can turn people off to you and make you seem distrustful. Instead, be yourself . . . no one does it better!

Motivational Moment

66 What would you do if you knew you couldn't fail? 99

Robert Schuller, American televangelist
and former host of The Hour of Power

- **Be sincere and respectful:** Begin your conversations by showing a genuine interest in others. Doing so draws people into conversation with you by allowing them the opportunity to talk about themselves. Ask questions to find out more information about their occupation and their goals. When you are genuinely interested in learning about other people and show them respect, the conversation will flourish. You will also come off as being more relaxed and more sincere. Soon enough the conversation will turn to you, and you will have the opportunity to share that you are in school and will soon be looking for a position.
- **Focus on listening:** As you network, you should listen to others with real focus to truly understand what they are saying. Do not try to think ahead of the conversation or jump in before another person has finished speaking. Instead, respond and react to the conversation you are listening to at the time.
- **Be on time:** Whether you are going to a social gathering, a professional event, or a family function, you should always be on time. Do not be afraid to be the first one to arrive either. Arriving on time gives you the opportunity to have quality time to talk with and meet new people before the room fills with others. If people perceive you as always being late, then they can only conclude that you will be late to work. This perception might influence whether they feel comfortable walking your resume into a hiring manager.
- **Avoid name-dropping without permission:** Although you want to take every opportunity you can to network, there is a right and wrong way to go about doing this. Maintain your integrity as you network by making sure that you do not do anything that you would not be proud of, such as name-dropping without permission. For example, do not call an employer and say, "I am friends with [fill in name]," as part of your introduction. Your contacts might not like you using their names without asking them first. Because it shows that you are trustworthy and loyal, your most valuable tool when establishing business relationships is your integrity.

Finding a Mentor

Now that you are gaining a foundation of education and skills through your program, you might find it useful to look for a professional mentor. Whether you realize it or not, you have probably already started to notice professional people in your area who work in the health professions. You might have even found yourself wondering what path they took to get where they are and achieve what they have achieved. You might also be noticing medical offices that you never noticed before you increased your medical knowledge. In fact, you may be surprised when you realize just how many medical offices there are in your local area. You might also surprise yourself when you realize that you actually know what a lot of those physicians do, whereas you might not have known before you started your education.

Your new education and experience have opened up a world to you that you previously might never have noticed. Navigating through this new world can be easier with the help and guidance of a mentor. What does a mentor do? A mentor:

- Gives you support by helping you to achieve your dreams.
- Offers advice when you want it and are ready to hear a new idea.
- Provides positive feedback that encourages you to keep moving forward.
- Offers constructive criticism to keep you grounded and help you improve on your skills.
- Presents a different perspective because he or she has been in the field and has experience to share.
- Listens to you and honestly answers questions.

A mentor should be someone you admire and respect because of the success that he or she has achieved in his or her field. Your mentor should also respect you in return, have the time to listen to your concerns, and be concerned about your success in your field.

So now you might be wondering, "How do I find a mentoring relationship in the health-care field"? Networking is a great way to meet potential mentors. Because it can take time to cultivate a mentoring relationship, you should start early, though. If you think a mentor might be beneficial to you, look at every networking opportunity as a possibility to find your new mentor. You might want to start by looking for and joining professional associations in your area and then attending meetings. These events are great places to meet and talk to professional people in your field of interest. Find the organizations and call them about their meeting dates and times. These organizations will soon be part of your professional life, so start now and get a head start on your professional career. Some organizations even have a mentoring list. Volunteer organizations are also great places to find a mentor. As you meet people, remember to ask for their business cards and, when you get home, add them to your networking notebook so you remember who they are, where you met them, and what their interests are in the health-care field or related fields.

Some people wait until they have their new career positions before looking for a mentor. That's okay, too, but you should remember not to ask your boss or someone else with authority over you to be your mentor. You need someone in the field away from your employment so that you have an honest, unbiased opinion when you need it. You might even have more than one mentor throughout your career, each one offering the guidance that you need at each level of your career. No matter when you are looking for your mentor, your goal will be the same: to find someone you are comfortable with who is willing and able to help you succeed in your career.

Once you find a person who you think might be a good mentor, just ask. The person might be very flattered to be asked to be your mentor. If he or she has the time, do not be surprised if he or she says yes to your request. But do not ask the first person you meet. A mentor serves an important role in your life, so you want to be sure that you pick someone who fits with your personality. Be sure to talk with several people before asking someone to be your mentor. Observe their personalities and watch how they interact with others. The more people you talk with, the better idea you will have about the type of person who will make a good mentor for you.

O N   T R A C K

You are on track if you can think of one person who you might want to ask to be your mentor. (Do not worry if you do not have anyone in mind yet, though, as your list will grow when you begin networking.)

1. _____

You should also be prepared for the possibility that someone might say no when you ask him or her to be your mentor. Do not take it personally. Mentoring is a big commitment, and some people are not willing or able to put in the time mentoring takes. You might also ask someone who is already mentoring another person. Even if someone turns you down when you ask him or her to be your mentor, keep looking. You will find the right person soon enough, and the benefits of having a mentor at your side on your journey will be worth the wait.

Motivational Moment

66 I was cut from my high school basketball team. 99

Michael Jordan, member of Basketball Hall of Fame

Mentor Moment

I was really nervous about asking my former boss to be my mentor. When she accepted, it was an "OMG moment" in my life. She wasn't in the medical field, but she was so easy to talk to and was always willing to find time to help guide me. I never forgot it. In fact, after being in the field for 7 years and becoming an office manager, I had a tear in my eye when a medical assistant called and asked me to mentor her. It was a great feeling to say, "Yes"!

Lisa from Oklahoma City, OK

Networking with a Mentor

In addition to networking on your own, you might also find it helpful to network with your professional mentor. You should ask your mentor for help only after you have followed all the steps in this chapter, however. Your mentor will assist you with guidance and support when you need it, but he or she will not do your work for you.

A mentor can help you network by doing the following:

- Telling you about professional organizations you can join and meetings you can attend.
- Taking you as a guest to a professional meeting.
- Introducing you to his or her professional colleagues.
- Informing you of some professional websites.
- Giving you professional magazines.
- Helping you review federal and state regulations in the health-care field.
- Giving you copies of medical alert memos he or she receives.
- Helping you analyze your marketing and networking experiences.

To keep yourself from being disappointed by your mentoring experience, you should ensure that you and your mentor are on the same page about what the relationship means. Make sure that your mentor has time to devote to mentoring by asking in advance and selecting a regular time for face-to-face meetings or phone meetings. These meetings can be informal; however, making sure they are on each of your schedules will help to ensure that you get the most out of your mentoring experience.

Success Journal

1. To increase your awareness, see if you can answer the following questions about your field. Try to provide at least three examples for each question. Remember that you can look to the television, internet, and print products for information that might help you answer these questions.

What are the new cutting edge ideas?

1._____

2._____

3._____

What new medical products are available?

1._____

2._____

3._____

What issues are currently being debated?

1._____

2._____

3._____

2. Create a Verbal Career Card for yourself that is appropriate to your current program level using the outline below.

1. Hello, my name is _____.

2. (Choose one of the introductory statements below, and mention your experience, skills, interests, education, or personal attributes that support your goal.)

Currently, I am a _____.

I am experienced in _____.

My skill is in the area of _____.

3. Currently, I am studying _____.

4. And I am looking for opportunities in _____.

3. Create a list of networking steps for your NAP.

1. _____

2. _____

3. _____

4. _____

5. _____

6. _____

BIBLIOGRAPHY

1. American Medical Association. About AMA. Retrieved May 20, 2010, from http://www.ama-assn.org/ama/pub/about-ama.shtml.

Resume Writing

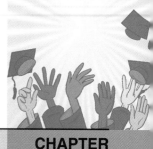

Learning Outcomes

After reading this chapter, the student will be able to:

1. Understand the importance of a professional resume.
2. Identify three common resume styles used in the health professions.
3. Explain how skills, qualifications, accomplishments, and experiences should be incorporated into a professional resume.
4. Create a professional resume.
5. Develop a professional cover letter.

Understanding the Importance of a Resume

Once you graduate, you will be ready to face the world with your skills. Remember that you are now preparing to market yourself for your new career, and your resume is your best tool for doing so because it informs others of your skill level and experience. Your resume is your marketing piece for you. It acts as an introduction to potential employers and professional contacts and helps you to get your foot in the door, so you must make sure that it properly represents the image that you want to convey. Some people feel shy when they think of their resume as a marketing tool. However, that is the reality. You are competing against other students from other schools, so you need to sell yourself. For some people, this is a really new experience. It may seem like boasting or tooting your own horn. Well, what better time to toot that horn than when you are looking to find a new position that will change your life for you and your family?

The words that you choose to put on your resume will reveal your personality, neatness, organization style, and even your level of confidence. Be sure to be positive in your tone and choose positive words for your resume to make sure that you are marketing yourself properly. This is a time to sell employers on why you should be hired for a position. If you have not yet infused the voice in your head with positive thoughts, there is no better time than when you start writing your resume to do it. The attitude you use to write your resume will be reflected in the way your present it.

What Is a Resume?

A resume is a document that summarizes your skills and experience. It is designed to act as your introduction to an employer and to other professionals in your field. By looking at your resume, a person should be able to tell certain things about you, such as the following:

- What jobs you have had
- How long you were employed at each job
- What responsibilities each job required of you
- What skills you learned on each job
- What other training you have received
- What awards you earned on the job
- How you helped each company reach its goals
- What projects you worked on during your employment

- Whether you served in any leadership roles
- Whether you acted as a trainer

This summary of your professional experience can prove beneficial whether you are looking for a practicum, looking for a position, or networking with people to make connections for when you are looking for a position in the future.

Motivational Moment

66 Resume: a written exaggeration of only the good things a person has done in the past, as well as a wish list of the qualities a person would like to have. 99

Bo Bennett, author of Year to Success

When Will You Need a Resume?

As mentioned in previous chapters, your resume will be a versatile tool that will benefit you throughout your educational experience and new career. It will serve as an important marketing tool for you for at least three different situations:

1. **Networking:** Your resume will be an important tool to make your first impression before you are officially a graduate and are searching for full-time employment. First, you will use your resume to make connections when you are marketing and networking yourself. (See Chapter 7 for more information on marketing and networking.)

2. **Practicum:** Later in your program, about 2 to 3 months before you graduate, you will prepare your resume to be a tool to help you to lock up a practicum. Whether it occurs in a medical office, hospital, clinic, or some other clinical setting, your practicum not only gives you experience working in the health professions field, it also often opens a doorway for you to future employment (see Chapter 11 for more information on practicums). As for your future career position, you will apply for your practicum with a resume, and you will undergo an interview process. Practicum sites choose who they want to interview and select to fill the practicum position based on the resumes they receive.

3. **Career search:** Perhaps one of the most well-known uses of a resume is its role in job searches. Employers generally review resumes to screen candidates during the hiring process. Your resume is the tool that gets you an interview. A person's resume tells the employer whether the person has the skills and experience that are required for the position. Therefore, the information you include in your resume, along with your cover letter (see the section later in this chapter for more information about cover letters), will determine whether you are placed in the candidates-we-want-to-interview pile as opposed to the candidates-we-do-not-need-to-see pile. Remember, you have only one chance to make a first impression in this scenario. The potential employer initially scans your resume for only 20 to 30 seconds; if something on your resume catches the person's eye or piques his or her interest, then your resume may get an additional 2 to 3 minutes of review. This brief examination of your resume can determine whether you go to the next step and get an interview. *Although your resume is the employment search tool that will get you an interview, it will not get you the position.* Once your resume serves its purpose for the employer, the hiring process continues to the next step: the interview. (See Chapter 9 for more information on interviewing.)

Motivational Moment

66 It's not enough that we do our best; sometimes we have to do what's required. 99

Sir Winston Churchill, former prime minister of the United Kingdom

Creating a Professional Resume

To make sure that your resume can best serve its purpose, you must take the time to create one that includes all of the necessary information and also looks professional. That means creating a resume that highlights your qualifications, experience, and accomplishments; is easy to read; and is free from errors. With modern technology, you now have available to you every tool you will need to create such a resume. To understand the importance of your resume, you need only to remember the popular saying, "you only have one chance to make a first impression." Your resume could make your first—*and only*—impression if you do not take the time to make sure that you prepare a document that looks professional and puts your best foot forward by highlighting your best skills.

Understanding the Parts of a Resume

The first step in making sure that your resume is professional is to understand the parts of a resume. Most resumes include some common elements:

- Heading
- Objective
- Education

- Qualifications
- Work history
- References
- Other personal information.

You will decide which of these factors fit on your resume and how to present them based on your experience and what you want your resume to say about you.

Heading

Your heading is the identification portion of your resume. It appears at the top of your resume and includes your name and various contact information, such as your street address, home phone number, cell phone number, and e-mail address.

You will have many choices to make about how you want your heading to look, including which font to use, which letter size (point) to use, and where to position your heading. These choices can be used to achieve some individuality and make your resume stand out. However, they will also determine the style for the remainder of your resume, so you should be sure that your heading presentation is clean, clear, and professional. (See Fig. 8.1 for some formatting options for your resume.)

Although you can make your heading look however you want it to, the consensus is that it should be centered on the page. This placement means that as a person flips through a stack of resumes, he or she will need to bend your resume to see your name, which will also allow the person to briefly glance at a few of the other items on your resume. Even if you choose not to center your heading, you should use an attractive font that is in a readable size. One tip is to stay away from fonts that use tails (an added curve or extension of a letter) because these tails can blur into one another when your resume is printed or faxed, making it hard to read.

Objective

An objective is a short sentence that explains what your professional or career goals are and how you want to use your skills in your new position. You might also see it labeled as "professional objective" or "career goals." An objective can help you when you are looking for a position by establishing your professional identity, making your resume stand out, and emphasizing what you have to offer an organization. To be effective, your objective should not be too general or too vague.

Some people disagree on whether an objective is necessary, though. One thought is that a resume need not include an objective because the objective in

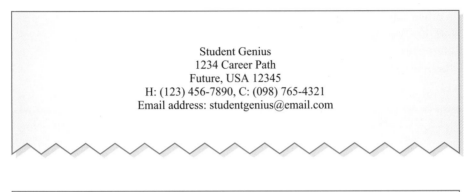

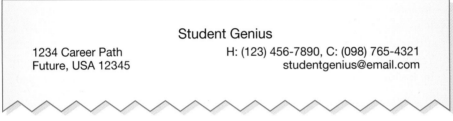

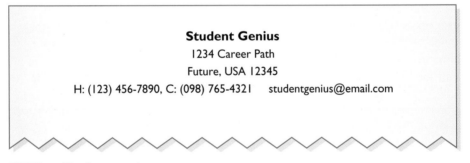

FIGURE 8.1 Heading examples.

submitting a resume to an employer is to be hired for a specific position. Others feel that including an objective can help you tailor your resume to a particular position by showing an employer the following:

- You know what you want.
- You are familiar with the field.
- Your career goals support the organization's goals.
- Your goals are about the position you are seeking, not your personal needs.

In addition, for an entry-level resume, your objective identifies your skill level.

When you are ready to create your resume, you might want to check with your career services department about the current trends regarding inclusion of an objective statement on resumes in the health professions field. And remember, if you do decide to include an objective, it should be specific, simple, and to the point.

Objective Examples
- To use my skills to reach and exceed office goals in the position of medical assistant.
- To meet the qualifications of the position with accuracy, including good communication and customer service skills.
- To obtain a position as a medical assistant that will require me to expand my practical experience while providing quality health care to patients.
- To promote and implement the standards of billing and coding as established by the profession.
- To obtain a position as a surgical technologist in a health-care facility where I can use my technological training as well as my interpersonal skills to provide the highest level of care.
- To obtain a position as a medical assistant with a facility that will enable me to represent my employer professionally and provide the highest level of comfort and care to patients.

Education

The education section of your resume should list any formal educational training that you have earned beyond a high school level, including any previously earned degrees. You should list your most recent education at your current institution first. For each educational institution you have attended, you should include the name of the educational institution (college or school); its location (city and state); and the degree, certificate, or diploma you earned. You may also decide whether you want to include your graduation date or expected graduation date. Some people choose not to include this detail because doing so might provide information that the employer can use to determine a candidate's age.

In the education section of your resume, you can also list any honors or awards that you received during your education, such as attendance awards, as well as certifications you have received and national examinations you have passed.

Qualifications

Qualifications are the skills that you have acquired through your education or work experience that make you capable of handling a job and its responsibilities.

In addition to your skills, the qualifications section of your resume will also include your experience and accomplishments. Experience is knowledge that you have acquired not from formal education but from real-life interactions and observations. It shows that you have the ability to reason, evaluate, and perform tasks. One of the most important components of your experience on an entry-level resume will be your practicum. The real-life training you gain in the field during your practicum by performing or observing processes and procedures translates as valuable transferable skills. Accomplishments are tasks that you performed or acknowledgments you received as a result of your knowledge, skills, and abilities. Examples include awards (e.g., attendance awards) and certifications (e.g., HIPAA, cardiopulmonary resuscitation [CPR], and first aid).

Depending on what you want to highlight in your resume, you may use any of these terms "qualifications," "skills," "transferrable skills," or "experience"—to head this section. No matter what you call it, though, this section will be a large and important component of your resume. If you are designing an entry-level resume, this section might be the most important part because you might not have an extensive and detailed work history. On the other hand, if you are "age experienced," you might feel like you are having trouble fitting in all of the skills you have acquired over time. Luckily, various resume styles are available that will allow you to showcase what you feel is most important in your resume (see the section entitled Choosing a Resume Style later in this chapter for more information).

You should be prepared to include all of the skills you have gained through your postsecondary education, including your practicum once you have completed it, as well as your work experiences. Although you might feel at a loss when it comes to listing the skills you have, you must remember that your education has just equipped you with a completely new set of skills. For example, if you are in a billing and coding program but you were cross-trained in medical assisting, your skills could include front office skills, such as telephone triage, medical records, billing and coding, medical terminology, scheduling, and authorization of referrals, and back office skills, such clinical skills.

A good place to find the skills with which your education has prepared you is your school's program brochure. Even if you have not achieved all of those skills yet, you will reach that skill level by the time you reach graduation.

As a recent graduate with an entry-level resume, you might also want to include some of the courses that you have taken in your program.

- Medical history and fundamentals
- Medical office administration
- Anatomy and physiology
- Medical career skills and response training

Including these courses shows prospective employers that you have a certain level of skill and knowledge and also helps to fill out your resume if you do not have much other information to include.

Your list of skills should not stop with those you have recently acquired in your education. To be sure that you include all of your skills, also consider your experience in the following categories:

- Computers (possibly divided into hardware and software skills)
- Leadership roles
- Medical skills
- Lab skills
- Customer service
- Accounting
- Military service (if applicable)

If you think that you do not have any skills in one or more of these areas, think back on the responsibilities of your previous jobs. Ask yourself these questions:

- What were the responsibilities of my job?
- What were the tasks I needed to accomplish?
- What skills did I use to accomplish my tasks?
- What did I use (equipment, methods) to accomplish my task?
- How did each of my tasks and responsibilities help the department, help the customer, or bring in money?
- Did I directly interact with customers in any capacity during my job? If so, how?
- What was I trained to do in my military service (if applicable)?

Also consider what personal responsibilities you have that relate to these skill areas. If you are still having trouble developing this portion of your resume, you can also consult with someone in your career services department. (See Box 8.1.)

Mentor Moment

When I first started school, I didn't even know how to turn on a computer because we didn't have one at home. Luckily, the director of education at my school was willing to help. She worked with me before class twice a week and taught me how to save files, print documents, use the toolbars, and so much more. By the time I graduated, I could input data on an insurance form with no errors. I was much more confident in my computer skills, and it paid off after graduation.

Sharon from Boston, MA

O N   T R A C K

You are on track if you can list three or more skills you learned from your past employment positions.

1._____

2._____

3._____

4._____

5._____

BOX 8.1 HEALTH-CARE EMPLOYERS' WISH LIST OF SKILLS

To begin to understand what skills you should list on your resume, start by considering the following list of skills that are valued by employers.

- **Human relations:** As a health professional, you will work closely every day with other people, including patients and coworkers. Therefore, your human relations skills should be high on your resume. Good terms to use when describing these skills include "communications" and "customer service." Including your human relations skills on your resume will show an employer that you can contribute to patient retention and recruitment.
- **Problem solving:** At the entry level, you will probably not be expected to make any major decisions that require problem solving. However, you will need to be able to think on your feet when it comes to making decisions about patients. You will also need to know when a decision must be referred to someone else, which is an important skill. Illustrating your problem-solving skills on your resume will show an employer that you have the ability and confidence to reach solutions when it comes to patient care.
- **Computers and information management:** No matter what specific field you are entering or what position you hope to achieve, employers will expect you to have a certain level of computer skills. Some positions require more skill than others (e.g., insurance paperwork and scheduling are now almost completely computerized), but all require some knowledge. Your ability to use a computer will also be closely linked with your ability to stay up-to-date on the latest information related to the medical profession. When describing your computer skills, be sure to include the names of specific programs you use as

BOX 8.1 (continued)

well as your level of proficiency in using them. If your computer skills are below par, you might want to consider some computer training classes.

- **Science and math:** Science and math skills are at the core of many health careers. For example, employers might expect potential employees to be able to operate a calculator, measure medications, and calculate bills. As a health professional, you should also maintain and express an interest in advances being made in the fields of science and medicine, such as new procedures. The more knowledgeable you sound on your resume, the more separation you will create between you and other candidates.

- **Money management:** Although money matters are usually handled by a special department in the health-care field, including money management skills on your resume shows potential employers that you have the ability to be organized and responsible. Remember to look to all of your transferrable skills in this area, including any experience you have cashiering and balancing a cash drawer.

- **Teaching or training:** You might think that the health professions field does not require many teaching and training skills, except for positions in a classroom setting. However, as a health professional, you will commonly instruct patients on how to take medications, perform certain exercises, and follow certain requirements for medical testing. Later in your career, as a higher-level employee, you might also be asked to train new staff members or assist with training. Therefore, you should include on your resume all teaching and training skills you have.

- **Business management:** Although you might not typically think of the health-care field as a business, it is one. The product offered in the health-care business is service to patients (customers). Therefore, any business management skills you have should be highlighted on your resume. Employers will value that you understand the concept of business and the importance of retaining customers.

- **Vocational-technical:** In the health-care field, vocational-technical skills refer to your ability to work with medical and office equipment. Although you are still building your medical skills and experience working with medical equipment, you probably have other skills that you take for granted that might be appreciated by an employer, such as the ability to load paper into a copier or unjam a fax machine. Although you might not even consider such abilities as skills, they are keys to keeping an office running smoothly.

- **Foreign language:** Being able to speak a second language is a highly valued skill and could increase your hiring potential in most areas of the country. Some positions even require knowledge of a second language. Even if you are not fluent in another language, the ability to communicate common words and phrases, such as "yes," "no," "thank you," "good morning," and "the doctor will be right with you," is typically valued by employers because it enhances your customer service.

Work History

The work history or work experience section of your resume should include a list of your previous jobs, going back no more than 5 years, if possible. For each job, you should include the name of the company, the title or titles you had on the job, and the months or years you worked there. You might also want to include this information:

- Your supervisor's name, which adds credibility
- Any awards you won on the job, such as employee of the month, which show your work ethics
- Your salary, which reveals increases you received in your pay rate
- Some of your job responsibilities, which can reflect your excellent customer service skills

The following format is one way to accomplish this task.

Work History

Company	Position/Title	Dates	Awards
Taco Bell	Assistant Supervisor	Nov. 2010–Present	
McDonalds	Cashier and Trainer	Feb. 2009–Oct. 2010	Employee of the Month

This format is a quick and simple way to present your work history. Later in this chapter, you will discover different resume formats that will give you more options for designing your resume style. If your work history is not very impressive, you might want to gravitate toward a simple style. However, if you have an extensive work history, you might want to choose another style that emphasizes your responsibilities at each of your previous positions, such as the one shown here:

McDonalds, Cashier and Trainer, February 2009–October 2010

- As lead cashier, responsible for the audit of seven cash drawers and responsible for daily reports of seven cashiers
- As trainer, responsible for training new employees on cash drawer management, customer service, and customer problem-solution communications

If you have a gap in your work experience due to a layoff, pregnancy, child rearing, or disability, you might find it in your best interest to explain these gaps on your resume. Here is option for how you can present this information in your resume:

McDonalds, Cashier and Trainer, February 2009–October 2010
Pregnancy Leave, November 2010–January 2011

Motivational Moment

66 Courage is fear holding on a minute longer. 99

George S. Patton III, U.S. Army general

References

References are those people who have the knowledge and ability to speak about your professionalism and responsibility in a positive way. Through your connection with them, your references have first-hand knowledge of such important aspects about you as your work ethics and personality. As a general rule, for an entry-level position you will probably want to find three to five people to serve as references for you so that you can include them on your resume or on a references page. Although your references page might seem like part of your resume, it is really an extension of it. For that reason, most resumes include a line at the bottom that reads, "References available upon request." You will probably also need to supply these references to the employer as part of the employment application. Applications commonly ask how many years you have known each reference, so be ready to answer this question.

So, who should you include as a reference? The people you choose as your references can be a mix of business and personal contacts:

- Past employers or supervisors
- Teachers
- Religious and volunteer group leaders
- Community group associates
- Day-care providers
- Friends

Remember, anyone who knows you well and can vouch for your ability to contribute to an organization would make a good reference.

Start by asking the people you contacted for letters of recommendation, including supervisors, managers, and coworkers from your past and current positions. When you ask these people to write a letter of recommendation for you, also ask them if they would mind being listed as a reference. Let them know what you are studying and how you are performing as a student, as well as when you will graduate. Keeping in touch with these people so that they are aware of your situation is helpful so that they will be ready to field a telephone call on your behalf.

The following format is one way to list your references.

Name	Phone Numbers (work and cell)
Company	E-mail address (if you have permission to list)
Position	
Work Address	
City, State, Zip	

Examples

Mr. Supervisor	Work: (123) 456-7890
Taco Bell	Cell: (098) 765-4321
Manager	mrsupervisor@email.com
123 Taco Bell Way	
Chalupa, Universe, 12345	

Ms. Supervisor	Work: (789) 123-4560
McDonalds	mssupervisor@email.com
Manager	
123 McDonald's Pkwy	
Burger, Universe, 12345	

O N   T R A C K

You are on track if you can name at least three people you could ask to be a reference for you.

1. _____

2. _____

3. _____

Other Personal Information

At one time, including hobbies, family status, and other personal information in a resume was a popular trend. However, it is unlawful for a prospective employer to ask you personal information related to race, religion, marital status, and number of children, and you should not include such information in your resume.

Hobbies can help to show that a person has a well-rounded personality, and they also help to fill up space. However, employers do not hire you for your hobbies; they hire you to gain more customers, make money for the company, or meet department goals. Therefore, including your hobbies on your resume is no longer recommended. If your employer is interested in that aspect of your life, you will see a question about it on the employment application or you will be asked about it during the interview process.

One type of personal information that you might want to include in your resume is military experience. You can add this information toward the end of your resume, unless you earned your education through the military or gained specific skills that are worth noting. Remember that your military experience has taught you certain skills that you can highlight on your resume, such as the ability to be punctual, the ability to follow orders, and attention to detail.

Motivational Moment

66 Anyone who has never made a mistake has never tried anything new. 99

Albert Einstein, German physicist and Nobel Prize winner

Choosing a Resume Style

Now that you understand what information you need to include, you are probably getting excited to write your resume. However, before you begin writing, you should ask yourself, "How do I want to showcase my skills?" The answer to this question will determine which resume style you use.

There are several resume styles. The most common and popular in recent decades have been chronological, functional, and achievement. Because you are preparing your resume for an entry-level position, one of these standard resume styles might work best for you.

Chronological Resume

A chronological resume focuses primarily on one area: work history. If you have not had any holes in your work history, then this style is an excellent choice for showcasing how employable you have been throughout the years. In a chronological resume, you list your work experience in chronological order, which is where the style gets its name. In other words, you list your current job first, with all of the relevant information (position or title, dates, and responsibilities), and then work backward for about 5 to 10 years, depending on your age and the number of positions you have held. The style of this resume focuses the reader's attention on the dates of the work history so that a potential employer can easily see your work experience and titles of responsibility.

Although a chronological resume focuses on the work history, it should include all of the resume elements previously described. However, because the work history is the focus and takes up a considerable part of the resume, skills are typically listed under the education heading, if they are included at all. As a result, the style of a chronological resume might cause some potential employers to overlook your skills and achievements, which is a drawback to this style. (See Figs. 8.2 and 8.3.)

Name
Address
City, State, Zip
Phone (home and cell on separate lines if possible)
E-mail address

Objective: (optional)

Work History:

From–To (usually "Present" for first entry listed)	List title or position, company, and responsibilities
From–To	List title or position, company, and responsibilities
From–To	List title or position, company, and responsibilities

Education:

From–To	List college or school name; city; degree, certificate, or diploma; expected graduation date; and honors

Skills: (optional)

References:

	Include as a separate references page or state "Available upon request"

FIGURE 8.2 Sample format for chronological resume.

Student Genius
1234 Career Path
Future, USA 12345
Home: (123) 456-7890
Cell: (098) 765-4321
studentgenius@email.com

Objective: To utilize my skills in radiography, which will allow me
to meet your department goals.

Work History:

2010–Present   Radiologist, Kaiser Hospital, Denver, CO
Responsible for all admission X-rays in the
emergency department and supervised on weekends

2008–2009   Radiologist, Kaiser Hospital, Santa Clara, CA
Responsible for physician X-ray orders, with some
experience in E.R.

2006–2008   Radiologist, Sunrise Hospital, Las Vegas, NV
Responsible for physician X-ray orders as part
of practicum

Education:

2004–2006   ABC College, Anyplace, USA
Certificate in Radiology
Dean's list
Field experience: 2 years
Excellent attendance awards

Computer Skills: IBM compatible; MS Windows, Word, and Excel; and
Internet Explorer

References: Available upon request

FIGURE 8.3 Chronological resume example.

Functional Resume

The emphasis of a functional resume is job titles and experience. If you
have had different jobs with impressive titles and have learned many skills,

then this style could be a good choice for highlighting your work history, skills, and experience. Unlike a chronological resume, with a functional resume you list your job titles in order of their importance rather than by date. This resume style points out your transferable skills to a potential employer. If you are in the process of a career change, this style can accent your level of responsibility and the skills you bring to a new position. This style is also a little more forgiving of gaps in your work history, so it might work well for you if you have had to take some time off from work for any reason. (See Figs. 8.4 and 8.5.)

The drawback to this resume style is that you might highlight that you have had responsibilities and titles that were higher than the entry-level position for which you are applying at this time in your career. As a result, some employers might view you as being overqualified for a position. However, you can tailor the responsibilities you include to fit the position for which you are applying and present them as strong transferrable skills. The ones you do not include you can present later on during your interview as leadership qualities.

Combination Resume

The combination resume style is currently a popular choice because it offers the best of two other resume styles: chronological and functional. The chronological format style lists the work history at the bottom of the resume, listing previous positions in order by date, including title and company. The functional format style lists the skills and experience as the focus in the combination resume. (See Figs. 8.6 and 8.7.)

This resume style is an excellent choice for someone who has been a health professions school student. It allows you to focus on your education, which includes your training and lab skills.

Achievement Resume

An achievement resume highlights just what you would expect: your achievements. Your achievements include your skills, abilities, and accomplishments on projects, sales, and presentations. This style might work well for you if your list of achievements is more impressive than your work history or job titles. For example, if you have a short work history or your time spent in different positions was brief, you can use this resume style to highlight stronger aspects of your experience. (See Figs. 8.8 and 8.9.)

An achievement resume might not be the best choice for an entry-level position because your experience might not leave you with many achievements

Name

Address   Home phone
City, State, Zip   Cell phone
                                   E-mail address

Objective: (optional)

Education: (Summarize briefly, including degree, certificate, or diploma; expected
                    graduation date; and name of school or college.)

Personal Summary (or Personal Profile for "age experienced" student)
List skills, core values, professional interests and accomplishments,
and certifications. (Note that the "Personal Summary" can sometimes
replace the "Objective.")

Skill Summary
List skills you have learned through your education and experience, possibly categorizing
them under headings.

**Work Experience (or Professional Experience
for "age experienced" student)**
List date (more recent first), company, title or position, and responsibilities.
List date, company, title or position, and responsibilities.
List date, company, title or position, and responsibilities.
List date, company, title or position, and responsibilities.
List date, company, title or position, and responsibilities.

References
Include as a separate references page or state "Available upon request"

FIGURE 8.4 Sample format for functional resume.

to highlight. In this case, your resume might have too much white space on the page, which makes it look thin or skimpy. Be sure to choose this resume style only if it is in your best interest to highlight your achievements over your work history.

Student Genius

1234 Career Path   Home: (123) 456-7890
Future, USA 12345   Cell: (098) 765-4321
                              studentgenius@email.com

Objective: To obtain a long-term growth position as a medical assistant, which will
              allow me to meet and exceed department goals.

Education: Will graduate in June 2011 with a diploma from ABC College
              and national certification. 3.5 GPA.

Personal Summary

Multitasker, Dependable, Self-starter, Quick learner
Proficient in MS Windows, Word, and Excel and Internet Explorer
Certifications: CMA, HIPAA, CPR, and first aid

Skill Summary

Front Office   **Back Office**
• Telephone triage   • Triage
• Medical records   • Injections
• Medical terminology   • Venipuncture
• Scheduling   • Urinalysis
• Referrals   • EKGs

Work History:

August 2009–Present   Cashier   Dollar Store, Anyplace, USA
                             Experienced in handling money
                             Balanced out register
                             Proven ability in customer service

July 2005–August 2009   Waitress   ABC Pizzeria, Anyplace, USA
                             Food service in fast-paced environment
                             Customer satisfaction
                             Stocking and inventory control

References
Available upon request

FIGURE 8.5 Functional resume example.

Other Resume Styles

Although the previously described resume styles are most commonly used in
the health professions field, some other resume styles have merit, and your

Name
Address
City, State, Zip
Phone (home and cell on separate lines if possible)
E-mail address

Objective: (optional)

Personal Summary: List skills, core values, professional interests and accomplishments, and certifications. (Note that the "Personal Summary" can sometimes replace the "Objective.")

Skills: List skills you have learned through your education and experience, possibly categorizing them under headings.

Education:

From–To

List college or school name; city; degree, certificate, or diploma; expected graduation date; and honors

Work History:

From–To
(usually "Present" for
first entry listed)

List title or position, company, and responsibilities

From–To

List title or position, company, and responsibilities

References:

Include as a separate references page or state "Available upon request"

FIGURE 8.6 Sample format for combination resume.

knowledge of them will assist you in choosing the resume style that is best for you based on your experience and preferences:

- **Imaginative resume:** This carefree style of resume takes advantage of imagination and creativity. However, using an unconventional format could bring

Student Genius
1234 Career Path
Future, USA 12345
Home: (123) 456-7890
Cell: (098) 765-4321
studentgenius@email.com

Objective: To utilize my skills as a massage therapist to help people find relief from physical pain and discomfort and feel healthier both in mind and body.

Personal Summary: A caring, proficient massage therapist who excels in deep tissue and hot stone therapy. Experienced in working on a team to reach team goals and with little supervision when working on my own. Nevada state licensed.

Skills
• Outstanding in deep tissue and hot stone massage
• Proficient in Swedish massage
• Great body wrap and scrub techniques
• Excellent skills in table shiatsu
• CPR certified
• Familiarity with most current office equipment
• Front desk customer service skills and experience working a multiline phone

Education:

2010–2011	ABC College, Anyplace, USA
	National certification in massage therapy
	Attendance honors
	GPA of 3.5

Work History:

Team Member, ABC Retail Store	2010–Present
Bank Teller, ABC Bank and Trust	2008–2009
Cashier, ABC Supplies	2007–2008
Cashier and Customer Service Representative, ABC Gas Station	2004–2006

References: Available upon request

FIGURE 8.7 Combination resume example.

unconventional results. If it is done well, an imaginative resume could attract the eye of a potential employer; however, if done poorly or the style is not appreciated by the potential employer, you might lose the opportunity for the employer to see your skills and experience. This style is not generally recommended for an entry-level position in the health professions and better lends itself to positions in the creative arts, such as designers and artists.

Name
Address
City, State, Zip
Phone (home and cell on separate lines if possible)
E-mail address

Objective
(optional)

Background Information
(or Personal Profile for "age experienced" student)
(optional)
List skills, core values, professional interests and accomplishments,
and certifications. (Note that "Background Information"
can sometimes replace the "Objective.")

Education
Summarize briefly, including degree, certificate, or diploma; expected graduation date;
and name of school or college.

Summary of Accomplishments
List examples of projects completed, goals met, and multitasking
experience as well as examples that illustrate your ability to be
dependable, a self-starter, and a quick learner.

Technical Qualifications
List computer qualifications if you have extensive ability
as well as knowledge of office equipment.

Career History (or Professional Experience for "age experienced" student)
(optional)
List most impressive title or position, company, responsibilities, and dates.
List next most impressive title or position, company, responsibilities, and dates.
List next most impressive title or position, company, responsibilities, and dates.
List next most impressive title or position, company, responsibilities, and dates.

References
Include as a separate references page or state "Available upon request"

FIGURE 8.8 Sample format for achievement resume.

- **Targeted resume:** A targeted resume directs the objective and skills included to a specific position for which you are applying. It showcases all of your education, work history, and achievements in such a way as to impress a potential employer and capture a certain position and title. As you gain experience in the health professions field, you will be able to develop a more targeted resume that can assist you in moving up into more advanced positions.

Student Genius
1234 Career Path
Future, USA 12345
Home: (123) 456-7890
Cell: (098) 765-4321
studentgenius@email.com

Objective
To obtain a long-term growth position as a biller and coder
that will allow me to meet and exceed department goals

Background Information
A hard-working, reliable person who works well on a team or individually

Education
Graduated in 2011 with a diploma from ABC College,
national certification, and a 3.5 GPA

Summary of Accomplishments
Billing and Coding Skills
• National certification
• HIPAA certification
• CPR and first aid certification
• Extensive training in billing and coding
• Outstanding filing skills
• Excellent skills in co-pay collections
• Mastery of several database scheduling systems
• Fast and detail oriented with insurance authorizations

Technical and Related Qualifications
Computer Skills: MS Windows, Word, and Excel; and Internet Explorer
Training Experience: Trained new employees on company policies and procedures
Customer Service: Worked with the public for the last 4 years
Accounting Skills: Balanced a daily cash drawer with few errors

Career History

1/2010–4/2010	ABC Hospital Anyplace, USA
	Biller and Coder
7/2008–3/2009	XYZ Urgent Care Anyplace, USA
	Coder
3/2006–7/2008	ABC Candy Company Anyplace, USA
	Sales Representative

References
Available upon request

FIGURE 8.9 Achievement resume example.

O N   T R A C K

You are on track if you can identify two resume styles that you think might work for you at this time:

1. _____

2. _____

Making Your Resume Look Professional

Almost as important as the information you include on your resume is how your resume looks. If your resume does not look professional or is hard to read or understand, it will most likely be tossed in the trash can. Your resume is going to speak for you, so it needs to look like you. It needs to be *confident* like you and be *neat* like you. If your resume does not represent these aspects of you, then you may not get called in for an interview. If you do get a call, then you know that your resume is doing its job.

To make your resume look professional, you should type it on a computer using an attractive and readable font and should print it on a quality printer. A laser printer offers the highest printing quality. You have many choices when it comes to the style of your resume; however, you should follow certain guidelines.

- The font size you use should be large enough to read but not so large that it looks bulky or overwhelming. Font size 10, 11, or 12 is usually appropriate for titles and bullets.
- The information on your resume should be well organized, with identifiable headings. Headings may be placed in a larger font, in bold, or in all capital letters to make them stand out from the rest of the resume.
- The margins on your resume should not be too large or too small. A 1-inch margin is standard for the top and bottom of your resume page, and a 1.5-inch margin is standard for the sides.
- When your resume requires changes, such as when you have a new address or phone number, you should make the changes on your computer and print out new copies of your resume. You should not cross out information in ink or use liquid correction fluid to make changes.
- You should use a light-colored paper; white is preferred, especially if you are going to fax your resume. Soft colors with matching envelopes can be appropriate when you are sending out your resume by mail.

No matter what resume style you choose, you must be sure to design a resume that looks professional. That means making sure that the information on it is readable, easy to understand, and quick to review. Your resume needs to be designed to get you the call for an interview.

Another way to make sure that your resume looks professional is to make sure that it fits on one page (for an entry-level position) and is not overwhelmed with words. One way to do this is to use short bullet points and phrases rather than full sentences whenever possible. When you remember that an employer spends only about 20 or 30 seconds reviewing your resume, you will understand the importance of presenting your information in quick, easily accessible points. The employer will not take the time to read long sentences, so you want to be sure that your most attractive traits are hard to miss on the page. Bullets also allow more information to be viewed in a small space. Entry-level resumes generally have more bullets, but you may need to add some longer phrases or sentences as your experience grows. (See Box 8.2 for more tips on designing a professional resume.)

Motivational Moment

66 Perhaps the most valuable result of all education is the ability to make yourself do the thing to do when it ought to be done, whether you like or not. 99

Thomas Huxley, British anthropologist

BOX 8.2 TIPS FOR DESIGNING A PROFESSIONAL-LOOKING RESUME

You have choices in how you design your resume. No matter what you decide, re-member that your resume is an extension of you. Make sure it represents you well.

- Font: If you are familiar with your word-processing program, you have proba-bly realized that you can change the style of the type that you use. This is known as the "font." Fonts differ in their looks as well as their size. Some fonts are very professional looking, whereas others are more fun and have flair. Some fonts are easier to read than others. You want to use a font that has clear, clean, and crisp letters that do not touch one another. The default font on a computer is usually Times New Roman. Therefore, many resumes use this common font. Arial is another popular font because it is easy to read; how-ever, Ariel Black does not work as well because faxing resumes that use this font can blur the letters. When designing your resume, you can choose from any of the available fonts on your computer. Using an interesting font might be one way to help your resume stand out. However, no matter what font you

BOX 8.2 (continued)

choose, you should make sure that the letters are readable, and you should use that same font for the entire resume.

- **Font size:** The size of the font you use is just as important as the style you choose. Because of their design, some fonts naturally look smaller or larger than others. Choose a font size that is easy to read, but is not too large, because overwhelming type can make your resume look very unprofessional. Most professional resumes use font size 11; however, size 10 or size 12 might also work for you depending on the font you use. Many times, people play games with the font size in order to get their resumes to fit on one page. People who do not have enough information to fill their resumes tend use a larger font size, such as 14, whereas others with too much information tend to use font size 9. Employers can see through this game, and therefore there is no advantage to it. Instead, play with other elements of your resume to keep it looking professional.

- **White space:** When you first start your resume, you are facing a blank page that can seem daunting. However, white space can be an important component of making your resume look professional. The right amount of space in between the lines of your resume can make it more readable, and the right amount of space between the sections of your resume can help draw the reader's attention to important sections. Single-spacing is recommended between bullets and other resume information, and double-spacing is recommended between sections. White space around your resume—in the form of margins—can also help your layout look clean and professional. Play with a margin space of 1 inch on the side and 1/2 inch on the bottom for starters. Then you can adjust any of these elements of white space to fit your resume.

- **Alignment:** Alignment refers to the placement of your text on the page. Many people choose to center important information, such as their personal heading and section headings. However, text can also be aligned on the left-hand or right-hand side of the page along the margin (this is known as "justified" text). To determine which alignment will work best for your resume, watch the amount of white space on your page as you play with different alignments. Your eye will guide you. Remember that whatever is most readable will work best.

- **Font characteristics:** The use of such font characteristics as **bold,** *italics,* underlining, and CAPITALIZATION can be a good way to make important information, such as section headings, stand out on your resume. You should be careful using these attributes if you expect to have to fax or scan your resume because they can make it hard to read; however, most resumes are now submitted electronically, and the use of these attributes causes little trouble. You should generally stay away from using color on your resume, though, because most employers will print your resume in black ink, negating the affects of colored fonts.

(box continues on page 258)

BOX 8.2 TIPS FOR DESIGNING A PROFESSIONAL-
LOOKING RESUME (continued)

- **Bullet style:** If your resume has bulleted points, the bullet style you use is another design choice you will have to make. Depending on your personality and
  career field, you might want to choose a straightforward style that highlights
  your professionalism or a more creative style that shows off your creativity and
  flair. Here are some examples:

  - Straightforward
  - Design
  - Flair 1
  - Flair 2

  You should avoid using icons such as smiley faces as bullets because they are
  not professional.

Making Your Resume Sound Professional

Once you overcome the hurdle of getting a prospective employer to look at your
resume for longer than 30 seconds, you must make sure that you grab the employer's full attention by using words that make your resume read as strong and
professional. At every opportunity, you should elevate the vocabulary in your
resume to the highest level because you never know who will be reviewing it.

In the health-care field, the person reviewing your resume might be a human resources director, office or department manager, supervisor, or physician.
Using words that catch this person's attention, such as buzz terms and action
words, will help to ensure that your resume receives more than a cursory glance.
You should also avoid using pronouns, such as "I," in your resume.

Using Buzz Terms

One way to make your resume sound professional and get noticed is to use
health-related buzz terms, such as "record," "triage," and "EKG," which can help
employers to quickly identify whether you possess the skills required for a position. Many companies and even large clinics and hospitals use technology and
other searching methods to swiftly screen resumes by scanning for such words.
These buzz terms can help to quickly identify candidates that meet certain requirements of the job. In some cases, these organizations hire other people or
companies to perform these initials scans, significantly narrowing down their list
of candidates. If your resume does not include the right buzz terms, it might not

even make it past this initial round to move on to the review by the organization that is actually looking to hire. Although this hiring practice might not be as common for entry-level positions, you should be aware of the importance of buzz terms for your future resume.

Another type of buzz terms that will be important for you to include on your resume are those that represent your core values, work ethics, and professionalism. (See Box 8.3.) These adjectives help make your resume sound stronger and more professional and also offer a glimpse into the type of person you are. Employers scan resumes for these words to determine whether you have the core values and are competent to make on-the-job decisions that will promote the health-care field's goal of helping others and making a difference in the world.

O N   T R A C K

You are on track if you can list three personal buzz terms that you would like to include on your resume.

1._____

2._____

3._____

BOX 8.3 LIST OF PERSONAL BUZZ TERMS

Ambitious	Articulate	Assertive
Calm	Caring	Cheerful
Compassionate	Confident	Congenial
Conscientious	Considerate	Consistent
Cooperative	Courteous	Creative
Dedicated	Dependable	Determined
Diligent	Eager	Efficient
Energetic	Enthusiastic	Flexible
Genuine	Goal-directed	Helpful
Honest	Independent	Industrious
Intelligent	Intuitive	Knowledgeable
Leader	Listener	Motivated
Open-minded	Optimistic	Orderly
Organized	Persuasive	Poised
Positive	Prompt	Productive

(box continues on page 260)

BOX 8.3 LIST OF PERSONAL BUZZ TERMS (continued)		
Punctual	Quick	Reliable
Resourceful	Respectful	Responsible
Self-reliant	Sharp	Sincere
Strong	Supportive	Task-oriented
Tolerant		

Using Action Words

Action words are verbs that put energy into the meaning of the bullet points you list in your resume to describe your skills. They show action (which is why they are called "action words") and give your potential employer information concerning your qualifications, experience, and accomplishments. Although you can use adjectives such as "good," "excellent," and "outstanding" on your resume, these words cannot stand alone and do not explain anything. You need to use a strong action word that describes what you can do. Potential employers will be looking at how your current skills can transfer to their company, department, or office. Action words are the best way to show them that you have the right skills. (See Box 8.4.)

BOX 8.4 LIST OF ACTION WORDS		
Accomplished	Achieved	Administered
Analyzed	Arranged	Assembled
Assisted	Balanced	Built
Complied	Composed	Consolidated
Coordinated	Created	Delegated
Designed	Encouraged	Established
Examined	Expanded	Identified
Illustrated	Inspected	Installed
Maintained	Managed	Monitored
Operated	Organized	Performed
Prepared	Processed	Purchased
Recommended	Recorded	Regulated
Remodeled	Repaired	Scheduled
Solved	Supervised	

You will find many places to use action words on your resume. Any task that you performed on a job can be turned into a strong action word. Remember that every job has its own standards and expectations, even employment at a fast-food restaurant. You need to think of your job performance as meeting goals, solving problems, and achieving other higher level goals. In some cases, you just need to use some creativity to recreate your job tasks and responsibilities using strong action words, elevating your job skills to a new level for your resume (see Box 8.5). Although you have many actions words from which to choose, you should select words that pertain to an entry-level resume.

O N   T R A C K

You are on track if you can describe three of the skills you learned from your past employment positions or personal experience using strong action words.

1. _____

2. _____

3. _____

BOX 8.5   TURNING JOB EXPERIENCES INTO RESUME SKILLS

Using action words in your resume can help you turn your past job experiences and tasks into strong resume skills. Here are some examples.

Job Tasks	Resume Skill
Answering phones	Screened calls to schedule appointments
	Maintained office schedule
	Assisted with customer service
Cashiering	Contributed to smooth operation of front-end of retail store
	Balanced cash drawer
	Provided customer assistance
Filing	Managed office files
	Developed file-keeping system
	Illustrated ability to be detail oriented

(box continues on page 262)

BOX 8.5 TURNING JOB EXPERIENCES INTO RESUME SKILLS (continued)

Stocking shelves	Prepared inventory for display
	Inspected goods for quality
	Performed job task with little supervision
Waiting tables	Fulfilled customer needs to their satisfaction
	Performed in a fast-paced environment
	Utilized problem-solution skills
Writing letters	Composed legal and customer correspondence
	Displayed excellent communication skills
	Maintained the high quality of communication

Identifying Weaknesses in Your Resume

Above all requirements, a professional resume must be error free. That means there are none of the following

- Spelling errors
- Grammar errors
- Font inconsistencies
- Formatting errors, such as inconsistent spacing or margins
- Informational inaccuracies

You must correct all errors because they can hinder your chances of receiving an invitation to interview. Errors just seem to jump out when an employer is quickly reviewing your resume, and if a resume error is the first thing an employer sees about you, you might not be given the opportunity to show that you have more to offer.

Here are some ways that you can approach finding and correcting some common resume errors:

- **Finding misspelled words:** Using a spell-checker to find misspelled words might seem like a given when you write your resume; however, many people rely just on a spell-checker and do not thoroughly review their resumes once they are written. Remember that your computer's spell-checker will only catch misspelled words not *incorrectly used* words that are spelled correctly.

- **Clarifying gaps:** Make sure you have identified and explained any employment gaps in your resume. Because the recent economy has led to many layoffs, most companies are not surprised to see some unemployment on resumes. However, more and more, employers want to know the reason someone was unemployed.

- **Avoiding overstatements:** Although you always want to be confident and highlight your best attributes, you should make sure that you do not stretch the truth when it comes to your qualifications. Overstating or misrepresenting your skills, experience, or education will not serve you well as it usually reveals itself during the interview process. When this happens, you end up making yourself look untrustworthy or deceitful, as opposed to confident and positive. In addition, if you have not been factual on your resume, your new employer's expectations of you might be higher than you can handle, creating more stress than you deserve to have in your first position.

Creating an error-free resume might seem almost impossible; however, it is within your reach. It just takes time, patience, and careful proofreading. Once you have finished writing your resume, you need to proof it and proof it and proof it again. You are likely to find at least one mistake each time you review your resume. Having someone else look over your resume for errors is also a good tip. After working on your resume for so long, you are likely to miss obvious mistakes that someone else might see. So, when you think that you have finalized your resume, you should ask a friend or classmate to proofread your resume. You should also be sure to bring a copy to your career services department for review. Someone there might see something that you and others have missed.

Mentor Moment

I once advertised for an administrative assistant position at our college campus. I couldn't believe it when I received 400 applications! However, once I removed the resumes with spelling errors, I was left with only 67 resumes to review. Any resume that had a spelling error just wasn't worth my time.

Thomas, Director of Education, from Middletown, DE

Keeping Your Resume Updated

You must realize that your resume is a document in progress. You will continue to alter and add to your original resume as your experience and skill levels change. Think of your resume as a "living and growing" product of your brief history of life and work experiences. You should not create a resume and lock it in stone. Your resume should always reflect your most current level of skill. You should keep an electronic copy of your resume on your home computer or someplace else that is easily accessible so that you are able to make any necessary changes at any time.

Entry-level resumes are typically one page in length, which is a standard in the business industry. As you gain experience with different medical equipment, increase your skills, earn new titles through promotions, and change positions, you must update your resume to reflect these changes. If you learn to use new office or medical equipment on the job, make sure to add it to your resume. Also include any awards and special recognitions you earn, committees you lead, seminars you attend, and additional classes you take. When you do so, your resume might increase to two pages in length. However, the actual length of your resume is not as important as making sure that your resume always reflects the highest level of experience that you have achieved.

Creating a Professional Cover Letter

Although you might think that your resume is the first thing an employer will see, most employers expect that your resume will come with a cover letter. In fact, many position advertisements will ask you to include a letter when you submit your resume. Whether you are mailing, e-mailing, or faxing your resume, it should be accompanied by a cover letter. A cover letter is a business-style letter addressed to a potential employer that serves as a form of introduction for you and your resume.

Understanding the Importance of a Cover Letter

Think of your cover letter as an opportunity. You get a chance to reveal something more about yourself to employers by addressing them in paragraph form, rather than in the short, bulleted points they will see on your resume.

Your cover letter should grab the attention of the reader and make him or her want to read your resume. It should also include two important facts:

1. Why you want to work for this particular health-care organization or office
2. The strengths you have, based on your skills, experience, and work ethics, that will most benefit the company

Think of your cover letter as another chance to make a good first impression. It highlights for the employer the most important points about you and gives you a chance to explain why you are the best candidate for the job. Do not worry about repeating information from your resume in your cover letter. Just make sure that, like your resume, your cover letter puts your best foot forward so that you maximize your chances of getting an interview. That means making sure that the quality and professionalism of your cover letter match those of your resume. Your cover letter must be well written and *error-free* to make the best possible first impression.

Understanding the Parts of a Cover Letter

Like your resume, your cover letter will start with a heading that includes your name, address, and contact information. Unlike your resume, your cover letter will include these components:

- The date
- The contact person's name, title, company, address, and department, if you know it
- A greeting or salutation, such as "Dear Employer," "Manager:" or "Ms./Mr." (If possible, you should call or check the position advertisement for the name of the person to whom you will be submitting your resume so that you can use the person's actual name in the salutation.)

This information will be followed by several paragraphs that state your interest in the position and your strengths:

- The first paragraph should include the purpose of the letter, the position of interest, and even the lead source, if applicable.
- The next paragraph should explain your interest in the position and should indicate what you have to offer the company, including your education, training, and experience. It should also include a specific request for an interview; keep this request brief by limiting it to one sentence.
- The last paragraph should state that you have enclosed a resume for review and should thank the potential employer for his or her time and consideration. It should also indicate that you plan to follow up in a few days.

You should end your cover letter with a formal closing, such as "Sincerely," "Best Regards," or "Respectfully." Include your name in typewritten letters beneath your closing, but be sure to leave room for your signature. Use only blue or black ink for your signature. Blue ink is best because then the original will not look like a copy. Avoid such colors as red, purple, green, and orange because they do not look professional.

When you are including other documents with a professional letter, such as your resume, you should add the word "Enclosure(s)" after your name to indicate that the letter is accompanied by other documents. (See Figs. 8.10 and 8.11.)

Motivational Moment

66 There are eight things people want most in life: to be happy, healthy, reasonably prosperous, secure, have friends, peace of mind, good family relationships, and hope. 99

Zig Ziglar, motivational speaker

Name
Address
City, State, Zip
Phone (home and cell on separate lines if possible)
E-mail address

Date

Addressee's Name
Title
Company
Address
City, State, Zip

Salutation (e.g., "Dear XXX," "Dear Employer," "Manager:" or "Ms./Mr.")

First Paragraph: Introduction, purpose, position of interest, and place where you found or heard about the position.

Second Paragraph: Interest in the position, list of your strengths, and request for interview.

Summary Paragraph: State resume enclosed, follow-up information, and thank you.

Closing (e.g., "Sincerely," "Respectfully," or "Best Regards")

Signature (in blue ink if possible)

Your typed name

Enclosed (in smaller font): (e.g., "Resume," "Letters of Recommendation," "References Page")

FIGURE 8.10 Sample cover letter format.

Student Genius
1234 Career Path
Future, USA 12345
Home: (123) 456-7890
Cell: (098) 765-4321
studentgenius@email.com

September 2, 2011

Mrs. Teri M. Erhardt, Office Manager
ABC Family Practice
1234 Health Professions Ave.
Anyplace, USA 12345

Dear Mrs. Erhardt:

I was very excited to discover your opening for a medical assistant, as advertised in the *Medical Assisting Review Journal.* Your advertisement caught my attention because I am familiar with your clinic's reputation and the quality of service you provide.

I recently graduated from a comprehensive medical assisting program at ABC College, and I am proud to say that I graduated with a 3.5 GPA. During my education, I also won several attendance awards. Now, I am looking for exactly the type of position your organization is offering to utilize my various skills as a medical assistant. I have experience with medical terminology, triage, medical records, and vitals. I am a great multitasker, a self-starter, and a quick learner. I think these skills, along with my experience and certifications, make me the perfect candidate for your position. My strong work ethic would make me a reliable and dependable employee on your staff.

Thank you for taking the time to consider me for this position. The enclosed resume further outlines my qualifications for this position. I am very excited about this opportunity, and welcome the chance to discuss how I would be a benefit to your office and patients. I look forward to speaking with you when your time permits.

Respectfully,

Student Genius

Student Genius
Enclosed: Resume

FIGURE 8.11 Example cover letter.

Success Journal

1. List five personal "buzz terms" to describe yourself and that would be good to convey to a potential employer.

   1. _____

   2. _____

   3. _____

   4. _____

   5. _____

2. List five job responsibilities you have had, and for each, list one to three action words you can use to describe those responsibilities as skills on your resume.

Skill	Action Words
_____	_____
_____	_____
_____	_____
_____	_____
_____	_____

3. List three courses you have taken in your program, and then list the skills you learned in each of those courses.

Course	Skills Learned
1. _____	_____
	_____
	_____
	_____
	_____

2. _____   _____

_____

_____

_____

_____

3. _____   _____

_____

_____

_____

_____

4. Begin to compile the information for your resume by completing the following information.

Personal data (name, address, phone numbers, and e-mail address)

_____

_____

_____

_____

_____

Objective:

_____

_____

_____

(continues on page 270)

Success Journal (continued)

Education (name of each educational institution, degree earned, skills developed)

_____

_____

_____

_____

_____

_____

_____

_____

_____

Work history (name of each company, your title, employment dates, salary, and job skills)

_____

_____

_____

_____

_____

5. List three to five people you could ask to be a reference. For each potential reference, include the person's name, position, and contact information; whether your relationship was personal or professional; and the length of your relationship.

1._____

_____

_____

_____

2._____

_____

_____

_____

3._____

_____

_____

_____

4._____

_____

_____

5._____

_____

_____

_____

Interviewing Skills

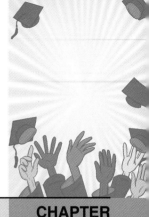

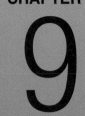

Learning Outcomes

After reading this chapter, the student will be able to:

1. Identify different interview styles.
2. Describe how to behave professionally during an interview.
3. Answer some common interview questions.
4. List interview mistakes to avoid.

Preparing for an Interview

If your resume makes a good first impression, then you might be given the opportunity to make a second impression during the next step of the hiring process: the interview. In some ways, the interview is the most important component of the hiring process because it gives you the opportunity to show the employer that you would be the best fit with the company's policies, with the other employees, and with the customers. How you answer questions during your interview, how you showcase your personality, and what impression you leave could significantly impact your chances of getting offered the position. Remember that your resume is the tool that will help you get the interview, but it is up to you in the interview to get the position.

In some cases, the interviewing process begins with a quick telephone interview. This telephone interview is used to further screen and weed out candidates who do not meet the company's standard of employability. Some employers use this form of interview to make sure that they are spending their time with only the top candidates for the in-person interviews. Not all organizations use telephone interviews to screen candidates; however, you should be sure that you are prepared for this possibility.

Once you reach the in-person interview, you need to be physically and mentally ready to present yourself to the employer as the best candidate for the position. That means preparing for the interview by making sure of the following:

- You understand the employer's needs
- You look professional (see Chapter 10 for more information on looking professional)
- You can anticipate what might happen during the interview process, including what might go wrong
- You come equipped with the right tools, including multiple copies of your resume (see Chapter 8 for more information on preparing your resume), a small purse or work bag, a notebook, two pens, and your portfolio
- You are prepared to answer any possible interview questions you might be asked, including those related to your salary requirements

You must remember as you prepare for your interview that you are in competition with graduates from your school and also those from *other* schools. If your resume has the same top qualities as another candidate, your interview could be the deciding factor in whether you are made an offer. The more prepared you are for the interview process, the more confidently you will be able to express to the potential employer that you are the right person for the position.

Motivational Moment

66 All our dreams can come true if we have the courage to pursue them. 99

Walt Disney, American animator, entertainer, and philanthropist

Understanding the Employer's Needs

One way to prepare yourself for the interviewing process is to understand the employer's needs, which begins by understanding what the employer is looking for in a candidate. The first way to determine this information is to revisit the position posting, which usually explains the qualifications and, sometimes, the traits the employer is looking for in a candidate. You should look over these requirements and be prepared to discuss with the hiring manager how your skills and experience meet the organization's needs and are transferrable to the position in question. To save yourself and the medical organization time, you should not apply for any position for which you obviously are not qualified. A good rule is that you should be able to do 75% of what an employer is requesting in the posting. If you meet this requirement, you should apply for the position.

To better understand what the employer is looking for in a candidate, you should also find out more information about the organization by doing some research. Investigate the company's goals, competitors, and type of customers. You should also visit their website. Most websites include information about the organization's history, and some also include the organization's mission statement. Sometimes, an organization's website will also give you some hints as to the salary range for different positions. The more information you have about a prospective employer, the more prepared you will be to understand that employer's needs and the more knowledgeable you will sound during the interview.

Most people think that the reason for an interview is to select the top candidate; however, the employer is really looking for the person who will be the *best fit* for the office, hospital, or clinic. If most of the candidates for a position have graduated from a postsecondary educational institution, then the student who has the strongest academic record, had outstanding attendance, and is *the best fit for the office* will be hired.

Each organization has a different corporate culture, and employers usually want to hire new people who will fit into that existing culture. Do not be surprised if, as you are interviewing, you feel as though you might fit in at one organization but not at another. The interview process is about both you and the employer finding the right match. That's why putting your best foot forward—and also being yourself—are so important when you interview.

Mentor Moment

During my career search, I found a position I was interested in, but I did not meet all of their requirements. The only thing I could not do was type 60 words per minute. My typing skills were accurate, just not fast. I decided to apply anyway, and they called me in for an interview. During the interview, I made sure to mention that my typing skills were more accurate than fast and that I felt accuracy was more important with insurance forms. I was myself, and they made me an offer.

Lynette from Ontario, Canada

Understanding Different Types of Interviews

The next step you need to take to prepare for your interview is to anticipate the possibility of undergoing different types of interviews. For an entry-level position, you will most likely experience a one-on-one interview. However, you should also be aware of and be prepared to undergo any of the other interview types because you never know when you might experience them along your career path:

- **One-on-one interview:** In a one-on-one interview, you will meet with only one other person, usually the human resources (HR) director, hiring manager or supervisor, or office manager, but possibly even the physician. The advantage of a one-on-one interview is that you might feel more relaxed and comfortable because you are being questioned by only one person. In addition, because one-on-one interviews are the most common type, you will probably also feel more prepared for this type of interview because you will get the most practice with it. The disadvantage of a one-on-one interview is that you are the only person in the room with the interviewer, so all of the attention will be on you.
- **Telephone interview:** As previously mentioned, the telephone interview is usually part of the selection process used to determine who should come in for an in-person interview. It usually takes between 10 and 15 minutes. The person conducting the telephone interview will most likely ask you some of the same questions you will be asked in your in-person interview. The goal is to determine whether you are qualified for the position.
- **Screening interview:** This type of interview is closely related to the telephone interview; however, it occurs after an employer has determined that you are qualified for a position. The goal of the screening interview is to save time by eliminating candidates and selecting only the best candidates for the interview process. The questions you are asked during a screening interview might seem tough to answer because the interviewer is trying to gauge your ability to think quickly. For example, you might be asked to answer scenario-related questions

that put you on the spot. Only top candidates should emerge from this process. This type of interview usually lasts between 30 and 45 minutes. No matter how the screening interview is performed, you must treat it like an official interview and be sure to mind your professional etiquette manners. Do not become too casual during the interview because doing so might cost you the opportunity to make it to the next interview.

- **Group or committee interview:** In a group or committee interview, you are usually questioned by a panel of three to five people. The group might be composed of people in the hiring department, such as a potential supervisor, the office manager or supervisor, and coworkers. In a more official group, such as a committee, the interview might be conducted by department heads or the director of the organization. Each member is allowed to ask you questions according to their field of interest and expertise.
- **Stress interview:** The stress interview is more of a technique that is used during the interview process than it is an actual interview type. For some positions, particularly managerial and higher positions, the ability to handle a high-stress environment is a requirement. Therefore, the interviewer will ask you questions to gauge how you react to stress in real-life case scenarios. The questions are almost always behavioral and require you to think on your feet.
- **Lunch interview:** A lunch interview is usually a one-on-one interview that is conducted over a meal during lunch hours. Some employers use this type of interview to save time or to fit interviews into their busy schedules. Others might use this technique to relax candidates and better gauge their true personalities. The questions asked during a lunch interview are typically standard ones, such as those used to gauge your strengths and weaknesses. If you are asked to participate in a lunch interview, remember that your table manners become just as important during the interview as your professional interview etiquette. For an entry-level position, this type of interview is not the most common.

No matter what style of interview your hiring process includes or how many people you meet with, the best way for you to prepare for your interview is to practice answering basic interview questions in a calm, well-thought out manner (see the section Being Prepared for Common Interview Questions later in this chapter).

Determining Your Salary Requirement

Although money is a prime motivating factor for people who are seeking a new career, many people go into an interview unprepared to answer the question "What are your salary expectations?" or "How much are you looking to make?"

This could be because candidates anticipate that the employer will already have a set salary for the position. Although it is true that most organizations have salary ranges for certain positions based on their budgets, knowing your own salary requirement and being prepared to state it at your interview might determine whether you start in the position at the bottom or top of that salary range. Consider this, an employer will be looking to find the best candidate possible for the best price. If you do not know what your own salary requirement is, you might be given the lowest offer. Although this question might not come up until the second interview, you should be prepared to answer it before you even begin interviewing.

So, how should you determine your salary requirement? You need to add up your bills and expenses and determine what you need to make to be able to get through each month. Remember, though, that the stated salary will not be what you take home in your paycheck. Out of each paycheck, you will need to pay for taxes, benefits, and other items (see Chapter 13). Other factors that you must consider when you are calculating your salary requirement include the organization's location. Time spent traveling and the cost of transportation might lead you to consider taking a job at a lower pay rate than you intended if the company, office, or hospital is close to your home or your children's schools.

Chapter 1 presents some sample salaries for common health professions. However, to build your knowledge and confidence in the area of salary, you should research health care–related salaries in your state or local area and keep your salary requirement range near the standard for your area in order to increase your chances of being hired.

No matter what, you need to be realistic about the salary levels for entry-level positions. However, you should also keep in mind that your salary might change. Some organizations have 3-, 6-, or 12-month probation periods during which they evaluate your performance and after which you might be given a pay increase. In this case, you might want to consider accepting a position that has a lower starting salary because you can expect that, with optimal performance, you will be given an increase in the near future.

One mistake you do not want to make is to base your salary expectations on your current job. You know—and you should make sure a potential employer knows—that your current salary probably does not represent your value or potential. An interviewer might even ask you, "What did you earn in your last job?" However, the answer you provide to this can be misleading. You need to be ready to tell the interviewer that your current position search is a career change for you and that the salary at your last job reflects only your determination to work and make money so that you could go to school during the day.

O N   T R A C K

You are on track if you are able to answer the following salary-related questions.

1. How much do graduates at your school typically make? _____

2. What is the least amount of money you need to make to pay your monthly bills? _____

3. What salary range will you request when you are ready to look for a career position? _____

Getting There on Time

The last way to make sure that you are prepared for the interview is to make sure that you arrive on time. Being late for an interview not only makes a bad first impression, but it will also distract you and leave you stressed out by the time you get into your interview. The result of this will be that you are thrown off your "A game" and come off as less confident during your interview.

One way to ensure that you arrive on time is to pay attention when you are scheduling your interview. Write down the date and time, and do not be afraid to repeat the information back to the person scheduling the interview to confirm that you have gotten the correct information. When it comes to an interview, you are better off arriving too early than arriving late. To be safe, you should plan to arrive about 10 to 15 minutes before your appointment. If you arrive earlier than that, you can always wait in your car, go to the restroom, or look around the waiting room for information about the organization. You can use any information you find to improve your answers during the interview itself.

One way to ensure that you arrive on time is to know where you are going. Using a GPS or looking up the directions online using a directions website such as MapQuest or Yahoo Maps can help you to make sure that you know where you are going and how much time you will need for travel. You can confirm your directions by calling the office before you leave for your interview. Remember to allow extra time for lights, traffic, and other unexpected delays during your commute. Also make sure ahead of time that you have enough gas so that you will not need to make an unexpected stop along your way. You might even want to take a test drive to the office a day or two before your interview at the same time of day as your scheduled interview time so that you will know exactly where you are going and what the traffic will be like. If you make every effort to be on time but something goes wrong and you still end up being late, be sure to call ahead and let the interviewer know that you have been delayed.

Mentor Moment

I never really had any problems with interviews—until that day! For most of the interviews I went on, I was pretty comfortable talking about myself and my qualifications. I usually left my interviews feeling as though I had made a good impression. But one day, I was interviewing for a job in the city, and I completely underestimated how long it would take me to get there with afternoon traffic. I showed up at least 15 minutes late. The whole last 15 minutes of my ride, I wasn't even sure that the hiring manager would still see me for the interview. She did, but I was so frazzled by the time I got in there that I gave the worst interview of my life. I was not at all surprised when I didn't get called back for a second interview with them.

Sasha from Orlando, FL

During an Interview

The skills that you will require during an interview actually begin when you arrive at the location. One key to a successful interview is making a good first impression and maintaining that impression throughout the interview process by being friendly, courteous, and professional to everyone you meet.

Making a Good First Impression

You might think that your interview begins when you sit down with the interviewer; however, you will begin making your first impression as soon as you arrive. In fact, if you arrive late for your interview, you could start making a bad impression *before* you even arrive. Instead, make sure to begin with a good first impression by being on time for your interview. Then, continue building on that good first impression by acting professional while you wait for your interview in the lobby. Do not smoke, chew gum, or use your cell phone to call or text while you are waiting. In fact, if you have not done so already, now is a great time to turn off your cell phone. Consider that someone (such as a vice president or HR director) might be observing your behavior at any point during your interview process, even while you wait. An employer might observe how you greet and treat the receptionist to measure your capacity for customer service and to see how well you will fit into the working environment. In this way, your interview begins the moment you walk in the door and so should your professionalism.

Mentor Moment

I once had a job as a receptionist at a very elite company. At one point, the company was interviewing for a new vice president to oversee one of the divisions. As the receptionist, I greeted candidates and asked them to wait in the lobby. One day, after a gentleman had completed his interview and left the building, the president of the company came over to me and asked, "What did you think about him?" I was really surprised that he wanted my opinion, but it always stuck in my head after that point that the receptionist is part of the interview process.

Terry from Atlantic City, NJ

Keeping Your Cool While You Wait

Even if you prepare thoroughly and arm yourself with the proper tools, you might still feel nervous as each interview approaches. If this happens, remember that even the best athlete is probably a little nervous before a big game. In fact, some athletes *want* to feel this nervousness before a game to keep them on the edge of excitement and encourage them to perform their best. If you think of this nervousness as energy, you can turn it around and use it to your advantage. You need to work like an athlete to achieve a high level of performance and win at the "interview game."

You should remind yourself as you go into your interview that you are one of the top candidates for the position; otherwise, you would not be there for the interview. Your qualifications, work experiences, and accomplishments are as high as or higher than any of the other candidates, and if you have properly prepared, you will have your portfolio with you to back up these qualifications and accomplishments. Reminding yourself that you have worked hard and deserve to be where you are will go a long way toward helping you stay relaxed while you wait for your interview.

Motivational Moment

66 Confidence has a lot to do with interviewing—that, and timing. 99

Michael Parkinson, English broadcaster and journalist

Here are some other techniques that will help you to remain calm while you wait for and perform your best during your interview:

- **Smile:** Greeting the front desk person with a smile will relax you and will put you in the proper positive frame of mind for heading into your interview.

- **Warm up:** Like stretching before a big game, you can release some of your nervous energy while you are waiting for your interview by walking around the lobby. You can use this time to look at any informative material on the walls, such as plaques, pictures, awards, and medical information. Doing so will help you release some of the energy stored in your legs, will take your mind off of your nerves, and might also provide you with some useful information. Stand or walk around for as long as you can before taking a seat. When you do sit down, you can continue to warm up by gently swaying or tapping your foot to the music in the office.
- **Breathe:** Once you finally take a seat, you might experience that nervous feeling in your stomach again. If so, you can sit up tall and practice some calming breathing exercises. Breathe in very deeply through your nose and then out through your mouth. Breathing will help you to relax and release more of your nervous energy.
- **Change the scenery:** If sitting and waiting makes you more nervous, ask to use the restroom. The walk to the restroom will help to release some of your nervous energy, and the change of scenery might keep your mind from worrying. If you use the restroom beforehand, you will not need to worry about having to go during the middle of your interview.

Another thing that might help to take your mind off the interview while you wait is the employment application. In some cases, you will be asked to complete the application before you go in for your interview. The application is important because it is likely to cover some aspects of your personal history that are not reflected in your resume. (See Chapter 12 for more information on completing the employment application.)

If you can keep yourself calm and focused before the interview, you will be ready to be confident, positive, and polite during your interview. Once the interview begins, you probably will not feel as nervous because concentrating on the interview questions will help you to quickly release the energy and tension in your body.

Acting Professionally During the Interview

When your wait it finally over, you will enter the most important part of the interviewing process, where you need to make your *best* impression. This section outlines some of the basics of interview etiquette. Following these suggestions will help to ensure that you make a good first impression and carry that good impression throughout your interview. Of course, part of making a good first impression is being yourself. That means putting your best foot forward while you showcase your personality, knowledge, skill level, and patient care techniques.

Show Your Confidence with Eye Contact

In many cases, the person who will interview you will meet you in the lobby and then lead you to the interview room. As the interviewer greets you, you should be sure to make eye contact. You need to say hello with your eyes and make direct eye contact with confidence. Holding your head down or looking anywhere other than at the interviewer comes off as disrespectful and insecure, which could make for a very short interview.

Make a Strong Impression With a Strong Handshake

As the interviewer greets you, he or she may also extend a hand for a handshake. A strong handshake builds on the respect and confidence that you begin to form with your eye contact. Extend your hand firmly and energetically with a straight, open palm to connect with the interviewer's hand. As your hands meet, close your fingers around the interviewer's hand with a firm and confident grip and shake hands for approximately 3 to 5 seconds. Your grip is important because no one wants to shake hands with a limp, spaghetti-fingers hand, and no one wants to shake hands with someone who squeezes so hard that the blood to the fingers stops flowing.

Another thing your handshake should be is dry. If you are worried about having sweaty palms, then you should hold a tissue while you wait or wipe your hands on your pants or skirt before you get up to greet the interviewer. You want to be sure to avoid extending a sweaty hand for this important handshake.

Make the Most of the "Longest Mile"

The path from the lobby to the interview room can be referred to as the "longest mile." When you hear your name called in the lobby, you might immediately be ready for the interview to begin. However, what do you say to the interviewer during the walk between the lobby and the interview room? Although the interview has not officially begun, the interviewer might ask you a casual question or strike up conversation with a simple comment, such as "Tell me where are you from" or "Did you have a hard time finding us?" You should be prepared for some of this small talk by anticipating some common questions (see Box 9.1). What you say during the longest mile and how you say it are important because they will begin to form the interviewer's first impression of you.

You can also show some self-confidence by taking control of the conversation a little during the longest mile, such as by asking the interviewer the first question or following up with a question after you are asked one. For example, if the interviewer asks you "Did you have a hard time finding the office?" you might answer, "No, I have lived in this area for a few years," and then you can

BOX 9.1 QUESTIONS YOU MIGHT BE ASKED DURING "THE LONGEST MILE"

- What can you tell me about yourself?
- Did you have any trouble finding the office?
- How long did it take you to get here?
- Are you originally from this area?
- Do you follow any sports?
- Have you been watching (insert name of popular television program)?
- Did you see (insert name of recent movie)?
- How long was your health professions program?

follow up by asking, "How long have you lived in this area?" Another good question you can ask is, "How long have you been with this company?" Questions such as these express your interest in the interviewer as a person. They also invite the interviewer to talk about himself or herself a little bit and focuses the attention on the interviewer instead of on you, which gives you a chance to relax and might help you to feel more at ease when you get into the more formal portion of the interview. Be sure to stay away from sensitive topics, though, such as politics and religion.

Mentor Moment

I wanted to be calm during my interview so, as I waited, I strolled around the lobby. This walk proved to be very informational, though, as I ended up reading plaques, brochures, and other information that I found concerning the company. On one brochure, I found a picture of the vice president who was going to be interviewing me. It had a little biography that stated that he grew up in Colorado. Later, as we walked from the lobby to the interview room, I asked the vice president whether he was a skier since he had grown up in Colorado. He spent the entire time of our walk talking about Colorado, and I could relax and not say a word. I just listened. You never know how you will be able to use the information you find to your advantage.

Carroll from Houston, TX

Take the Lead from the Interviewer

Paying careful attention to how the interview acts toward you can give you some cues to how you should act with the interviewer. For example, if the interviewer introduces himself as "Richard Blake," you should refer to him as "Mr. Blake" until he gives you permission to call him by his first name. If he simply introduces himself to you as "Richard," then you can probably call him by his first name, although you might want to ask for permission first in case the interviewer accidentally forgot to mention his last name. If the interviewer is a woman, then use the term "Ms." and her name to be polite.

You can also take the lead from the interviewer when it comes to the quality, tone, and volume of your voice during the interview. If the interviewer has a soft or quiet voice, you should also use a soft or quiet voice. You should try to match the volume of the interviewer as well.

Listen Carefully

Although you will feel as though you have to do most of the talking during an interview, one important key to a successful interview is to listen carefully. When you ask a question, you should patiently wait for an answer and pay attention to the response. If you do not listen carefully, you might miss important information or you might seem as though you are not interested.

When you are asked a question, you should listen carefully to make sure that you understand what is being asked. If you are not sure that you understand the question, ask the interviewer to repeat it and listen carefully again. Even though silence can sometimes be uncomfortable, you will find it is in your best interest to take the time to make sure you understand each question, clearly answer each question, and then wait for the next question.

Here are some other tips to help you listen carefully, which will help keep you focused on the conversation and remain calm:

- Do not think of what you want to say while the person is talking.
- Do not interrupt or try to talk over the interviewer.
- Pay attention and enjoy the conversation.
- Be courteous and respectful.

Communicate Clearly

Just as important as listening during an interview is communicating clearly. Your potential employer is looking for someone who has communication skills and can use these skills to bring in and retain customers or patients. When it is your turn, you must be able to speak up during an interview to talk about yourself and respond to questions. You cannot just sit and let the interviewer do all the talking because doing so will not give the interviewer a good sense of who you are and why you are the right person for the position.

If you have listened carefully and take time to think about what you want to say before you respond, you should be able to clearly and succinctly answer each question in a professional manner. Some candidates lose a position because, instead of clearly answering an interviewer's question, they ramble to the point of being unfocused, incoherent, and even annoying. Thinking about what you want to say before you respond will ensure that you do not stumble over your answers or say something embarrassing that could damage your reputation.

Another component of speaking clearly is to use correct English with proper grammar. Avoid using slang terms during your interview, as they sound unprofessional and their meaning might not be clear to the interviewer. You should also try to make sure that you speak at a normal conversational speed. Do not let your nervous energy lead you to speak too quickly, but also do not speak too slowly because you could put the interviewer to sleep!

Watch Your Posture

The way in which you carry yourself, also called your posture, is an important part of how you present yourself to a potential employer. Using proper posture, such as sitting up and walking straight, surrounds you with an air of confidence to which the interviewer will respond. Many people do not realize that they slouch when they sit in a chair or lower their shoulders when they walk. These improper postures give the impression of a lack of self-confidence. To make the best impression, you should be aware of how you carry yourself and make every effort to ensure that your posture matches the sense of positivity, self-assurance, professionalism, and belief in yourself that you want to put forth during your interview.

Relax and Be Yourself

One of the best ways to ace an interview is to relax and be yourself. If you are nervous, try not to let it show. During an interview, any gesture that is repeated over and over comes off looking like nervousness. Be aware of your own nervous habits and curb them before your interview.

O N   T R A C K

You are on track if you can list three of your own nervous habits here and can prepare yourself to cope with them if you become nervous before an interview.

1. _____

2. _____

3. _____

Even when you are nervous during an interview, you can take some small steps to look more relaxed. For example, maintaining good eye contact and keeping your hands open in your lap, instead nervously clenching your fists, will give you the appearance of looking natural and relaxed. You should also avoid the following:

- Crossing your arms
- Talking too fast
- Swinging your leg or foot
- Biting your lip
- Clicking your pen
- Tapping your pen on your notebook
- Chewing gum

Being prepared for your interview will also help to give you the added confidence you need to eliminate the appearance of these nervous habits.

Motivational Moment

66 The way I work, the interview never becomes larger than the person being interviewed. 99

Ken Burns, American documentary film producer and director

Being Prepared for Common Interview Questions

The interview process should not be a surprise to you. If you have done your homework, you will know what types of questions to expect to answer during your interview and will have prepared some answers (see Box 9.2). Remember, the process of interviewing is not bigger than your personality, accomplishments, and skills. As long as you prepare for your interview, you will be ready to answer interview questions in a confident, conversational manner.

Now that you know about and understand the different types of questions you might be asked during an interview, you are ready to tackle some specific questions. Listed here are some general and specific questions you might be asked during your interview and how you can prepare for them.

- *What can you tell me about yourself?* Many interviews begin with this question or some form of it (e.g., "How would you describe yourself?" and "Tell me about yourself"). As previously mentioned, you might hear this question as you walk to the interview or it might be the question the interviewer uses to "break the ice" during the interview. In any case, you should be prepared to answer it by deciding what information you first want to reveal to the interviewer. You

BOX 9.2 TYPES OF INTERVIEW QUESTIONS

Listed here are some common types of questions you might be asked in an interview.

- **Getting-to-know-you questions:** These types of questions are sometimes used as an ice breaker to make the interview seem more relaxed. They allow you the opportunity to speak about your strengths and core values.
- **Work history questions:** These types of questions help the interviewer understand the journey you have taken to get where you are now. They can reveal information about transferable skills that you have learned that will help you in your next position.
- **Work style questions:** These questions reveal whether you are able to work well by yourself with little supervision. They might deal with your ability to independently complete a project and meet deadlines.
- **Work interest questions:** These types of questions tell the interviewer whether you like a front office, back office, or emergency department environment. They provide the interviewer with an idea about which area you would excel in if you were hired.
- **Educational diploma and degree questions:** These questions are generally fairly straightforward questions that inquire about your specific degree and certifications. They might also involve more specific details about your education, such as what you learned and practiced in the lab portion of the program and where you did your practicum.
- **Behavioral questions:** These questions are becoming very popular during interviews, and sometimes an entire interview will be composed of just this style of questions. They demonstrate to the interviewer how you would react in different case scenarios, such as those related to patients, coworkers, and supervisors.
- **Personality questions:** These questions are meant to determine whether you have an energetic customer service personality that will enhance the organization.
- **Relocation questions:** Many times, office, hospitals, and clinics share employees and need to know whether you are mobile. The willingness to relocate might or might not be a requirement for being hired.
- **What-can-you-contribute-to-the-organization questions:** These types of questions offer you the opportunity to showcase your unique and individuals skills. To be able to answer them, you need to know your strengths, weaknesses, values, and work habits—in other words, you must know what you have to offer the organization as an employee. Employers will be looking for candidates who are versatile and have a can-do attitude that can benefit the organization in various situations, such as when someone is out sick.
- **Salary questions:** Although questions about salary usually wait until a second interview, you might be asked about your salary expectations or requirements during your first interview—or even during a screening interview. (See the section Determining Your Salary Requirement.)

should use this opening to talk about your core values and strengths. This might also be an opportunity for you to use your Verbal Career Card, which summarizes for people what you want them to know about you (see Chapter 7). Just make sure that if you do use your Verbal Career Card you can relate it in a conversational tone.

- *Can you walk me through your resume?* You should enter your interview assuming that your interviewer has only glanced at your resume. Even if this is not the case, the interviewer might want you to be able to relate a summary of your resume, including your experience and skills. As you summarize your resume, you should focus on your strongest aspects and be sure to explain how your skills are transferrable and can contribute to the organization (see Box 9.3). You can also use this question as an opportunity to show the interviewer your portfolio.

- *How would your instructors describe you?* This question is just another way for the interviewer to find out more about you as a person and a potential coworker. You can use this type of question as another opportunity to showcase additional skills that you have. For example, you might disclose that your instructor would say that you work well with others: this fact illustrates your ability to work as a team player. Or, you might relate that your instructor felt you provided an excellent example for your fellow classmates: this detail illustrates your potential to be a leader or future supervisor.

- *What did you learn while in school? What academic subjects did you like best?* These questions offer you the opportunity to show some enthusiasm by speaking about your favorite subjects, courses, labs, or class projects. If you have not done so already, these questions easily lead into the opportunity for you to show your portfolio with pride. Use the sections of your portfolio that

---

BOX 9.3   CONVERSATIONAL WAYS TO RELATE YOUR TRANSFERABLE SKILLS

- I learned attention to detail when working with paperwork and accounting.
- I learned to help people and enjoyed working with the public.
- I opened the store every weekend, so I learned to be a morning person.
- I am a high-energy person, and I like to be busy.
- I understood the sales process, so I made a good trainer.
- I worked with cash for 7 years, so I can balance accounts.
- I became a manager after a few months, so I am a quick learner and good leader.
- I was a waiter/waitress for 3 years, so I know how to talk to the public and solve customer problems.

include test papers, lab paperwork, and awards to support your response to these questions. However, keep in mind that a potential employer might also like to hear that you enjoy a challenge, so use that opportunity to explain why you also liked the subjects in which you might not have earned perfect scores.

- *What motivates you?* To answer this question, you can look inside yourself and tell the interviewer why you wanted to work in and be a part of the health-care field. You should be prepared to explain what gets you up in the morning, why you want to help people, and how important it is to you to make a difference in someone's life. Be real and honest, and let your sincerity be visible during the interview.

- *What led you to choose the career for which you are preparing?* This question might be another way the interviewer asks about your motivation. It might also be the interviewer's way of gauging what you know about your chosen field. Be prepared to explain from your heart why you choose your given field over all of the other options, including details about the responsibilities of that field. You might also add why you switched career fields if that is true for you.

Mentor Moment

When I was interviewing for jobs as a surgical technologist, I had no trouble talking about what led me to choose that career. My brother was born with a hole between the two chambers of his heart, known as a ventricular septal defect. Even though I was only 8 at the time, I was amazed at how the surgeon helped my brother to live a longer life and I wanted to become a part of making that happen for other people.

Mike from Honolulu, HI

- *What are your strengths? What are your weaknesses?* You have probably heard these broad questions before; however, you need to take time and have short answers prepared for these interview questions. If you do not, you will probably end up rambling and might come off *exhibiting* weaknesses instead of *talking* about them. Your strengths are usually easy to define. You might be an organized person, someone who pays attention to details, or someone who has excellent customer service skills. However, talking about your weaknesses could be a little tougher. You must be willing to admit your weaknesses, but in some cases you can present them in such a way that they do not come off sounding negative (see Box 9.4).

O N   T R A C K

You are on track if you can write down two of your best strengths and two of your weaknesses.

Strengths

1. _____

2. _____

Weaknesses

1. _____

2. _____

BOX 9.4 ADDRESSING POTENTIAL WEAKNESSES
IN A POSITIVE WAY

Weakness	Positive Approach
Overly energetic	I am persistent and hard working.
Overly neat	My attention to detail is outstanding.
Overly social	I get along well with people and have excellent customer service skills.
Quiet	I have always been a quiet person, but I enjoy talking to patients because I know I am helping them.
Slow	Although I was never a really fast worker before, I am fast at filing because I love working with my medical skills.
Unorganized	I use to be unorganized; however, my new medical training has taught me to be organized at the front desk.

- *How do you evaluate success?* You should think carefully before you answer this question and be sure to remember the principles of the health-care field. The health-care field is about making people feel better. In your new position, you will be working in a team environment, and your actions will reflect on the organization for which you work. For example, a potential employer might want to know that you are a team player, that the patients' interests come first for you, that you are there to help the physicians see as many patients as possible, that you value the importance of documenting accurately on patient records, and that you will show respect to patients.

- *What skills do you have that will make you successful?* Hearing this question should prompt you to remember all of the skills listed in the admission brochure for your academic program. These are the same skills from your cover letter and on your resume. You can feel certain that the interview time you have is well spent if you can confidently answer this question by listing the skills you have learned in your health professions program and learned through your previous work experiences.

- *What can you contribute to our organization? Why should we hire you? Why do you want this job? Why do you want to be in this field?* These questions are all similar and yet different. However, if you can answer one of these questions, you should be able to answer all of them. The goal of these questions is the same: for you to show your confidence, reveal your passion for the field, and speak up about your abilities. These questions offer you the opportunity to explain why you will be a better match for the organization than any of the other candidates. When an interviewer asks, "Why should we hire you?" or "Why do you want this job?" he or she is not looking for your personal goals in your new career. Therefore, you should not answer by saying, "I need the money" or "I want to buy a new car." Instead, focus on what you have to offer the organization and why your skills make you the right person for the position. Helping others and making a difference in the world could be the foundation for your answer.

Mentor Moment

I was interviewing with a physician and he asked me why I was the right person for the position. I told him that I would be there with him until he saw his last patient. I guess the physician wanted to know that I would be dependable and he could count on me because I got the job.

Coraline from Papillion, NE

- *What relationship should exist between a supervisor and subordinates?* Organizations in the health-care field, especially in hospitals and clinics, usually have many layers of managers and supervisors. By asking a question such as this, the interviewer might be looking for you to acknowledge your ability to show respect, seek help with a problem, and follow the chain of command. Be sure that you do not give an answer that sounds immature. For example, instead of responding "I like to be friends with everyone I work with," you might consider a more appropriate answer, such as, "I believe in following the chain of command and respecting all leadership positions in an office."

- *How would you handle office politics?* Most people are aware that office politics can be found in every workplace and are almost impossible to avoid. However, your employer will want to hear that you have a strong commitment to doing your job and completing your assigned tasks despite these politics. When you answer this question, reassure the interviewer that you plan to be respectful of all of your coworkers by remaining focused on your responsibilities.

- *How often were you absent from school?* As mentioned in previous chapters, your dedication to school, as evidenced by your class attendance, might be questioned during your interview. If you have an excellent attendance record, you can show the interviewer the attendance awards in your portfolio and be proud of your response. If, on the other hand, your attendance was not perfect, try instead to focus on your strengths. For example, if you missed some classes but you were still able to do well and get good grades, you should focus on that. You can point out that your attendance was good (rather than excellent); however, you had a high grade point average. Just be sure that you do not come off sounding cocky. And do not mislead the interviewer or misrepresent yourself by avoiding the question or offering false information. You are better off being honest and then focusing on your strengths. If your attendance was poor due to a personal or family emergency, a job change, public transportation, military orders, or some other valid reason, you should briefly explain the reason and then remind the interviewer that, despite that hardship, you were still able to graduate with a passing average. Remember to be honest about any hurdles that challenged you during your program but then quickly change the subject to talk about what skills you have and how you can contribute to the organization.

Motivational Moment

❝ You can't build a reputation on what you're going to do. ❞

Henry Ford, founder of Ford Motor Company

- *How do you plan your time?* or *Can you meet deadlines?* The health-care field is filled with timelines, deadlines, and target dates. An employer will want to know that you are an organized person who can manage his or her time well and understands the importance of time management. Your experience with juggling school, work, a personal life, and possibly a family is a perfect example. Highlight your organizational skills and be proud that you have a schedule or system that works for you. Alternatively, think about a specific time when you had to meet an important deadline and the lengths to which you went to accomplish that goal. Take this opportunity to highlight not only your persistence in getting a job done but also to explain your attention to detail and your dedication to reaching department goals.

O N   T R A C K

You are on track if you can describe two occasions where you needed to meet important deadlines and you did!

1. _____

_____

_____

2. _____

_____

_____

_____

- *How would you describe your ideal position?* Be careful about how you address this question. You should be sure to list some of the qualities of the position for which you are applying, but you should also include a few qualities found in an upper-level position. Doing so indicates your desire to fit into and learn from the current position in order to advance yourself and your qualifications to a higher-level position in a few years.
- *Who or what has been a significant influence on your life?* By asking this question, the interviewer hopes to learn about your core values. You might choose to talk about how your mentor, your study buddy or study group, an instructor, your spouse, a family member, a previous supervisor or coworker, or a best friend has influenced you in a positive way. Alternatively, you could choose to reveal a negative influence on your life that pushed you in a positive direction. No matter what influence you choose, you should take this opportunity to reveal more personal information about how and why you developed your current goals and values, such as how you became dedicated to the health-care field.

- *Do you consider yourself to be a self-starter?* Unlike many of the other questions you will be asked during your interview, this question has only one right answer: "Yes!" Your employer will be paying you to come to work to do a task, complete a project, solve a problem, or perform whatever duties are described in your position. Therefore, that employer will want to know that you are ready to do that responsibility and to do it with a smile. No employer wants to hire someone who needs to be pushed to do his or her work.

- *Do you think you are a little too old/too young for this job?* Although employers are not legally allowed to ask questions about your age, some might employ a question such as this one as a roundabout way of gauging this information. If you are asked this question or one like it, do not agree with this notion. Remember that age brings experience and transferable skills, whereas youth brings vitality and a path to create longevity in an organization. If you are tempted to agree with this idea even a little bit, then you must revisit your positive thinking because your uncertainty is more likely to be about your own self-doubts than it is about your abilities. Remind yourself of the energy and enthusiasm you felt for the health-care field when you first started your program.

- *What kind of people do you prefer to work with? What kind of environment do you prefer to work in?* Although these questions ask about your preferences, you should keep in mind that your answers will reveal information about yourself and your expectations of your workplace and coworkers. Answer professionally. Do not try to create ideal situations or expectations that cannot be met. When describing the type of people you prefer to work with, be realistic in acknowledging that each person has his or her own strengths and weaknesses. Focus your response on the kinds of skills that a potential employer would find desirable rather than focusing on personality traits with which you identify. Because most people describe themselves as the types of coworkers they most like to work with, an interviewer will carefully listen to the qualities you describe to learn something about you.

- *What are your career goals?* This question can be a little tricky, so think before you answer. You should be careful not to give the impression that you will be looking to leave the position or be expecting a promotion in a very short time frame. You need to balance your intentions to gain longevity in the position you are currently seeking with advancement in the field. An employer does not want to take the time to hire and train someone who will begin looking for another position right away somewhere else in the field. Although your long-term goals probably do include advancing into higher-level positions, at this point in your career you should focus on getting the entry-level position that will teach you the skills you need to advance. Reassure the employer that your goals include finding a position where you can learn new skills while building a long-term relationship with an organization that cares about people and where you will be happy.

- *What causes you to lose your temper? Do you have any pet peeves? Can you tell me about a time when you . . . ?* Questions such as these are sometimes known as behavioral questions. They can take all forms, but their general goal is to see how you react to challenging situations or scenarios. In addition to listening to your response, the interviewer will observe how you react to the question and how spontaneous you are in your answer. When answering a behavioral question, you should be sure to think through your answer before speaking, remain calm, and keep your answer short. The interviewer will not be looking to hear about personal issues that can set you off. Instead, try to think of a work-related situation in which people unfairly take advantage of their coworkers, such as taking too long for lunch or expecting others to cover for them.
- *Can you take instructions without getting upset?* Although this question might look like it is loaded, the interviewer will want to hear in your response that you are able to take orders and respect the chain of command. If you are not in charge, you will always be taking orders and instructions, and you must show the interviewer that you are okay with this role.
- *What outside responsibilities do you have?* Employers might ask a question such as this one to gauge your full level of responsibility as well as to determine your well-roundedness. You could answer this question by discussing your involvement in hobbies, church activities, and fitness activities, as well as some family activities.
- *Can we call your references?* As long as you have done your part by letting your references know that you are looking for a position and getting their permission to have a potential employer contact them, then you should feel confident in answering this question with "Yes, please feel free to call them."
- *Do you have any questions for me?* Interviewers commonly close out an interview by asking if you have any questions for them. If you are not prepared for this question, you might draw a blank, and your lack of questions could be misconstrued as a lack of interest in the organization or the position. Before you leave for an interview, you should prepare three to five general questions that you can ask the interviewer (see the section Being Ready to Ask Questions later in this chapter for suggestions on the types of questions you can ask).

Being prepared to answer these interview questions does not mean that you need to memorize your responses. Rather, it means being aware of some of the common questions you will encounter and being able to quickly, clearly, and confidently respond to them. No matter what questions you are asked during your interview, you should be sure to answer them with confidence. This is the time for you to show off your skills and "toot your own horn"—no matter how uncomfortable it feels. Know your strengths and accomplishments and commit them to memory so that you can discuss them in a conversational manner during your interview.

Motivational Moment

66 I want to live every moment totally and intensely. Even when I'm giving an interview or talking to people, that's all that I'm thinking about. 99

Omar Sharif, actor

Being Ready to Ask Questions

As previously mentioned, the interviewer might conclude your interview by asking whether you have any questions. You should come to the interview armed with three to five questions about the organization or the position. You can also close your interview by asking about when the position will be filled. The important thing to remember is that, at this point in the interview, the focus shifts to you, and you want to make a good impression by being ready to ask questions that show your interest in the position and the organization.

Here is a list of possible questions for you to consider asking the interviewer:

- What are the major responsibilities of the position?
- What are the major challenges for the department?
- What are the ideal qualities of the candidate for this position?
- How do my qualifications meet your needs?
- How are employees evaluated and promoted?
- What would be the career path?
- Who would I report to in the position?
- Do you offer any training or workshops?
- What types of equipment do you have?
- Am I one of the top candidates?
- When do you plan to make a decision?
- When can I expect to hear from you?
- Will you call me either way on the position?
- Would you mind if I call you on Monday to follow up?
- Is there any other information you need from me?
- Could I be considered for other positions?

Just be sure that you do not ask any questions that cover information you have already discussed in your interview because it might seem like you were not paying attention. You can, however, ask questions that follow up on information that you have already discussed. These types of questions will do the opposite; they will show that you were listening carefully during the interview and processing the information you heard.

O N   T R A C K

You are on track if you can choose three interview questions that you would feel comfortable asking at your next interview. (Note that these can come from the list or they can be your own!)

1. _____

2. _____

3. _____

Motivational Moment

66 Successful people ask better questions, and as a result, they get better answers. 99

Anthony "Tony" Robbins, American self-help author
and motivational speaker

Ending on a Good Note

As your interview comes to a close, make sure that the interviewer knows how to reach you. You might also consider asking about when a decision will be made about the position or whether the interviewer minds if you follow up in a couple of days. Then make eye contact, thank the interviewer for the opportunity, and exit with a positive and firm handshake. Do not be afraid to leave your interview with these words: "Thank you for your time and consideration. I want you to know that I would really like to work for your organization and assist you in reaching your goals."

Mentor Moment

When I went for my interview, I was nervous about what to say, but I thought my interview went really well. At the end, I asked the physician if I could follow up in a few days. My heart sank when he told me not to bother, but then he smiled and said I was the top candidate and I would be called tomorrow. What a nice surprise!

Caitlin from Tacoma, WA

Sending a Thank You Note or Letter

After your interview, you should also send a thank you note or letter to each person with whom you interview, thanking them again for their time and consideration. Even if you feel the interview did not go well, you should send a thank you and keep in mind that you might be considered later for another position.

You should keep your thank you note or letter short, with just a few sentences. (See Figs. 9.1 and 9.2.) Here are some sentences that you may include:

- It was a pleasure to meet you.
- I appreciate your courtesy in granting me an interview.
- I appreciate being given the opportunity to discuss my qualifications with you.
- I feel my training and experience meet your expectations for the position.
- I would like to assist you in reaching your goals.
- I am interested in working with you and look forward to becoming a part of your staff.
- Thank you again for your time and consideration.
- I look forward to hearing from you.

Whether you send a note or a letter depends on who interviews you and the position for which you are interviewing. You should send a letter, which is more formal, to an HR director or vice president. You can send a handwritten note or letter to an office manager or supervisor. The higher the position is for which you are applying, the more you should lean toward sending a thank you letter rather than a note. (See Box 9.5.)

Mentor Moment

During my interviewing process, I found a position that I really wanted and I thought was perfect for me. I was so happy to be brought back for a second interview, but I was even happier—and maybe even a little surprised—to see the thank you card I had sent after my first interview in my folder. I guess it really did make a difference!

Barbara from Des Moines, IA

Name
Address
City, State, Zip
Phone (home and cell on separate lines if possible)
E-mail address

Date

Format 1
Organization's name
Address
City, State, Zip
Attn: Contact's name (person to whom you are sending the resume)

Format 2
Contact's name (person to whom you are sending the resume)
Title
Company
Address
City, State, Zip

Salutation (e.g., "Dear XXX," "Dear Employer," "Manager:" or "Ms./Mr.")

First Paragraph: Introduction, reminder of position of interest and date or day of interview, appreciation of consideration.

Second Paragraph: Acknowledgement of qualifications for the position.

Summary Paragraph: Expression of continued interest and thank you.

Closing (e.g., "Sincerely," "Respectfully," or "Best Regards")

Signature (in blue ink if possible)

Your typed name

FIGURE 9.1 Sample format for thank you letter.

Student Genius
1234 Career Path
Future, USA 12345
Home: (123) 456-7890
Cell: (098) 765-4321
studentgenius@email.com

September 12, 2011

Mrs. Teri M. Erhardt, Office Manager
ABC Family Practice
1234 Health Professions Ave.
Anyplace, USA 12345

Dear Mrs. Erhardt:

Thank you again for meeting with me regarding your medical assistant position. I appreciate your consideration and genuinely enjoyed meeting you and the members of your staff.

The interview convinced me even more of how much I want to be in the medical field. Because my training has prepared me for dealing with patient care both in person and over the phone, I feel that I would be able to assist you in reaching your goals.

Once again, it was a pleasure to meet you! I look forward to hearing from you regarding your decision.

Respectfully,

Student Genius

Student Genius

FIGURE 9.2 Thank you letter example.

BOX 9.5 AVOIDING INTERVIEW BLUNDERS

Here are some common interview blunders and how you can avoid them.

1. It is a blunder to apply for a position for which you are not qualified just because you want it. Make sure that you meet 75% of the qualifications for a position before applying.
2. It is a blunder not to prepare for the interview. Make sure you understand what the employer is looking for and do your homework on the organization.
3. It is a blunder not to understand the information that is given or asked by an interviewer. Listen carefully and make sure that you understand what is being said before you respond.
4. It is a blunder to talk too much or too fast during an interview. It is also a blunder not to talk enough. Make sure to communicate in a conversational tone.
5. It is a blunder not to look professional. Be sure to look clean and dress nicely when interviewing for a position in the health professions field.
6. It is a blunder to be late for an interview. Plan to arrive early and make sure that you know where you are going and how long it will take you to get there.
7. It is a blunder to chew gum during an interview.
8. It is a blunder to have poor eye contact and a weak handshake. Look the interviewer in the eye and offer a firm, confident handshake.
9. It is a blunder to show a lack of enthusiasm. Get excited about the interview and let that excitement show.
10. It is a blunder to bad-mouth past employers or coworkers. Make sure to make your best impression by focusing on yourself during the interview.
11. It is a blunder to be ill-mannered and not show appreciation for the interviewer's time. Be courteous at all times during the interview.
12. It is a blunder not to ask the interviewer questions toward the end of the interview. Be ready to ask three to five questions about information that was not already covered during the interview.
13. It is a blunder to turn in a poorly written application. Take your time with the application and be neat.
14. It is a blunder not to send a thank you note or letter. Follow up on the opportunity to remind the interviewer of your interest and thank the interviewer for his or her time.
15. It is a blunder to be defeated after your interview. Believe in your skills. Do not give up! Learn from your interview.

Evaluating the Interview

After an interview, you will probably feel nervous, wondering how well you did and speculating on whether you will be called back for a second interview or, even better, made an offer (see Box 9.6). In some cases, you will have a good

BOX 9.6   WHEN TO EXPECT AN OFFER

After an interview, you will probably be wondering when you should expect to hear back about the position. How long it takes to receive an offer really depends on a number of factors, including the following:

- The position
- The organization, including its hiring practices, budget, and pay schedule
- The number of candidates who must be interviewed
- Scheduled orientation and training dates

Generally, you can expect to hear back about the position within 10 working days.

Although health-care organizations hire all year round, on any day of the week, some trends do emerge in health professions hiring. Depending on when you interview, you might receive an offer on the following schedule:

- Before the holidays, so you are trained and ready for the new year
- After the holidays, so you can begin working under the new year's budget
- At the end of the first quarter, after the year-end reports
- In April, to meet accreditation standards and ensure you receive training before July
- In May or June, so that the organization ensures that they have extra help to cover the vacation time of other employees
- In July or August, so the organization can get ready for the rush of students going back to school
- In September, so that you can be trained and ready for the flu season
- In October, so that you will be counted as an employee during the current year to justify the new budget proposal in November.

sense of whether the interview went well, but in others, you might feel clueless. You might be wondering how well you answered the interviewer's questions, what the interviewer thought of you, and whether you made a good impression. To get a better sense of how you did during your interview, you should think back over the interview and evaluate how it went. As part of this process, you should make a note of any mistakes you made and questions you were unprepared for so that you can improve on these areas in your next interview—if a "next interview" is even necessary.

Knowing Whether the Interview Went Well

Knowing whether an interview went well can be difficult. You are relying on your own memory to help you make this judgment. However, many people have a tendency to be their own worst critic; therefore, you might harshly judge how well you performed during your interview. On the other hand, some people come out of an interview feeling so great that they are in shock when they are not made an offer; if this happens to you, then you might not be able to go back and clearly analyze what went wrong during the interview or why you did not get the offer. Keep this fact in mind: you will probably never be as good as you think you are, but you will probably never be as bad as you think you are either. Reality generally lies someplace in between.

As you try to evaluate an interview, you can sometimes find certain indications that it went well.

- The interviewer gives you a clear timeline for when a decision should be made. For example, the interviewer says, "Someone should be contacting you by next Friday to let you know our decision."
- The interviewer asks about your timeline, other interviews you have scheduled, or your availability to start training. For example, the interviewer asks, "So, have you had many other interviews?" or "How soon would you be available to start training?"
- The interviewer tries to "sell" the position or company to you by talking about such details as the organization's benefits. For example, the interviewer says, "Our medical benefits are great, and they start in only 3 months."
- The interviewer spends a lot of time answering your questions. Your questions are answered with patience and at length to make sure you understand the information. You do not feel like you are being rushed out of the office for the next interview.
- The interview runs over the allotted time. For example, when you schedule your interview, you might be told to plan to be there for half an hour, and you spend an hour there on interview day.
- After your interview, the interviewer shows you around the workplace or introduces you to other people in the organization, such as the department manager overseeing the new position.
- The employer contacts your references or the interviewer tells you that he or she will be checking your references.

Learning from Your Mistakes

Even if an interview does not go well or you are not offered a position, you can make every interview count by learning from the mistakes you make. Ask yourself these questions about your interview experience:

- Was I prepared to answer all of the questions I was asked?
- Was I able to speak confidently about my qualifications and experience?

- Did I show I had outstanding medical skills?
- Did I show the employer that I have transferrable skills?
- Did I greet everyone I met with good eye contact and a firm handshake?
- Did I listen carefully to each question?
- Did I wait until the interviewer finished speaking before answering each question?
- Did I lose my thoughts when I was speaking?
- Did I say "um" too many times?
- Did I control my nervous impulses?
- Did I laugh at an inappropriate time?
- Did I smile and let my real personality show.
- Did I feel really uncomfortable?
- Did I ask the interviewer three questions about topics that we had not previously discussed?
- Did I offer a confident handshake and eye contact when I left?
- Did I ask when I would hear about a decision?
- Did I send a thank you note or letter?

Thinking carefully about each of these questions and answering them honestly will help you to identify possible areas for improvement in your interview skills. You might even want to jot down some notes right after the interview concludes so that you remember how the interview went, what went well, and what might have not gone so well. The more interviews you complete, the more your confidence will grow and the better you will become at interviewing.

You should try not to get upset or discouraged if an interview does not go well or you do not get an offer. In some cases, you might not get an offer, but the reason has nothing to do with how well your interview went. Remember that the employer is looking for the *right fit* for the position, not just the best-qualified person. You might do an excellent job during the interview of highlighting your skills, qualifications, and personality, but you just might not be the right fit for the position. In that case, you are sure to get an offer at another organization where the fit is better for both you and the employer. And remember, if you do make mistakes during your interview, turn those mistakes into opportunities to learn how to do better in your next interview. You might want to consult with the career services department at your school to get some advice on how you can improve.

Motivational Moment

66 Making mistakes simply means you are learning faster. 99

Weston H. Agor, American author and professor
of public administration

One way to learn from your mistakes *before* you make them during an actual interview is to complete some mock interviews. Have a friend, mentor, family member, classmate, study buddy, or someone from your school's career services or placement department pretend to interview you for a position. You can use the sample questions provided earlier in this chapter to practice. A mock interview should be as real as possible to simulate the actual interview process. You need to start from the beginning:

- Come prepared. Bring your portfolio, resume, and references as well as your notebook and pens.
- Dress for success and be professional. Greet the receptionist with a smile, friendly attitude, and respect. Greet the interviewer with good eye contact and a firm handshake.
- Stay relaxed and confident during the interview. Keep your entire body relaxed, but maintain good posture.
- Be ready for the first question, which will open the door for you to talk about yourself and experience.
- Be ready to answer other common questions.
- Be sure to close with a handshake and a thank you. If appropriate, ask when you can expect a decision.

By taking the mock interview seriously, you allow yourself the opportunity to make mistakes and learn from them before they cost you a position. If you are practicing with a classmate, you can each take turns being the interviewer and the interviewee. Doing so will give you an opportunity to learn from someone else's mistakes as well. The more you practice answering interview questions, the more comfortable you will be when it comes time for an actual interview.

Mentor Moment

When I was interviewing, I thought I would find a position right away because I was older than most other students, I had a lot of experience, and was very good at my skills. However, after more than eight interviews and no position, I found out through a mock interview with my director of education that my problem was that I spoke with a "chip on my shoulder." I answered questions with an angry tone, but my ears did not hear it. Once I learned what mistake I was making and knew what to improve, I had no problems landing a position.

Larry from Seattle, WA

Keeping a Positive Outlook

Interviewing can be tough. After an interview that went well, you might be on edge for a week or more, just waiting for the call to come in with the position offer. Unfortunately, the call sometimes never comes. It is easy to become discouraged and disappointed, especially if you do not get one or more positions that you really want. However, maintaining a positive outlook helps to keep your confidence high, which will come across during your interviews. Confidence is one of the first keys to receiving an offer.

You should also remember that the reason you might not receive an offer does not always have to do with you or your interview skills. Sometimes, organizations must impose a hiring freeze due to budget crunches or major restructuring, the person you interview with loses or resigns from his or her job during the hiring process or encounters a personal crisis, the department moves to another location, or something else happens that you do not know about. The point is, no matter what happens during your career search, you should remember not to get discouraged. Instead, be persistent in pursuing your goals. You must keep your momentum strong, keep your employment search moving ahead, and keep interviewing until you attain career employment success.

Motivational Moment

66 The only real mistake is the one from which we learn nothing. 99

John Powell, British film score composer

Always apply for more than one position at a time, and keep your momentum strong. You must keep your employment search moving ahead and keep interviewing until you win the interview "game."

Mentor Moment

During my career search, I found a position at an organization where I really wanted to work. I had an interview, but I did not get the job. Afterward, I called back every month to see if another position had opened up. After seven follow-up calls, I was finally called back and received a position. The interviewer told me he liked my determination and wanted people who really wanted to work at his office. Persistence pays off!

Patty from Marietta, GA

Success Journal

1. Describe why you want to enter the health-care field, but do so in a way that will appeal to an interviewer. Do not address personal goals, such as the desire to have more money or buy a new car.

_____

_____

_____

_____

_____

_____

2. Describe a past work experience that assisted you in becoming a better employee and explain why.

_____

_____

_____

_____

_____

_____

3. Give one example that illustrates your trustworthiness, honesty, and integrity.

_____

_____

_____

_____

_____

_____

4. Provide an example of a time when you faced an extremely stressful situation, including how you handled that situation successfully.

_____

_____

_____

_____

_____

_____

_____

5. Describe your ideal position.

_____

_____

_____

_____

_____

Professional Appearance

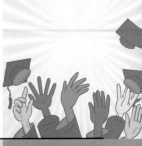

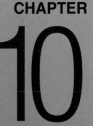

Learning Outcomes

After reading this chapter, the student will be able to:

1. Understand that a professional appearance begins with hygiene.
2. Explain how to "dress for success."
3. Select a basic interview outfit.

Understanding the Importance of a Professional Appearance

In today's society, you are surrounded by advertising that tells you how to dress, look beautiful, and be more masculine or feminine by using certain products. You probably see advertisements on television, buses, and billboards or in newspapers and magazines every day. New products are always coming on the market to make you look better or even younger: toothpastes that whiten your teeth, razors that give you the closest possible shave, lotions that defy the aging process. Looking your best is big business, and the manufacturers of these products want you to look your best so that they can get your dollars.

When the time comes for you to network, interview, or go to work at your practicum or new career, you must be ready by looking professional. You want to make sure that your new professional attitude is on a body that is groomed for success. Dressing for success in the health-care field is different from dressing for success in a sales or business position. Although wardrobe is one component of dressing for success, your professional appearance will begin with some basic hygiene practices. The focus in the health-care field is on the word "healthy." What you put on your body will be noticed only if it is on a healthy-looking body. Dressing for success is not about using the best product or most expensive product; it is about finding a routine for your daily hygiene practices and then wearing clothes and accessories that make you look professional and feel confident. When you look your best, you are more likely to approach every day feeling confident that you can "conquer the world."

Your appearance also helps you to make a good first impression, whether you are attending class, meeting new people, interviewing for a position, or caring for patients. In these scenarios, how you look can sometimes be as important as what you say:

- Your appearance should be an external reflection of your core values, skills, and strengths.
- Your healthy body should be a sign of your positive attitude and self-confidence.
- Your clothing and accessories should display the professionalism you have learned through your training and education.

Looking good will make you feel good, and looking professional will help you to embrace and be embraced by your new career.

O N   T R A C K

You are on track if you can name your most positive physical feature (e.g., eyes, cheekbones, hair, lips, figure, muscles, beard, eyelashes, smile).

Looking Healthy

When you think about what it takes to dress for success, you might be inclined to go purchase a nice new outfit, shoes, or a tie. However, dressing for success starts with looking healthy from head to toe. As a health professional, you must appear clean at all times, no matter your age or gender. Your new career will require you to deal with people up close and personal, so you must be able to show along every step of your journey to that new career that you have what it takes to look healthy and professional. Your commitment to looking healthy will reflect your commitment to your new career and will signify your respect for others and your field.

Looking healthy starts with making sure that you are including some basic hygiene steps into your daily routine. If you did not already have a daily routine, you have probably developed one since you entered your educational program. Your morning routine might include getting out of bed, getting dressed, eating breakfast, and going off to class or work. Your evening routine might include making dinner, studying, and, hopefully, finding a little time for yourself. Most people's daily routine also includes some time for getting ready to look their best. Each person develops his or her own personal hygiene routine, and that routine can vary based on the person's culture, customs, and personal circumstances. In addition, sometimes a person's routine does not go as planned due to time constraints, lack of motivation, or simple laziness. However, each health professional must make time in his or her daily routine for basic hygiene in order to look and feel as confident as possible at all times.

This section presents some important components of and suggestions for helping you to look your best. If some of the suggestions that follow are new to you, try to find a way to work each one into your daily routine. If the concepts that follow are already part of your regular routine, then use the following section as a checklist to confirm that you are doing everything you can to become professionally successful.

Hygiene Basics

Following basic hygiene practices ensures that you look clean and healthy every day. In the health-care field, you are required to perform tasks such as setting up equipment and performing procedures that will put you in the "personal space" of your patients. Because you will be working so closely with people, they will notice if you are not clean or if you have a bad odor. Bad odors can be offensive. Therefore, your hygiene practices should begin with getting a daily shower or bath. A daily shower or bath will wash dead skin cells from your body and help to keep you looking and smelling clean and fresh. In the health-care field, you are likely to come in contact with many people who are sick. You should use an antibacterial soap when you bathe to ensure that you are washing away your germs as well as the germs of all of the people with whom you come in contact during the day.

Mentor Moment

Studying in the medical field made me really aware of the prevalence of germs and the importance of keeping conditions sanitary. So when I started as a medical assistant, I developed a routine where I would arrive home, slip into a robe in the garage, and then immediately head to the shower and wash away any germs that I had collected during my day. I didn't want to bring any of those germs and bacteria from my day into my home, so this routine helped put my mind at ease.

Tony from Bar Harbor, ME

Here are some other basic hygiene practices you probably know are important and can follow to help your appearance and keep you healthy:

- Use an unscented or lightly scented moisturizing lotion on your skin after you bathe. Doing so helps to keep your skin supple and soft and prevents cracks from forming, where bacteria can enter your skin.
- Wash your hands with an antibacterial soap several times a day.
- Use a cotton-tipped swab or cotton ball to clean away hidden dirt from the outsides of your ears, a small detail that is often overlooked.
- Use deodorant or antiperspirant under your arms to prevent armpit odors. Try different brands until you find a deodorant that works for you. You are likely to be working closely with, and possibly reaching over, people all day, and using deodorant or antiperspirant can help ensure that you do not expose anyone to unsightly sweat stains or offensive odors.
- Don't wear strongly scented perfumes, colognes, or lotions because these products can irritate or make breathing hard for those with allergies, nasal congestion, or sensitive noses.

- Combat foot odor by using insoles, powders, or sprays designed to eliminate or reduce foot odor and wetness. Because you are on your feet all day, by the end of the day your feet might give off an unpleasant odor.
- Alternate between two different pairs of shoes during the week to give each pair a chance to air out between wearing.

Facial Care

Your face says a lot about you. It helps you to greet people, show your concern, and make your first impression. Therefore, facial grooming is an important component of your professional appearance. Depending on whether you are a man or a woman, your facial grooming routine may include cleaning your skin, moisturizing your skin, applying makeup, removing facial hair, and other steps. No matter what steps you take, the goal should be to ensure that your facial care routine helps you to put your best face forward by outwardly expressing your inner radiance and self-confidence.

Skin Care

Your skin is your face's canvas. To start, you should ensure that it has a clean and healthy glow by following a skin care regime. This regimen may range from simple and easy to complex and product laden, depending on your gender, the type of skin you have, and your preferences.

The skin care market is flooded with products that are designed to help you be clean, healthy, and young looking. Although many of these products are marketed toward women, more and more products designed specifically for and advertised to men enter the market because many men are also concerned about their appearance. When it comes to looking professional, the important thing to remember is that you need not spend a lot of money on expensive products to look good. A healthy professional appearance requires only that you follow a skin care regimen that keeps your face looking clean and vibrant. And remember that price does not always mean quality. Many different products are available on the market, and you are sure to be able to find the product that you need in a price range that fits your budget.

Good skin care starts with removing the dead skin cells and oil from your face and cleaning and preventing clogged pores. You can exfoliate dead cells from your skin using a facial scrub, cleanser, or soap. Following with an astringent can help to shrink your pores and give you smoother looking skin. After you have cleaned your skin, you might want to apply a moisturizer to condition it. Moisturizers vary greatly; some contain special ingredients such vitamin E and aloe, whereas others include the convenience of built-in sunblock. Some cleansers also have moisturizers built in. Be sure to read product labels and choose products that are designed for your type of skin (e.g., dry, normal, oily, or combination skin) and have the properties you need (e.g., blemish control, deep cleaning, moisturizing, hypoallergenic). If you have problem skin, you might want to consider consulting a dermatologist or using an over-the-counter medicated skin care product.

Optimally, you should clean your face twice per day. Think of this practice as washing away bacteria from your face and hands if you work with patients all day. An easy way to work skin care into your daily routine is by making it a part of your shower and nighttime rituals.

Motivational Moment

66 The expression a woman wears on her face is far more important than the clothes she wears on her back. 99

Dale Carnegie, American lecturer and author

Makeup

Once you have your clean and healthy canvas, you must decide what to do with it. For more women than men, that means deciding whether to wear makeup and, if so, what type of makeup and how much to apply. Some people find that a good skin care regimen is all they need to have a healthy appearance, whereas others feel better when they can use makeup to complement their features or hide their flaws. As with the other elements of your appearance, your goal for makeup should be to give you a healthy and attractive professional look.

Makeup is a complicated subject. Entire television programs, magazines, and websites are devoted to explaining how to use makeup to look natural, beautiful, and glamorous. Here is a summary of some different types of makeup products that are available and tips for using them that can contribute to your professional appearance:

- **Foundation:** Foundation is used as the base for makeup. Available in many different forms (e.g., liquid, cream, mousse, powder), foundation can help to even out uneven skin tones, minimize the effects of aging, control shine, and improve the condition of your skin. You should apply foundation lightly and softly to look more natural; remember that a little goes a long way. By using a sponge, brush, or other appropriate applicator, you can avoid the heavy foundation look. You should also choose a foundation color that blends with your natural skin tone. To select the right foundation color, match the color of the makeup to the skin on your wrist or neck.
- **Concealer:** Concealer is used to cover up blemishes, such as pimples and discolorations. You should select a concealer that blends with your skin tone and

apply only the amount necessary to cover the blemish. Use a little darker color to tone down redness and a lighter color to hide dark shadows.

- **Mascara:** Mascara can help to bring out your eyes by adding volume to, lengthening, curling, and defining your eyelashes. It can be a useful tool, especially if you have light hair or skin. You should apply mascara to your lashes lightly and softly, starting with a single stroke. If you are used to wearing mascara, you might want to apply a second coat; however, be careful not to apply too much. You should not feel the mascara on your eyes. Mascara should leave your lashes feeling soft and thick, not clumped and brittle. To get the most of your mascara, you may want to first curl your lashes with an eyelash curler. Sometimes, just a little mascara and blush is all you need to accent your features and create a healthy glow.
- **Eye liner:** Another way to make your eyes pop, especially if you do not have full eyelashes, is to use eye liner. Eye liner can help to define your eyes and make your eyes look bigger without the use of mascara by outlining them in a soft color. You should apply eyeliner smoothly and evenly in a very thin line at the base of your eyelash line. You should choose a color that is right for you, depending on your eye color.
- **Eye shadow:** Eye shadow can also be used to make your eyes stand out. When you are working, networking, or interviewing, you should choose soft, pale colors and apply your eye shadow lightly. Save your dark, frosted, and metallic colors for going out on the weekends. (See Box 10.1 for more information on how to make your eye makeup look natural.)
- **Blush:** Blush can help to give the cheeks a soft, radiant dab of color. You should apply blush to the apples of your cheeks (the round puffy parts of your cheeks that stand out when you smile) lightly and softly, starting with a single stroke. Most skin tones are enhanced by blush shades of light peach or pink.

BOX 10.1   MATCHING NATURAL EYE COLORS

To obtain a natural look, the makeup colors you choose for your eyes will depend on your natural eye color. Use this chart as a guide.

Eye Color	Mascara	Eyeliner
Blue	Light brown	Light brown
		Light gray
Brown	Brown	Brown
	Black	Plum
Green or hazel	Light brown	Light brown
		Dark plum

- **Lipstick:** Like most other makeup, lipstick can be appropriate as long as you choose a color that looks natural and enhances your look. Soft colors generally work best.

Although makeup trends change, the overall goal of your makeup look when you are interviewing, networking, or working in the health-care field should be a natural, professional look. If you feel that you need help creating this look, you might want to get a professional makeover. Getting a makeover can be easy. Many cosmetic counters in department stores perform free makeovers, or you can throw a makeover party at your home (e.g., Mary Kay, Avon). The people performing these makeovers will aim to sell you their products; however, you need not feel obligated to buy something. Take what you learn from your makeover and then apply it in your own way at home with your own products. You might also be able to get a free makeover at a local beauty school. Just make sure that you tell the person doing your makeover that you want a natural look.

See Box 10.2 for makeup mistakes to avoid.

Motivational Moment

66 I love the confidence that makeup gives me. 99

Tyra Banks, model and talk-show host

Facial Hair

Another component of facial care is grooming of facial hair. For men, that means completely removing facial hair using a straight-edged razor or using an

---

BOX 10.2   MAKEUP MISTAKES TO AVOID

- Avoid overapplying foundation as it will make your face appear caked with makeup.
- Avoid applying too much mascara, so that your eyelashes do not clump together.
- Avoid black, blue, and green eyeliners, as these colors are more appropriate for going out on a Saturday night.
- Avoid applying too much blush because doing so can make you look like a clown or make you look like you are coming from the gym.
- Avoid using old makeup, as it can irritate your skin and eyes.
- Avoid applying a darker foundation to create a tan because this gives you the appearance of wearing a mask.

electric razor to keep facial hair trimmed to a nice, clean look. Most men find it necessary to shave every day. Using a shaving cream, particularly one with a moisturizer, can help to minimize irritation and redness when you shave and can give you a closer, longer-lasting, smooth shave that helps to keep the "5 o'clock shadow" at bay. As with most skin care products, you might need to try several different razors and shaving creams before you find the one that is right for you. Some organizations have specific policies regarding facial hair, sideburns, and beards, so be sure to find out what rules apply to you.

Sometimes men also need to be aware of and trim nose and ear hair. In some cases, barbers will include these areas with a haircut.

Facial hair can also be a problem for women, especially those with thick, dark, or coarse hair. Facial hair grooming for women might involve shaping and defining the eyebrows. A set of tweezers and a mirror are the only tools required for this task, which might be the single step you need to make your eyes the real focus of your face. You can use the tweezers to pluck hairs that fall outside of the natural line of your brows. Examining your eyes in natural sunlight can help you to best see your natural brow line. You might also find unwanted facial hairs around your lip area or on your chin that can be removed using tweezers.

Alternatively, if you are up to it and your budget can afford it, you can have your facial hair waxed and shaped professionally once per month or every other month. If you choose to go this route, you can stretch your time between visits by removing stray hairs that pop up between your waxings. Professional facial waxing typically costs between $8 and $15. You might also be able to find a local beauty school where you can get it done for little to no cost.

Over-the-counter waxing products are also available, but you want to be careful using such products as they can sometimes cause hair root eruptions that lead to scarring. In some cases, over-the-counter bleaching creams or makeup can also be used to hide or soften the color of facial hair. Your local drug store will have several bleaching creams and upper lip hair removal products to fit your budget.

O N   T R A C K

You are on track if you can make a list of the skin care products and makeup you currently use or would like to try.

Skin care and shaving products

_____

_____

_____

(box continues on page 320)

Makeup (if applicable)

_____

_____

_____

Smile and Mouth Care

Once you have taken the time to ensure that you are making a good first impression with a clean and natural-looking face, you should turn your attention to your smile. In the health-care field, your smile is like a greeting card. Whether you are still in school, networking, interviewing, or working, you are meeting new people every day and greeting them with your smile. Properly caring for your mouth will encourage you to flash that wonderful smile everywhere you go.

Mouth care begins with making sure that your mouth is clean. That means brushing your teeth at least twice per day, preferably after meals, and flossing daily. You should also use a mouth wash or rinse after you brush to keep your breath smelling fresh. Carry breath mints or a travel toothbrush with you to ensure that you can maintain that fresh breath all day long. These steps will serve as the foundation for a healthy smile.

Once you make mouth care a part of your daily routine, you can begin to address any issues with or concerns you have about your teeth. For example, if your teeth are stained or discolored, you might want to consider using a whitening toothpaste, whitening strips, or another whitening product to help you to create a whiter and brighter smile. If you have more serious dental problems, you should consult with a dentist, if possible. If money is a concern, you might want to consider looking into whether any local dental schools offer free or minimal cost dental treatment.

Mentor Moment

I had 2 more months left in my program, but I had already started to develop my professional look. However, the alterations I made did not change the fact that I was missing my four front teeth. To help out, my director of education gave me an application for a local dental school, where I applied for care and got a free bridge. My smile and my confidence were both at 100% after that.

Robin from Billings, MT

Hair Care

Hair has always been a point of beauty and strength. The Bible tells us that Samson's strength was in his hair, and history tells us that Cleopatra's hair is known for being as dark as the night and as soft as a cloud. The way you wear your hair says a lot about you. Teenagers commonly use their hair to create fashion statements or keep up with current trends, such as by coloring their hair black, blue, or any number of other colors, or wearing Mohawks or buzz cuts. In the health-care field, you will also be using your hair to make a statement: I am a professional member of the health-care field who is neat, pays attention to details, and is ready to work hard to take care of patients.

Your hair will complement the first impression that you begin to make with your face. Therefore, it requires just as much care and attention as your face to ensure that it looks clean, styled, and well-groomed. As for facial products, there is seemingly no end to the number of products that are available for use on your hair. Cleansers, sprays, conditioners, straighteners, volumizers, gels, dyes, and other products are all marketed as ways that you can make your hair look more beautiful. When it comes to hair, your biggest problem might be choosing which product or products to use.

Having healthy, professional-looking hair begins with making sure that your hair is clean and shiny every day.For some people, that means washing it each day in the shower. Others can get away with washing their hair every other day or less frequently. The frequency with which you need to wash your hair for it to look clean and healthy depends on the type of hair you have and the products you use. Your hair should not appear oily or be caked with the previous day's styling products. Although these practices might be considered fashion statements in some environments, they will not be considered fashionable in the health-care field. In addition to being unattractive, oily or dirty hair is hard to manage, making it hard to style and control. If you have oily hair, you will probably want to wash it daily with a shampoo designed specifically for oily hair. On the other end of the spectrum, if you have dry or damaged hair, you might want to use a conditioning shampoo or separate conditioner to keep your hair and scalp moisturized.

Once it is clean, your hair should also be combed and styled. The style you choose will say a lot about how you want people to see you. For example, short hair typically emphasizes your eyes rather than your mouth and jawline. Be sure to choose a hairstyle that does not cover your eyes because making eye contact plays a large part in your communication skills. Some employers also have guidelines when it comes to hair. Be sure to know what rules apply to you when you are entering a new position.

The hair style that you choose might also determine how often you need to get your hair cut. Short hair typically requires more maintenance to keep it looking properly styled. If it has been a while since you have changed your hair style, you might want to choose a new style to go along with your new professional attitude. Look through magazines and watch television shows to find a style you like, and then visit a stylist and create your new style. Beauty schools also commonly offer new hairstyles at very reasonable prices.

Nail Care

When it comes to nail care, you need to nail it! In the health-care field, you will work with your hands a lot. Your fingernails are the focus of your hands, so they should usually be kept short (about 1/4 inch in length) and clean, whether you are male or female. In most cases, you should avoid wearing long acrylic nails. If you wear nail polish, choosing a clear or neutral shade, might be most appropriate. Dirty fingernails attract attention, whether you are interviewing for a position or caring for patients. The most important reason to have clean nails is because germs hide under the fingernails and can be spread to patients. That is why surgeons scrub up with a nail brush before surgery. Medical and dental assistants should frequently wash their hands and use a nail brush as well, especially after they come in contact with a patient.

Nail care policies vary, though. Some offices allow longer nails and brighter polish, depending on your position in the office and the equipment you operate. Once you are hired for a position, you can inquire about the specific policy of the office, hospital, or clinic where you will be working. However, while you are networking and interviewing and until you learn what is appropriate in your new position, you should keep your nails short and clean to give them a healthy, professional-looking appearance.

Dressing Professionally

By caring for your body and maintaining a healthy appearance, you set the stage for creating a strong first impression that says you are a health professional. The next step in making that first impression right is to choose the proper clothing, shoes, and accents to round out that professional look. You should be sure to choose a professional outfit that is comfortable and works for you, because how you feel in your professional outfit will determine the amount of self-confidence you exude and how well you make your professional statement. You want to choose an outfit that helps others focus on your talents and abilities, not your attire.

Motivational Moment

66 You have to perform at a consistently higher level than others. That's the mark of a true professional. 99

Joe Paterno, college football coach

Clothing

Because you have probably been wearing scrubs since you entered your educational program, you might not have given a lot of thought to the clothing you will need to find for your new career position. Your scrubs have become your attire and symbolized to people your commitment to reach your new career. Your scrubs are not a dress-down casual outfit; they are a uniform that identifies you as a member of the health-care field. Hopefully, you have worn that uniform with dignity and respect, making sure that your scrubs are neat and clean every day. Even in your scrubs, you want to make sure that you look professional and present yourself in a professional manner.

Mentor Moment

I wanted to stand out in my scrubs, so I would press a line down the center of my scrub pants like they were dress trousers. I liked the way it made me feel.

Charles from Little Rock, AR

Although you will most likely continue to wear those scrubs when you enter your new position in the health-care field, the fact is that you still need a formal professional outfit in which you can network and interview. You cannot go to an interview in scrubs, even for an entry-level position and even though you will most likely be entering a position where you will be wearing them. Now is the time to assemble a professional outfit that fits your new career.

You might want to begin by assessing the wardrobe you have in your closet and seeing what might work. Remember to try on each piece of clothing that you are considering to determine whether it still fits. Because your scrubs have been so comfortable and wide, you might find that you have put on a few pounds and your old jacket, suit, or slacks do not fit you. Once you determine what you already own, you can determine what you need to add to your wardrobe to complete your professional look. If you can afford it, you might even decide to buy a completely updated outfit, even if you have existing pieces that fit. Doing so gives you the opportunity to start with a fresh, new professional appearance that matches your new professional attitude.

O N   T R A C K

You are on track if you can list three items in your current wardrobe that you might be able to use to begin building your professional outfit.

1._____

2._____

3._____

Keep in mind when you are choosing your professional outfit that your clothing will be measured by how neat it is and how well it fits you, not by how expensive it is or where you got it. Your professional outfit does not need to break your bank. In fact, you might not need to buy anything, even if you do not have what you need in your own wardrobe; you might be able to find a friend or family member who could loan you some professional clothing. If you do not know of anyone who could loan you clothing, you should consider all of your shopping options, especially if your budget does not have much flexibility. Many discount stores offer new high-quality clothing at bargain prices, and you can often find good quality, lightly used clothing at thrift stores and nearly new stores. Buying your professional outfit one piece at a time to spread out your expense is also a good idea. Watch for special sales and coupons to save even more money when you are shopping. The goal when choosing your professional outfit is to find something that looks fantastic on you and to keep it looking its best (e.g., free from wrinkles) so that your self-confidence and self-esteem soar when you wear it. (See Box 10.3.)

O N   T R A C K

You are on track if you can list places you can go to find bargain prices on professional clothes.

1._____

2._____

3._____

BOX 10.3   CHOOSING A PROFESSIONAL OUTFIT

The goal in choosing a professional outfit will be to make sure that you look your best. That means choosing clothes that flatter your figure and hide your flaws. Here are some tips for how to do that.

For an **hourglass figure** (small waist with equal measure of hips and bust):

• Wear belts.
• Don dresses and coats with ties to show off your natural waist.
• Use flared pants to give you balance.

For a **top-heavy figure** (larger bust and shoulders):

• Avoid stripes that wrap around you.
• Wear V-necks for a more flattering look.
• Wear wide-leg pants.
• Wear A-line or full skirts.

For a **bottom-heavy figure** (more weight in and around the hips):

• Avoid tapered pants.
• Wear A-line skirts.
• Keep bottom colors dark.
• Use ruffles to bring more attention to your top half of your body.

For a **middle-heavy figure** (more weight in and around the middle with an undefined waist):

• Find a properly fitting bra to lift your chest and better define your waist.
• Wear items with an empire waist.
• Wear A-line skirts.
• Use a fitted blazer to flatter your figure.

For Women

Professional attire for women starts with some basics that will help you to look clean and stylish, such as a basic brown, blue, or black suit. Pantsuits are a popular choice. You might also choose to go a more traditional route and wear a dark skirt and jacket. Either of these options can be rounded out with a nice white or other light-colored blouse. White is a good choice because it is professional color that goes well with all dark suit colors and is flattering for all skin tones. If you choose to wear a skirt, it should come no higher that the top of the knee; thigh-high skirts and miniskirts are not the best choice for a professional look. Nylons are usually recommended to complete the look, especially if you are wearing heels or sandals. Fashion will dictate the need for nylons.

Once you have some of the basic wardrobe elements, you can look to the fashion industry to see how you can improve on and complement this look—or even create your own look. You might want to use color to accent your professional outfit and your personality, such as by choosing a red or gold jacket with your dark-colored skirt and white shirt or by choosing a brightly colored blouse to complement your dark suit. You might also consider choosing a floral or patterned blouse, as long as the pattern has a small print that is not too busy. (See the section entitled *Accents* later on in this chapter for more information about how to create your own professional style.)

Mentor Moment

I was always told to wear a blue suit for an interview. That was the basic uniform. However, I sometimes like to be different and so, when I was interviewing, I wore a black pencil skirt; white, tailored blouse; and a red bolero jacket that came to my waist. I was later told that all the candidates came in blue suits except me. I felt like I was hired because I stood out.

Christy from Mullan, ID

For Men

Professional attire for men starts with some similar basics, such as wearing dark brown, blue, or black. A suit is an easy way to take care of more than one piece of your outfit at the same time. However, if you do not have a suit, a dark pair of trousers, preferably slacks, and a matching or complementary sports coat will give you the same professional look. You can dress these over a white shirt to look sharp and clean. You may also choose to wear a colored shirt; just be sure to choose a color that complements the rest of your outfit and is in style. If you are unsure of what styles are currently in fashion when it comes to dress clothing, ask a salesperson. Choose socks that blend in with the rest of your outfit by matching the color of your trousers; do not use them to make a color statement. You do not want your socks to stick out like a "sore thumb" as you sit down to talk about yourself during an interview.

Finish off your look with a professional-looking but updated tie. Even if you choose basic colors for the rest of your professional outfit, you can add a splash of color and flair that will make you stand out by choosing an interesting tie. Just be sure not to choose anything too flashy. Your tie should not draw more attention than the personality you are presenting, but you can use this opportunity to show some originality and make an impression. Know the current styles for ties and choose an appropriate tie that works for you and looks professional.

Shoes

Another important part of your professional outfit is your shoes. When you meet people, they will quickly look you up and down, from your head to your toes. You want the first thing they see to be your shiny hair and glowing face and the last thing they see to be your nice, shiny shoes. You should choose shoes that are comfortable and sensible, but avoid casual shoes, such as tennis shoes, sandals, and sneakers. A leather shoe or a nice pair of loafers are good shoe choices for men. Women can wear heels as long as they are low to medium height and as long as they are comfortable to walk in. You do not want the first impression people have of you to be you falling down or walking funny in your high heels.

Your shoes should complement your interview outfit by matching in color and style. They should also be clean and in good repair. Scuffed shoes may signal to an employer that you lack attention to detail or a concern for your appearance. In some cases, simply wiping off the dirt might be all you need to have a nice pair of shoes for your professional outfit. You might also want to consider polishing your shoes with some polish or petroleum jelly if they need a little more attention.

If you do not have a nice pair of shoes, you might need to buy a new pair or borrow a pair from someone you know. As with clothing, you can often find good-quality, low-cost shoes at bargain stores and thrift stores. Try not to spend a lot on shoes, though, as you will probably only wear them while you are net-working and interviewing.

Motivational Moment

66 All mankind is divided into three classes . . . those that are immoveable, those that are moveable, and those that move. 99

Benjamin Franklin, inventor and statesman

Accents

Accents can help to make or break your professional outfit. Some accents will help you to stand out and be noticed, whereas others will distract from the professional look that you are trying to create. Make sure when choosing your outfit accents that you know what the recommendations are when it comes to such items as jewelry and accessories.

Jewelry

The right jewelry can help to complement your professional appearance. For example, the right necklace can help to accent and draw attention to your face and promote eye contact with the person with whom you are speaking. The rule is keep your jewelry simple, though. Your networking and interviewing opportunities are not the time for you to show off your jewelry; they are the time for you to show off your professionalism, skills, and personality. Make sure to pick jewelry pieces that are subtle and nice and complement your professional appearance. Also know that, while jewelry is an acceptable part of your professional look for networking and interviewing, it will not be part of your scrub outfit.

If you choose to wear jewelry to complement your professional outfit, choose jewelry colors that appropriately complement or contrast your outfit. For example, keep the following in mind:

- A green and blue necklace compliments a blue blouse.
- A gold necklace compliments but does not conflict with the power of a red jacket.
- A bold-colored necklace, such as red, contrasts a white blouse and dark jacket.

Some jewelry items should also be avoided. For example, you should avoid large hoop earrings and bracelets that dangle because they can make noise and become distracting during an interview or while you are talking with someone. You should also remove any large or flashy rings and watches. You can wear these items on the weekends, but they are inappropriate in a professional setting.

Another indiscretion when it comes to looking professional is facial jewelry. Facial studs, facial rings, and tongue rings and studs are generally not considered to be professional. Most likely, you have already had to remove these items to comply with your educational institution's dress code policy, so just leave these items out until you are through with your networking and interviewing. Then, you will need to check the policy at your new position to see whether such jewelry pieces are acceptable.

Tattoos

Although tattoos are considered decorative in some settings, they might not be appreciated in the health professions field. If you already have tattoos, you might want to consider covering them while you are interviewing, networking, and working. In some cases, you will even be required by your employer to cover them. If your tattoos become a problem, you might even want to consider having them removed.

Accessories

One of the most popular accessory items is a purse. Although most men do not carry a purse, some carry briefcases or small bags called "satchels." Although satchels are more common in Europe, some men in the United States carry them to professional events because they are a good place to store keys and other bulky items.

Many women carry purses everywhere they go, and those purses can sometimes be large enough to fit a person's entire medicine cabinet, desk, or apartment. However, when it comes to networking and interviewing, if you decide to carry a purse, you should choose one that is small and functional. It should be just large enough to carry your car keys, pens, and other absolutely necessary items. You might also choose to use a purse but not carry it with you into an interview or networking event; in this case, you should leave it in your car out of plain sight, such as in your trunk or under a seat. Even if you are used to carrying a purse, you can probably manage without one during these professional encounters.

If you choose not to carry a purse, satchel, or briefcase, you can carry your necessary items with you in your portfolio instead. Many portfolios include a small pocket where such items would fit. Alternatively, you can put your car keys in a jacket pocket and keep the other items in your portfolio.

O N   T R A C K

You are on track if you can list three items that you would like to acquire to make your current clothes or professional outfit look more professional.

1. _____

2. _____

3. _____

Just as important as what you should do to look professional is what you should not do. See Box 10.4 for tips on how to keep your professional outfit looking professional.

BOX 10.4   PROFESSIONAL OUTFIT DON'TS FOR MEN AND WOMEN

For Men

- Don't wear an ill-fitting jacket, in other words, one that is too short, too small, too long, or too large for you.
- Don't wear a flashy tie.

(box continues on page 330)

BOX 10.4 PROFESSIONAL OUTFIT DON'TS FOR MEN AND WOMEN (continued)

- Don't dress too casually. Save casual clothes, such as jeans, turtlenecks, and polo shirts, for the weekends.
- Don't wear tennis shoes or sneakers.
- Don't forget to iron your outfit before you wear it.
- Don't wear a large watch or chains.

For Women

- Don't wear a skirt that is too short or reveals too much thigh.
- Don't wear tennis shoes or sneakers.
- Don't wear nylons or stockings with prints or designs.
- Don't wear busy blouses that have large prints.
- Don't wear overly tight clothing, such as tight skirts, blouses, and sweaters.
- Don't wear low-cut blouses that accent your cleavage more than your personality.
- Don't forget to iron your outfit before you wear it.
- Don't wear too much jewelry.

Success Journal

1. Complete the chart below to determine what items you have in your wardrobe and what items you need or are in the process of purchasing to complete your professional outfit.

Item	Yes	No
Women		
Business suit		
Jacket		
Skirt		
Dress		
Blouse		
Shoes		
Nylons/stockings		
New hair style		
Manicured/polished nails		
Natural makeup		
Men		
Business suit		
Jacket		
Slacks		
Shirt		
Tie		
Shoes		
New hair style		
Cleaned nails		

2. Now create two complete professional outfits from what you have and what you want to purchase.

Outfit 1: _____

_____

_____

Outfit 2: _____

_____

_____

(continues on page 332)

Success Journal (continued)

3. Look at your calendar and commit to a date by which you will complete your professional look, possibly including getting your hair cut and styled, beard trimmed, and a makeover. Write the date here:

_____

Practicum

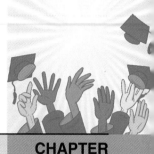

Learning Outcomes

After reading this chapter, the student will be able to:

1. Define the purpose of a practicum.
2. Identify and meet the nonclinical responsibilities and behaviors expected of a student during a practicum.
3. List common rules for succeeding at a practicum.

Looking Back at the Road to Your Practicum

Congratulations! If you are reading this chapter, you are probably about to enter your practicum—or maybe you just want a sneak peak at what is ahead of you. Before you move ahead to this important transition, you should take some time to look back at the road you have traveled to complete your program in the health-care field.

Can you remember when you first decided that you wanted to make a change in your life? You were probably unsure of what you wanted to do at first. Can you remember calling to speak with someone about your program? You were probably a little nervous that day and were not sure what questions to ask or where your conversation was going to lead you. Do those feelings still linger for you now? Probably not. You might not even remember them anymore. That is because you are not the same person anymore. You found the courage and determination to make it through and to be standing where you are right now in your program.

Do you remember all of the successes you have had since you started your program? Can you recall all of the challenges that you have overcome? If you have allowed this book to guide and support you, you have probably made many changes in your life that proved your dedication to your education and to your goals of making it to graduation and having a new career:

● Maybe you were challenged by your ability to accept that *you* control your mind. You now know how to feed your mind positive thoughts and control that "little voice" in your head, so that you will no longer be held back from achieving your goals.

Motivational Moment

66 A man is but the product of his thoughts. What he thinks, he becomes. 99

Mohandas Gandhi, Indian political and spiritual leader

● Maybe you were challenged by your ability to create and maintain a schedule that allowed you to have quality study time along with quality family and personal time. However, you discovered that time management and organization offered you the reward of filling each day with quality time, no matter what task you were performing.

- Maybe you were challenged by your fear of being able to connect with other students. However, you have most likely made long-lasting friendships with and learned from classmates whose nationalities, ages, religions, and other personal characteristics differ from yours.
- Maybe you were challenged by personal issues such as a lack of money, transportation, or child care. You confronted these challenges and found viable solutions that illustrate your ability to think critically and solve problems. In doing so, you proved your dedication to your goals by showing that you were not going to let anything stop you from succeeding.
- Maybe you were challenged by your fears of the lack of studying and test-taking abilities. However, you surprised yourself and others by learning new skills and excelling in ways that increased your ability to study, maximized your study time, and improved your grade point average.
- Maybe you were challenged by your lack of knowledge about marketing and networking. Now you have developed an arsenal of marketing tools that you are using to showcase your qualifications, skills, traits, and experience in a way that will impress interviewers and prospective employers. You also have the confidence and knowledge necessary to meet new people, make network connections, and provide a top-notch interview.

You will be able to carry with you into your new health profession all that you have learned from overcoming these challenges and achieving these successes:

- You should be very proud of yourself for successfully completing all of the course work in your health professions program.
- You have made the most of your time, and this should continue to be a priority as you balance your new career with your personal life.
- The new friends that you have made might feel like an "extended family" to you. They are now the foundation for a support system that will hopefully continue to help you throughout your career and your life.
- You will incorporate your ability to embrace diversity as you prepare to care for a diverse population of patients in the health-care field.
- You will transfer the studying and test-taking techniques you have learned to your health profession, where they will help you to stay organized and to complete projects and assignments.
- The people skills you have learned through your marketing and networking experiences will serve you well as you care for patients and interact with coworkers in your new position.
- The marketing materials you have developed will continue to represent you and showcase your skills as you update them to help you advance in your career.

Understanding Practicum Basics

With all that you have already achieved, believe it or not, you might now be about to face one of the most interesting parts of your health professions program: your practicum. Many, but not all, health professions programs require students to complete a practicum before graduation. A practicum is an opportunity for you to apply the concepts that you have learned from your clinical program to real-life situations and to learn even more. It is the culminating portion of your clinical program and will help to prepare you for your certification or national examination. If your program requires you to complete a practicum, you will not be able to graduate without successfully completing this major part of your program. If your program does not require you to complete a practicum, you will most likely gain the same experience, as in massage therapy, by completing hands-on labs or working in a clinic where you perform with actual clients.

Motivational Moment

❝ We keep moving forward, opening new doors, and doing new things, because we're curious and curiosity keeps leading us down new paths. ❞

Walt Disney, American animator, entertainer, and philanthropist

As you prepare for your practicum, you might be feeling a little nervous and uncertain. You might also be asking yourself some of these questions:

- What is a practicum?
- Will I know enough to be able to complete my practicum?
- How do I find a practicum?
- Can I handle being in a real-life health-care setting?
- What happens if I make a mistake?

This chapter answers these questions and provides some basic information that you will need to be successful in your practicum. However, the specific requirements of a practicum vary by specialty and educational institution. Most educational institutions develop practicum standards based on the guidelines of accreditation agencies, such as the Commission on Accreditation of Allied Health Education Programs (CAAHEP) or the American Association of Medical Assistants (AAMA). These standards outline the clinical skills required of you during your practicum and are specific to your program. Therefore, this chapter focuses on the nonclinical skills that you will need to be successful during your practicum.

What is a Practicum?

A practicum is the practical, hands-on portion of your program in which you will actually put your clinical knowledge and skills to work in the health-care field under the supervision of a qualified professional. Think of it as on-the-job training. Instead of going to class, you will report to a medical office, hospital, clinic, or some other off-campus setting, depending on your program. It is another step along your path to graduation, and the experience that you gain from it will help you to prepare for your certification or national examination.

You must successfully complete the required practicum hours for your program in order to be eligible to graduate and receive your diploma. Each health professions program requires students to complete a different number of practicum hours, which varies sometimes by state and the requirements of the accreditation agency. For example, medical assisting and billing and coding programs could have 4-week practicums that require students to work 8 hours a day, 40 hours per week, for a total of 160 practicum hours. However, one vocational institution requires students to complete *540 practicum hours* for their surgical technologist program. You should consult with an instructor or your institution's education department to find out the exact number of practicum hours required for your program.

Your practicum is an *extension* of your education, but it is considered part of your program. As such, you must continue to show your work ethic and a desire to be a medical professional by applying all of the knowledge you have learned as well as the skills you have cultivated throughout your program to your practicum experience. In addition, your attendance at your practicum will be monitored and recorded, just as it was while you were attending class. Maintain the high standards that you have set for yourself by completing all of your required practicum hours, attending your practicum on all scheduled days, and completing your practicum with professionalism, positive energy, and a smile.

Remember, if you stop now, you will *not* receive your diploma, certificate, or associate's degree. *Do not give up!* You need to reach the finish line, and you are almost there!

Motivational Moment

66 The best thing about the future is that it comes one day at a time. 99

Abraham Lincoln, 16th President of the United States

How Do I Find a Practicum?

In most educational institutions, practicums are established and coordinated by the education department. However, this varies depending on the size of the institution and available staff. For example, in some smaller institutions, the task may be handled by the career placement department instead. (For clarity, this book refers to the department that oversees practicums as the "education department." Be sure to find out which department handles practicums for your specific educational institution.) No matter its title, the department that oversees practicums identifies health professions sites, establishes contracts with those sites, and places all students at those locations for their practicums. It works directly with the sites and with students to ensure a positive experience for both parties while also ensuring that the practicum experience matches the instruction and materials presented in the educational program and adheres to safety standards and the legal scope of practice.

The person in charge of practicum assignments is commonly known as the "practicum coordinator," although he or she might also be called the "Director of Education," "placement director," or some other title. No matter the title, your practicum coordinator will be your point of contact throughout your practicum experience, not only placing you at a practicum site but also visiting you at the site, monitoring your progress, and evaluating your skills. You should direct any questions you have about your practicum to this person or someone else in the education department. If you have any concerns about or special arrangements you need to make regarding your practicum placement, you should speak with your coordinator as soon as possible. Although the coordinator will do his or her best to accommodate any special requests you have, you cannot expect to be able to choose where you do your practicum, and the coordinator cannot guarantee to fulfill all of your needs and preferences. The more time you give your education department to assist you with special arrangements, the more likely you are to be successful in reaching them.

Mentor Moment

When I was in school, I had to take one bus to drop off my kids at day care and then another bus to get to the campus. So, as my program was finishing up and I knew I would soon have to start my practicum, I made sure to let the education department know I preferred to be assigned to a site that was near public transportation. Luckily, my coordinator was able to find a place that worked perfectly for me and was easy to get to. I could tell that she was doing everything that she could to help me finish and graduate!

Theresa from Tacoma, WA

Although the education department assists in placing students at practicum sites, you must be accepted by the site before you are officially assigned to it. Here is how it works. Educational institutions typically send several resumes to each site, where someone reviews them and might request an interview with each candidate before making a choice. Like your future employer, the site will accept you based on the personality, skills, knowledge, and professionalism you present during your interview. (To make the best possible impression, you must be sure to follow all of the interviewing skills you learned in Chapter 9.) Once the site has made a decision, someone there will contact your educational institution to tell them who has been selected and when the person needs to report to the site.

Your resume will be submitted to several locations, and you might need to continue interviewing until you are selected for a site. If you are not selected after several interviews, someone in your education department might review your resume and counsel you on interviewing techniques to help you to improve your skills. Do not worry, though. The goal of education department is to place you at a site, and the staff will keep working with you until this happens. Once you have been selected for a practicum, the education department will give you the paperwork you need to begin.

O N   T R A C K

You are on track if you can answer the following questions:

1. How many total hours are required for your practicum?

_____

2. Who coordinates practicums at your campus?

_____

3. What special arrangements, if any, do you want to discuss with the education department?

_____

_____

What Should I Expect from My Practicum?

Your practicum will offer you the opportunity to watch and learn from other health-care professionals. Your first day will most likely be filled with a tour of the facility, basic training, and introductions as you meet and greet other staff members. However, you will quickly be expected to watch and learn from others.

When the staff feels you are ready to assist with certain tasks, they ill instruct you on what to do, and soon you will be performing tasks on our own.

Some general tasks that you might be asked to perform as part of your practicum include the following:

- Answering phones
- Making patient calls
- Seating patients
- Operating basic office equipment
- Performing housekeeping duties, such as cleaning equipment or removing waste
- Inputting data
- Inventorying medical supplies
- Taking payments
- Setting up patient rooms
- Taking patient histories
- Calling in prescriptions
- Filing

The specific clinical tasks that you will be asked to complete as part of your practicum vary depending on your health professions program, the type of setting in which you complete your practicum, and the legal scope of practice for your field. (See Box 11.1 for an example of some basic areas that might be included in your clinical tasks.)

Although some of the tasks you will be asked to perform during your practicum may seem menial, they are all necessary responsibilities that add to the

---

BOX 11.1 EXAMPLES OF CLINICAL TASK AREAS

As previously mentioned, the clinical tasks you will need to perform during your practicum are based on the guidelines of accreditation agencies. For example, CAAHEP requires students to meet certain standards in these basic areas related to patient care:

- Fundamental procedures
- Patient instruction
- Clerical functions
- Bookkeeping procedures
- General and clinical competencies
- Specimen collection
- Insurance claim processing
- Diagnostic testing
- Professional communications
- Legal concepts
- Operational functions

structure, maintenance, rhythm, and flow of the office. The office will be counting on you to carry out these responsibilities, and by doing so, you will begin to feel like a valued part of the team. You are depending on others, and more importantly, they are depending on you. This special hands-on interaction in the office is the best experience and learning opportunity you can have before you graduate, and you should make the most of it by completing each task with a positive attitude. How you think about the tasks you are asked to perform will have a lot to do with the success you have at your practicum site and the fulfillment you get from your experience there. For example, instead of focusing on the repetitive nature of a task, you can focus on the fact that your completion of the task helps to support the office staff, keeps the office organized, helps patients, and keeps patients happy by contributing to the office's organization and efficiency. A good attitude goes a long way and will be noticed and appreciated by the staff at your site.

Motivational Moment

66 The future belongs to those who believe in the beauty of their dreams. 99

Eleanor Roosevelt, former first lady of the United States

Your practicum experience can also be a great opportunity for landing a job after graduation. For example, you might be offered a position by the site or referred for an open position at another site. You can also ask the office manager, physician, or someone else from your practicum site to serve as a reference for you or to write you a letter of recommendation when you are ready to begin your career search. If you find someone you really connect with, you might consider asking that person to become your mentor. These reasons are good incentives for making sure that you impress your site manager with an ongoing positive attitude, professionalism, skills, and good work ethics.

How Much Does a Practicum Pay?

Students are *not* monetarily paid for their practicum hours. As previously mentioned, the work you will perform as part of your practicum is an extension of your program and classroom education. In essence, your site becomes your new classroom for the time you are scheduled to be there.

Although you do not receive monetary compensation for your practicum, it "pays" you in the sense that you are given the unique opportunity to learn from others in the health-care field and to become a real part of a health-care team.

- It allows you to practice your skills.
- It increases your customer service skills by offering you opportunities to interact with patients.

- It elevates your self-confidence by confirming the knowledge you have learned.
- It offers first-hand practice in working with patients that will increase your comfort level.
- It increases your awareness of your ability to contribute as a team player.
- It prepares you to pass your certification or national examination.
- It helps you to realize your potential as a new health professional.

In short, it prepares you for your new career. What you learn during your practicum and how you use the new knowledge and skills to make a difference at your practicum site will empower you to do your best and be proud to be part of the health-care field.

Motivational Moment

66 Education is the most powerful weapon which you can use to change the world. 99

Nelson Mandela, antiapartheid activist and
former president of South Africa

O N   T R A C K

You are on track if you can list three benefits that you expect to gain from your practicum.

1. _____

2. _____

3. _____

What Paperwork Do I Need to Complete?

Although each day at your practicum may be filled with various sorts of paperwork, you will likely be asked to complete additional paperwork for your educational institution. For example, you might be asked to report on your attendance each week using a chart, calendar, or some other form of time sheet. If so, at the beginning of the week you would give your attendance sheet to the site coordinator at your practicum. The site coordinator would fill in your hours throughout the week and then return the document to you for review at the end of the week. If you both agree to the recorded hours, you would then submit the paperwork to your educational institution. Depending on your educational institution, you may be asked to fax your time sheet or bring it in person to the education department at the end of your practicum. Most programs have a deadline for receiving this documentation, so be sure to know your program's regulations before you start your practicum. For example, you might be required to submit your hours before noon on Friday so that your hours can be recorded before the close of the workweek.

Your time sheet is important because it is a legal document. It serves as an official record of the number of hours you have worked, and it must be signed by the site coordinator to be official. Time sheet documentation is also important because it is used to show that you are in compliance with your financial aid regulations for your loans.

In addition to your time sheet, at the end of your practicum you will need to submit two evaluations to the education department: your evaluation of the site where you completed your practicum and the site's evaluation of you. Remember to submit all of your necessary documentation as soon as possible because you cannot graduate until this documentation has been received and processed.

Succeeding at a Practicum Site

Remember, your practicum is your final step in getting ready to graduate and perform effectively in your new career position. Therefore, you should aim to continue the success that you have achieved in your program at your practicum site. Because your practicum is an extension of your program, the same rules that you must follow at your school also apply to your practicum site. You will also be expected to follow the same office policies that the employees do; you need to look and act like an employee, even though you are not one. Remember, throughout your practicum that you are trying to make a good impression—not only because someone at the site holds your evaluation in his or her hands but also because this experience could lead to career opportunities. Be sure that you make a good impression from your first day to your last by looking and acting professionally.

Motivational Moment

66 Before everything else, getting ready is the secret of success. **99**

Henry Ford, founder of Ford Motor Company

Dressing for Your Practicum

Your learning institution or your practicum site will govern the dress code to which you must adhere at your practicum. You must follow this dress code in order to look professional and properly represent your institution. Although the required attire will differ from the attire you wear for interviewing, you should follow the suggestions for dressing professionally that were presented in Chapter 10, including the following:

- Maintaining proper hygiene
- Styling your hair so that it looks neat and stays out of your face
- Maintaining a natural makeup look
- Avoiding strong fragrances and scented lotions
- Steering clear of inappropriate jewelry

The proper attire for a student during a practicum is a pair of scrubs. Because you have been wearing your scrubs for several months at this point, you will probably need to buy some new ones to look professional for your practicum. If your budget can afford it, buy three new full sets of scrubs. If your budget is tight, you can try to use the bottoms from your college scrubs and buy only new tops. Ideally, you should choose scrubs with colors and prints that you can mix and match. However, your practicum site might require you to wear a specific scrub color and might specify that you cannot wear your college scrubs. Some medical offices wear certain colors on certain days. Be sure to find out what rules apply and what attire is considered acceptable for your specific location before you purchase any scrubs.

The shoes you wear need to be clean and comfortable. In addition, they should be sturdy and supportive because you will most likely be on your feet for the majority of your work shift. Adding gel cushions or extra padding to your shoes can make them more comfortable and supportive. The style of shoe you are permitted to wear varies by site. For example, a clean pair of tennis shoes might be acceptable at some locations, whereas other sites might require you to wear only white leather shoes.

During your practicum, you might also be asked to wear some form of identification (e.g., badge, special scrubs) that distinguishes you as a student to your coworkers and to patients. This is done for several reasons:

- To identify to your coworkers that you might need training or assistance with certain tasks
- To let patients in the office know you are in training
- To let patients know you will be assisting another staff member or another staff member will be assisting you

Conducting Yourself During Your Practicum

During your practicum, you are responsible for representing not only your educational institution but also the health-care site in which you are working.

Both of these parties have certain expectations about how you should conduct yourself. Here are some tips for adjusting to and meeting the expectations placed on you during your practicum:

- **Plan to adjust your schedule:** Your practicum might require you to put in more hours than was required for classes, and you also might need to travel farther to get there. You need to make sure that you plan for how you are going to accommodate these changes in your schedule before you begin your practicum, ideally at least 2 to 3 months in advance. If you have children at home, this adjustment could be particularly challenging, as you may need to make arrangements for getting your children off to school or picking them up. If you are an evening student, you might also find this adjustment to be more challenging because most, if not all, practicums are offered during the day. If possible, work with your education department and practicum coordinator to find a site that best accommodates your existing schedule and situation.

- **Volunteer with respect:** Although you will be working hard at your site and that work should benefit the organization, you must realize that the site is doing *you* a big favor by allowing you to *volunteer* as a guest at its facility. The organization and its employees are spending their time to expand your knowledge and skills so that you can become a trained health professional. As a student, you should be very respectful and appreciative of this opportunity.

- **Behave professionally:** Behaving professionally means making good decisions on the job and carrying yourself in a manner that reflects your level of confidence and professionalism. You should arrive at your site on time (or early), put in a full day, and show up every day. If you must miss a day due to an illness or emergency, be sure to call the site and your learning institution to let them know. Make sure in advance that you have the office's phone number and know who to contact. You should also be courteous, friendly, and respectful to everyone you encounter. If you act unprofessionally in any way toward anyone, you could be released from the site. (See Box 11.2 for more tips on behaving professionally at your practicum.)

Mentor Moment

I helped to place a student once at a practicum in an obstetrician's office. On her third week at her site, the student asked to borrow a pregnancy test. The office manager said no, but later found out that the student had taken the pregnancy test anyway. The student failed to realize, I guess, that "borrowing" a pregnancy test was stealing a pregnancy test, and sadly she had to be let go from the site and from the program.

Paulette, practicum coordinator from Northfork, WV

BOX 11.2   OTHER TIPS FOR ACTING PROFESSIONALLY AT A PRACTICUM

- Be sure to know and follow all of the office's policies. (You might even consider reading the employee handbook during lunch on your first couple of days.)
- Practice good etiquette, such as by offering a firm handshake when meeting someone new; maintaining good eye contact when speaking with people; and using simple courtesy words and phrases, such as "please," "thank you," "you're welcome," and "excuse me."
- Provide the highest level of customer service possible. For example, ask patients for permission before touching them or performing procedures such as taking a blood pressure measurement.
- Avoid using slang terms and inappropriate language.

Exchanging Inappropriate Terms for Appropriate Ones

Slang	Preferred Alternatives
Yeah	Yes
Nope, Naaah	No
This sucks.	This is not very good.
I hate this.	This is not my favorite.
This does not work.	I need help to fix this.
This messes with my head.	I'm confused.

- Maintain positive body language (e.g., good posture, confident smile).
- Do not stand around idle. Offer to help others until you find or are given additional work.
- Keep your cell phone and other electronic devices off while you are at work.
- Be sure to adhere to the site's smoking policies.

- **Follow directions:** Put simply, do as you are told by your supervisors. If you do not understand what you are being asked to do or you need to know how the office performs a specific procedure, politely ask. Each office is a little bit different. Asking about the office's policies and procedures shows that you respect and want to follow the rules. When you do ask a question, though, pay attention to the answer, and write it down so that you do not need to ask again.
- **Learn from your experience:** Remember, your practicum offers you the opportunity to watch and learn from other health professionals. You should be prepared to learn on your first day and every day after that by paying attention and listening to others. When appropriate, take notes so that you need not ask others to re-explain something that you have already been taught. And remember to document all the skills that you learn throughout your practicum so that you can add them to your resume.

Motivational Moment

66 He who asks is a fool for five minutes, but he who does not ask remains a fool forever. 99

Chinese proverb

- **Follow your educational institution's standards of practice:** Remember that your practicum is an extension of your education. Therefore, you should not forget anything that you have learned, and you should apply the techniques and ethical and safety standards learned during your educational program.
- **Leave your personal problems at the door:** Remember that your practicum site is a professional atmosphere. You should not carry your personal troubles into the workplace or discuss them at work. Such details commonly travel the office "grapevine" and might make their way to the hiring manager.
- **Maintain a good attitude:** The more positive your attitude, the more confidence you will show and the more responsibilities the office manager and staff will allow you to take on. If you bring a poor attitude to your practicum, you could be released from the site. Remember that the site is doing you a favor by allowing you to volunteer there; there is no rule that they need to keep you, and they will find it easy enough to place a new student from another school.

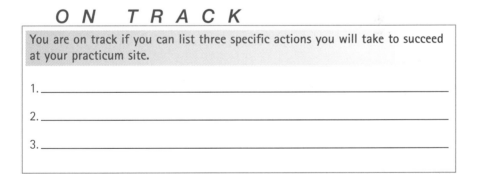

O N   T R A C K

You are on track if you can list three specific actions you will take to succeed at your practicum site.

1. _____

2. _____

3. _____

If you encounter any problems or incidents at your site (e.g., witness inappropriate behavior toward a coworker or patient, are asked to complete a task that is not appropriate or is unethical, encounter a problem with an employee, make a mistake), you should report them to your practicum coordinator and, together, develop a plan of action. Communication is key, and failure to follow this protocol may result in withdrawal from your program. Your institution and its staff do not want to see you give up now that you have made it this far. Make sure you give them the opportunity to help you be a graduate by communicating any issues and working things out together.

Although you need to communicate problems at your site to your practicum coordinator, you should not leave your site until your shift is up. Wait until your lunch break or after your shift to contact your coordinator. In addition, you must have the approval of your practicum coordinator before terminating your experience with a site. Remember that your practicum coordinator is there to assist, advise, and help you work through any issues or difficulties you have. In many cases, a call from the coordinator to the office manager can clear up an issue to everyone's satisfaction.

Successfully Completing Your Practicum

Once you have completed your required number of hours, you should have a feeling of accomplishment. Your self-confidence should be soaring because you will have a clear understanding of how a medical office, hospital, or clinic functions to serve patients and you will have learned new skills that will enhance your resume and serve you in your new career. Maybe you will have made some new friends or found a mentor. You should be sure to leave your practicum site in a professional manner and leave a good impression behind you that reflects the good experience you have had.

Although you have no guarantees that your practicum site will hire you, leaving behind a good impression is the best type of marketing. Here are some tips for how to do this:

- **Leave a copy of your resume:** If your experience was a positive one, be sure to leave several copies of your resume at the office for future reference and, if applicable, express your interest in a position at the organization if one is available. Even if the organization currently has no open positions, you never know when one will become available. You might also consider asking your practicum site to pass your resume along to other offices on your behalf. If you have worked hard during your practicum and taken every opportunity to learn, then you have showed the staff at that site the potential that you have to be a good employee. Hopefully, even if your site cannot hire you, someone there can write a recommendation letter for you or recommend you to another office.

- **Say "thank you":** You should show your appreciation for being given the opportunity to learn by sending your site supervisor a thank-you note. If it helps, think of your practicum as an interview that has lasted about 160 hours, and then follow all the same courtesy procedures.
- **Follow-up:** Before you leave, you might want to ask whether you can call to see how things are going and to find out if the site has or knows of any open positions.

Last but not least, to officially complete your practicum and be considered a graduate, you must complete and turn in all your paperwork. You should bring all original documents to your school's education department the day after you complete your last practicum hour, including the following:

- **Your original time sheets signed by the office manager or site supervisor:** These documents become part of your official attendance record and transcript.
- **Your evaluations:** Usually, you are required to turn in two evaluations. The first is the evaluation that someone at the practicum site completes on you that relates how you performed. The second is your evaluation of the site. Both forms vary from institution to institution and based on your accreditation requirements.
- **Any other paperwork required by your institution:** In order to meet state and accreditation agency requirements, you might have to complete some additional forms for graduation.

After visiting the education department, you might also need to visit the financial aid office to complete an exit interview and fill out some more paperwork.

Congratulations, you are almost a graduate! Once your registrar has recorded your attendance and you have met all graduation requirements for your program, you will have reached your goal of becoming a graduate. Your next step is to pass your certification or national examination and begin your career search.

Motivational Moment

66 The quality of a person's life is in direct proportion to their commitment to excellence, regardless of their chosen field of endeavor. 99

Vince Lombardi, former NFL football coach

Success Journal

1. In what type of facility would you like to complete your practicum?

   _____

   _____

2. What special requests or considerations, if any, do you have for your practicum coordinator?

   _____

   _____

3. What questions do you think you will have for your site when you start your practicum?

   _____

   _____

   _____

   _____

   _____

   _____

4. What challenges will you and your family face when you start your practicum and how will you approach these challenges to ensure that you will be successful?

   Challenge _____ Solution _____

   _____ _____

   _____ _____

   _____ _____

   _____ _____

   _____ _____

Career Search Strategies and Preparation

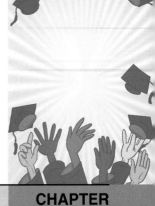

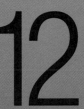
Learning Outcomes

After reading this chapter, the student will be able to:

1. Understand and define career search strategies.
2. List the priorities in planning a career search.
3. Identify ways employers learn about employment candidates.

Making Your Career Search Successful

Each month that you are in your educational program, you move closer to your goal of graduating and finding a career in the health professions. Think of how much you have already achieved. You have learned how to do the following:

- Visualize the future you want
- Develop a positive attitude to keep you on track and motivated to reach your goals
- Structure your schedule so that you have quality time for school, work, yourself, and your family
- Overcome challenges that might keep you from making it to graduation
- Improve your studying and test-taking skills
- Use your practicum experience to study for your certification or national examination
- Successfully market yourself and network with people to find opportunities in your field
- Create a resume that will help you to stand out
- Make the best possible impression during an interview
- Dress for success

Because you have come so far, you are now ready to look at what it takes to actually find your new career.

Motivational Moment

66 Don't wait until everything is just right. It will never be perfect. There will always be challenges, obstacles, and less than perfect conditions. So what? Get started now. With each step you take, you will grow stronger and stronger, more and more skilled, more and more self-confident and more and more successful. 99

Mark Victor Hansen, American inspirational author and speaker

Because of the demands it places on you, a career search can be overwhelming. You might find yourself quickly becoming discouraged if you do not see results coming in fast enough. However, you must be committed and patient. Remember that you are looking for *the right offer*. Making your career search successful instead of stressful takes a positive attitude and a solid plan.

Mentor Moment

I tend to be stubborn in nature and am not one for planning and following directions. When it came to my career search, though, I knew I had no time to waste and I knew that I didn't know everything I needed to know. So I took the time to develop a plan, and I stuck to it. Now that I am working as a biller and coder, I am so glad I did. I love my position and the office in which I work.

Bernice from Aurora, IN

Devising a Plan

Like most other undertakings, a successful career search begins with a plan. Looking for your new career position requires your full attention and will be a full-time job. Without a proper plan in place, you are likely to waste time doing things that will not help you in your search or you might just sit around worrying and feeling sorry for yourself. Unfortunately, you have no time to waste. The process of doing a career search, interviewing, and accepting a position can take anywhere from 1 to 4 months. One popular perception is that for every $10,000 you want in your salary, you might need to do 1 month of searching.

Here are some action steps that you might want to include in your career search plan:

- Update your resume.
- Make copies of your resume.
- Create or update your portfolio.
- Make sure that you have an interview outfit.
- Make sure you have a professional look (hairstyle, manicure).
- Practice answering basic interview questions.
- Alert your references that you are ready to begin your career search and that they might be contacted by a potential employer.
- Spread the word to others that you are ready to look for a position in the health professions.
- Choose the career search strategies that you will use and add them to your plan.

As you develop your plan, remember that you are seeking an entry-level position that can offer you the opportunity to earn experience.

Mentor Moment

My career search reminded me of when I planted a garden as a kid. I planted the tiny little seeds and then had to wait for the sun and water to nourish them until they grew into vegetables that were big enough to eat. It seemed like it would never happen, but I kept my hopes high and waited. My heart leapt with joy when I finally saw them sprout. I felt the same way when I finally got the right job offer after endless hours of "nourishing" my career search.

Nancy from Savannah, GA

Continuing Your Marketing and Networking Strategies

Remember, networking never ends. You must continue to implement your marketing and networking strategies throughout your career search. In fact, even after you find your new position, you will still need to network because most people will hold five to seven different positions within their lifetimes. Continuing to network throughout your career will help to ensure that you continue to make connections that advance you as far as you can possibly go in your new career. In addition, the further along in your career you are, the more others will be turning to you for networking opportunities. For now, though, you should focus on the strategies that will help you to find your new *entry-level* position.

Motivational Moment

66 You gain strength, courage and confidence by every experience in which you really stop to look fear in the face. . . . You must do the thing you think you cannot do. 99

Eleanor Roosevelt, former first lady of the United States

The marketing and networking strategies that you began to develop earlier in your educational program will now grow into a full-blown advertising campaign for your career. You should prepare yourself to market the message that you are soon going to graduate or have recently graduated and are ready—and qualified—to begin your career. You should begin by making sure that your marketing materials (e.g., business cards, resume, portfolio) are up-to-date. You want to be sure that your resume highlights all of the skills that you have learned throughout your educational program, including those you learned during your practicum. Also be sure that you have added any certifications you have earned or national exams you have passed since you originally created your resume.

You should also be sure to double-check that all of the information on your resume, including address, contact numbers, and all dates, are correct.

Once you have ensured that your marketing materials are ready, you will be ready to kick your advertising campaign into high gear. Now is the time to tell people you are ready to graduate or have already graduated and are looking for a position in the health professions. When it comes to your job search, do not be shy. Contact everyone you know and enlist them in your search, including current and former classmates, family, and friends, as well as the connections you have made through networking. You never know who or where your next lead will come from, so you should be sure that everyone you know is aware of your goal of finding a new career position. Be sure to take advantage of all of your networking outlets, including posting the news online, sending e-mails to personal and professional contacts, and sending out text messages on your cell phone. Remember that these marketing opportunities are a unique way to spread the news to hundreds of people in just a few minutes.

Motivational Moment

66A lobster, when left high and dry among the rocks, does not have the sense enough to work his way back to the sea, but waits for the sea to come to him. . . . The world is full of human lobsters; people stranded on the rocks of indecision and procrastination, who, instead of putting forth their own energies, are waiting for some grand billow of good fortune to set them afloat. 99

Orison Swett Marden, American writer and founder of Success Magazine

Understanding Career Search Strategies

If you had to look for a part-time job while you were taking classes, then you are probably already familiar with some of the most common and popular ways to approach your career search. Now is the time to take what you know about looking for a job and apply it to your career search. Although some of the steps are similar, hopefully you will find your career search more fulfilling because you now have the medical knowledge and skills required to pursue your dream career, the confidence and preparation needed to win over an interviewer, and the focus and drive to reach high and achieve your career goals.

Using the Search-and-Apply Method

The most simple career search method is the search-and-apply method. With this popular method, you search advertisements for open positions and then send your resume to prospective employers. At one time, the print media were the giants in this market, and you could limit your searching to the classified ads in local newspapers and in free employment papers. However, you must now broaden your scope to include online outlets (see Boxes 12.1 and 12.2). In fact, many local newspapers and free employment papers also have websites with online classified advertisements. Printed newspapers are generally available at convenience stores and supermarkets, if you do not have one delivered. Free employment papers are sometimes found in boxes near public transportation sites, such as bus stops and train stations. You can also find position postings on general websites, such as Google, Yahoo, and Craig's List; on job market websites such as Monster.com, CareerBuilder.com, and JobCentral.com (most have sections devoted to health-care jobs); and on medical job market websites (see Box 12.3).

O N   T R A C K

You are on track if you have identified when the employment listings are printed in your local newspapers and free employment papers.

Newspaper _____ Day_____

Newspaper _____ Day_____

Free employment paper _____ Day_____

BOX 12.1 CONDUCTING AN ONLINE CAREER SEARCH

Today, position postings are not just found in newspapers, they are found at your fingertips on your computer. This fact changes how you must conduct your career search. Although you might be able to find more openings and will have an easier time finding positions if you are planning on or willing to relocate, you will also likely be competing with hundreds of applicants for each job. An online search also requires you to take certain precautions when it comes to protecting your personal information.

Here are some steps that can help you to conduct a successful online career search:

- Start by checking with your school's placement office to see if they have a list of recommended websites for your program.
- Use a major search engine, such as Google, Yahoo, or Bing.
- Surf several different websites and explore all your options. The opportunities are endless on the internet.

BOX 12.1 (continued)

- Try to keep your patience. Hunting for sites can be frustrating, especially because some websites move or disappear and others make you sift through advertising to find what you are looking for.
- Sort through the junk and be critical of the information you are viewing.
- Change your key words if you are not finding many position openings when you conduct your search.
- Print out information you find to keep a record of your search.
- Write down website addresses or add them to your favorites list to save time the next time you search.
- Share information you find (such as good search sites) with your classmates so that they might be more willing to share such information with you. Although you might be competing with your classmates for positions, sharing information can help to improve the efficiency of your career search.
- Do not be afraid to ask for help and get some fresh ideas on key words and resources.

If you find an interesting position online and want to apply, you might be asked to fill out an online application or to cut and paste or upload your resume and cover letter. As always, your resume should be clean, neat, and error free before submitting it to a potential employer. Be sure to investigate employers as much as you can, however, before providing them with your personal information.

BOX 12.2 PROTECTING YOUR IDENTITY

Identity theft is on the rise. Some identity thieves are able to achieve their goals by hacking into personal or business computers and stealing personal data, the type of data that you must supply to an employer when you apply for a new position. If your identity is stolen, you might have to spend hours defending your credit record and disputing unauthorized purchases.

Although applying for positions online is now standard practice, you must be sure to do all you can to protect your identity when you do so. Here are some tips for protecting your identity during your job search:

- **Research each company before you apply:** Make sure that you research a company before providing any sensitive information about yourself online. Start by researching the organization's website to find out certain information about its history and structure (e.g., how many years it has been in business, how long it has been located in your area, how many employees it has, what

(box continues on page 358)

BOX 12.2 PROTECTING YOUR IDENTITY (continued)

benefits it offers, what medical specialty areas it employs). You can also research some businesses through the Better Business Bureau (www.bbb.org) and U.S. Federal Trade Commission (www.ftc.gov). One drawback is that these organizations only provide information about businesses that have applied to be members. However, you should consider whether you want to apply o work at a business that has not applied to be a member of one of these organizations.

- **Protect your Social Security number:** Supplying some personal information on an online application is fine and necessary; however, you should protect your Social Security number because this special identifier can be used by others to steal your identity. For this reason, most companies will not ask you to provide your social security number on online applications. **Know your rights:** Certain personal information, such as your age, religion, and marital status, are not considered legal inquiry for employment. In other words, employers cannot ask about or base their hiring decisions on these candidate attributes.
- **Report potentially fraudulent postings:** If you suspect that you have found a fraudulent job posting on a major job market site, you should try to contact the site's administrator to report it. You can also contact local authorities

BOX 12.3 MEDICAL JOB MARKET WEBSITES

- 4 Allied Health Jobs: *http://4alliedhealthjobs.com/*
- Absolutely Health Care: *www.healthjobsusa.com*
- AllHealthcareJobs: *www.allhealthcarejobs.com*
- AlliedHealthCareers.com: *http://alliedhealthcareers.com/*
- BMJ Careers: *http://careers.bmj.com/careers/hospital-medical-healthcare-doctors-jobs.html*
- Health Career Web: *www.healthcareerweb.com*
- HireHealth: *www.hirehealth.net*
- MedHunters: *www.medhunters.com*
- NationJob: *www.nationjob.com/medical*
- PublichealthJobs.net: *http://publichealthjobs.net/*

If you know of a particular organization where you would like to work, you can also search for open positions directly on the organization's website. Some organizations post positions on their own websites before, or instead of, posting them on job market sites. This search method can also help you save time because you can research the organization at the same time that you are applying for a position.

When you are searching for your career position, also remember to visit the career services department at your educational institution. This department might keep classified listings on hand or have position postings of its own to help students who are searching for positions.

Once you find one or more positions that interest you and for which you are qualified, move to the next step and apply by submitting your resume or filling out the application (see Fig. 12.1 for a sample employment application). Some employers require you to submit a resume *and* complete an application. That's because the employment application usually provides information to the employer that cannot be found on your resume (i.e., more information on your personal background) and streamlines the process by asking specific questions of interest to the employer. For example, you might be asked about your high school education, any criminal charges, gaps in your employment, and reasons for leaving previous positions. Having this information can help employers save time by choosing only the top candidates for interviews.

The "apply" portion of the search-and-apply method is important because employers do not know that you are interested in a position until you apply. Depending on which search strategies you use and the employer's specifications, you might be asked to mail, e-mail, or fax your application or resume or to submit these documents online. In some cases, you are asked to complete the employment application only after you have been brought in for an interview. This practice varies by organization.

Here are some tips on how to make the search-and-apply method work for you.

- **Schedule a time and place to search for positions:** Just as you plan when you will get up in the morning, you should plan time in your day to seek out career opportunities. To truly make your career search part of your schedule, you can devote the same each day to your search and have a dedicated space in which you conduct your search. Like reporting to work, you should plan to be at your career search location at a particular time every day and should spend that time working hard.
- **Know how to read the classifieds:** The classified section lists jobs in alphabetical order, sometimes grouping them by field. You should start by quickly scanning the sections that apply to your experience (e.g., health care) and circling any postings that stand out to you or list positions that interest you. Then go back and read each posting carefully.
- **Keep an open mind:** Look at employment listings with an open mind, allowing yourself to see each listing that fits your qualifications and skills as an opportunity.
- **Know whether you are qualified:** The best way to determine exactly what an employer's needs and expectations are for a position and what the employer is looking for in a candidate is to carefully review the position posting. The

---

APPLICATION FOR EMPLOYMENT

PERSONAL INFORMATION

Date: _____

Name: _____

Address: _____

City: _____ State: _____ Zip: _____

Phone # (H): _____ (W): _____ (C): _____

Email: _____

Social Security #: _____

Are you at least 18?   Yes   No

Are you a U.S. citizen?   Yes   No

If you are not a citizen of the United States, are you eligible for
employment in this country?   Yes   No

Position applying for: _____

_____ in the field of health professions

_____ Full Time
_____ Part Time (include hours available) _____
_____ Temporary

Approximate salary desired: $_____ /year

If employed, when can you start? _____

Have you ever been convicted of a felony?   Yes   No
If yes, please explain the circumstances:

_____

_____

Are you related to anyone employed here?   Yes   No
If so, who? _____

Were you previously employed here or at another division of this company? Yes   No
If yes, where? _____

FIGURE 12.1 Sample employment application.

EDUCATION HISTORY

List any educational instruction, past and present, including business, trade, technical, or vocational school; and extension, correspondence, or evening courses.

Name and Address	Major Course of Study	Diploma/ Degree	Date Attended From	Date Attended To
High School				
Business or Trade School				
College or University				
Graduate/Professional				
Other				

Specialized training:_____

_____

_____

_____

Apprenticeships and skills:_____

_____

_____

_____

Extracurricular activities:_____

_____

_____

_____

Honors received: _____

_____

_____

_____

FIGURE 12.1—cont'd

Continued

<u>REFERENCES</u>

Please provide contact information for three personal references (for example, coworkers, teachers, professional acquaintances).

Name and Address	Occupation	Telephone # and Email Address	Years Known	Relationship	May We Contact This Person?
					Yes No
					Yes No
					Yes No

Submit an extra page to state additional information you feel would be helpful in considering your application, such as your interest in this company and any special experiences, skills, and community service.

<u>EMPLOYMENT HISTORY</u>

Employer name_____ Phone #_____

Address _____

Job title _____ Supervisor _____

Reason for leaving _____

Responsibilities _____

Employed   From_____ To_____ Hourly rate/Salary_____

Employer name_____ Phone #_____

Address _____

Job title _____ Supervisor _____

Reason for leaving _____

Responsibilities _____

Employed   From_____ To_____ Hourly rate/Salary_____

May we contact the employers listed above? Yes   No
If no, which employer do you wish us not to contact? _____

FIGURE 12.1—cont'd

posting usually explains the qualifications and, sometimes, the traits the employer is looking for in a candidate. As a general rule, if you have 75% of the qualifications and skills on the employer lists, then you should apply for the position. Remember that the position posting is the employer's wish list for a candidate. The employer will interview candidates who do not meet all of their qualifications and might even appreciate a candidate who does not exactly qualify based on the requirements but shows courage and tenacity by applying anyway.

- **Do not waste your time.** Making the most of your career search time means knowing what *you* are and are not looking for in a position. Do not waste your time looking at positions that are located too far away from where you live. If transportation is a concern, you should look for positions that are located near your home or near public transportation so that you never have to worry about whether you will be able to make it to work. You can also save yourself time by eliminating positions that list a salary that is not worth pursuing.
- **Keep track of positions that interest you.** (See the section Keeping Your Career Search Organized later in this chapter.)
- **Tailor your resume and cover letter to each position you apply for.** This means making small changes to gear these items to the employer's needs. For example, you might need to modify your objective, highlight certain medical skills over others, and clearly explain how your work history and skill set match the exact requirements of the position. Tailoring your resume and cover letter will require a little work on your part; however, doing so could make all the difference in getting that invitation to interview.
- **Be professional.** Make sure your resume, cover letter, and references page all look professional. If you are faxing your application or resume to an employer, you will also need a professional-looking fax cover sheet (see Box 12.4).

Motivational Moment

66 Some desire is necessary to keep life in motion. 99

Samuel Johnson, English author

BOX 12.4 CREATING A PROFESSIONAL FAX COVER SHEET

If you are going to be faxing your resume, you will need to create a fax cover sheet. Here is a sample cover sheet format that you can use to design yours.

Name
Address
City, State, and Zip

FAX

To: Contact name at prospective employer

From: Your Name

Fax: Prospective employer's fax number

Fax: Your fax number or school fax number

Phone: Prospective employer's phone number

Phone: Your phone number

Subject:

Pages:

For Review

For Consideration

Comments:

Using the Walk-and-Talk Method

Another popular career search method is the walk-and-talk method. That means going door to door to local offices, hospitals, and clinics and getting your message out there. Many politicians use this basic method when they are running for office; they go to neighborhoods to speak to small groups because it offers them an opportunity to personally introduce themselves to people and convey their message in a more personal manner than that allowed by television ads and other outlets. The message you are trying to convey is that you are look-ing for a position in the health-care field and you have something to contribute to an organization. Another goal of the walk-and-talk method is for you to have in-formation interviews in which you talk to people in and gather facts about each organization.

Here is how the walk-and-talk method works:

- Walk to offices, hospitals, and clinics near your home. To maximize your time, also visit office complexes, which usually contain multiple offices in one building.
- When you arrive, ask to speak to an office manager, hiring manager, or someone in the human resources department.
- If you are granted the opportunity to meet with one of these people do the following:
  - Introduce yourself (possibly using your Verbal Career Card).
  - Pass along the message that you are looking for a position in the health-care field.
  - Present the person with your resume and references.
  - Ask about any available opportunities at the organization.
  - Be prepared to answer some interview questions on the spot.
  - Ask for the person's business card. If you do not receive a business card, make sure to at least get the person's name and contact information before you leave.
- If you do not get the opportunity to speak with an office manager, hiring manager, or human resources employee do the following:
  - Ask the person at the front desk or whoever you do get to speak with any questions you have about the organization.
  - Leave your resume with that person and ask him or her to pass it along to the appropriate person.
  - Make sure to get the name and contact information of the person you would like to see.
  - Ask whether you can make an appointment with the appropriate person for another day.

- Call the next day to make sure the appropriate person received your resume. If not, ask whether you can fax it.
- No matter what happens during your time at the organization, remember to keep a smile on your face and thank everyone for his or her time. Your posture, eye contact, and smile are your calling cards when you meet someone for the first time. Maintain a professional demeanor no matter what happens to ensure that you make the best possible first impression.

If the walk-and-talk method works for you, you could be granted an impromptu interview on the spot. Be prepared for this possibility by being ready to answer some common interview questions (see Chapter 9, Interviewing Skills).

Motivational Moment

66 Success is not the key to happiness. Happiness is the key to success. If you love what you are doing, you will be successful. 99

Herman Cain, American newspaper columnist,
politician, and radio talk-show host

The walk-and-talk method has several advantages:

- You limit your search to your local area. Thus, if you find a position, you know it will be close to your home, which will be convenient and save you time and gas.
- You ensure that you are more than just a name on a resume. The people with whom you meet can see and hear you and will be able to form a better first impression of you than is possible by just reviewing a resume.
- You have the possibility of being hired on the spot, if the hiring manager interviews you that day.
- You might be reaching out to an untapped segment of the career market if you visit small offices, which commonly have a small staff and do not have a large budget to pay for advertisements.

The hardest part of this method is that it takes time, patience, and practice. You must enter each organization ready to impress, which means dressing professionally, being prepared to ask questions, and being prepared to answer interview questions. This method takes confidence because you need to "walk the walk" and "talk the talk."

Mentor Moment

I was looking for a position as a medical assistant, and I noticed that some new medical offices had opened up not far from my home. Hoping that new offices meant new open positions, with resume in hand, I walked into each office and introduced myself. Each time, I tried to make a good impression with whomever I spoke to, but I didn't hold on to much hope that I would get a call. I was really shocked 2 months later when I did get a call and was hired at one of the offices.

Kristin from San Juan, PR

Attending Career Fairs

Career fairs, also called job fairs, are events at which representatives from different organizations gather to meet prospective employees and explain the opportunities available in their businesses. Each organization has a booth with the company's name. The booth might look like a small carnival booth, or it might just be a simple table labeled with the company's name or logo. The booth is usually manned by one or more people who are recruiters or representatives from the organization's human resources department. These people hand out literature about the organization and are available to talk with potential candidates to provide them with more information. Some organizations also offer small gifts, such as pens, notepads, and candy, to draw people into their booths.

For a person such as yourself who is looking for or will soon be looking for a health professions position, career fairs are wonderful opportunities because you can find out about the employment availabilities at many different organizations all at one time. You also have the opportunity to meet the organizations' representatives face to face so you can make a strong first impression in person.

You might encounter several types of career fairs:

● **Campus-sponsored career fairs:** These career fairs are the most popular type and are a great use of your marketing time. They are often sponsored by specific academic departments as a way to show off recent graduates who have been hired by major companies. This type of career fair offers you a unique opportunity to talk with students who were recently in your shoes, to ask them questions, and to hear about their experiences as well as the companies for which they now work. The best part is, if these companies hired these former students from your campus, then they could also hire you.

- **Commercial entry-level career fairs:** These career fairs, which are commonly community sponsored, attract many companies from various fields as well as large crowds of attendees. The major attraction of this type of career fair is that the companies are there to hire specifically for entry-level positions.
- **Commercial specialty career fairs:** These careers fairs cater to a particular field of interest, such as health care, computers, or engineering, and are commonly sponsored by major companies within that industry. The advantage of this type of fair is that you do not have to waste time visiting or sorting through booths that are completely unrelated to your field.

So, how do you find a career fair? Depending on the type of career fair you are looking for, the fair might find you. Campus-sponsored fairs are usually advertised on campus bulletin boards, in the career placement center, and by instructors. Commercial career fairs are typically advertised in the classified ads, on local morning news programs, and on the internet. You might even learn about career fairs at other local schools in this way.

Once you decide to attend a career fair, you must prepare yourself. This starts by ensuring that your resume is up-to-date and ready to be distributed. To keep your resumes looking their best, you should carry them in your portfolio or in a briefcase or computer case. Bring a lot of copies of your resume with you to the career fair, especially if it is a large fair. One guideline is that you should bring two copies of your resume with you for each organization that will be represented at the fair. This is because you might start out talking with one person and then end up talking to another person from the same company; you should be able to hand each person with whom you speak a copy of your resume. Thus, you could need as many as 50–100 copies of your resume, depending on the size of the career fair. When it comes to the number of resume copies you bring with you, you are better off being overprepared than underprepared. You do not want to encounter a great opportunity at the end of an event, only to have to tell the representative that you have run out of resume copies. Doing so will not make the best first impression. Even if you do not get the chance to hand out all the resumes, you should be prepared with more copies than you need so that you can make the most of every opportunity.

Being prepared with your resume is only the first step. You must also be ready to put your best foot forward with the right attitude and professional appearance (see Chapter 10). You must be sure to put forth the impression that you have the attitude and skills that will make you an excellent employee. Your body language needs to say, "I want to be hired!" Remember that a confident posture, good eye contact, and a strong smile are some of the best accessories you can wear when you are dressing for success. The booth representatives are trained to quickly size up candidates and determine which ones meet their standards, so they will be judging you before you even have a chance to speak with them. In fact, many times, representatives will mark the top corner of your resume with an "A," "B," or "C" after you hand it to them to sum up how they judged you. An "A" means that you are a top candidate and might receive a call from the company within a few days. Dressing and acting professionally the entire time you are at a career fair is your best way to make a strong first impression.

Being prepared also means being ready to answer some common interview questions (see Chapter 9). When you meet the booth representatives, you will likely be given a mini-interview that helps them to finalize their judgment of you. Although it is unlikely that you will be given a formal interview at a career fair, during this mini-interview you might be asked some of the same questions that you would be asked during a formal interview. The way in which you answer these questions is the next best way to make a good first impression and increase your chances of being contacted by the organization.

Many people leave career fairs disappointed because they do not walk out with a new position. However, just as many leave real career opportunities inside the doors of a career fair because they do now know how to work the fair. Because career fairs can be large and overwhelming, you must approach them in such a way that you make the most of your time. Here are some key tips to ensuring that your time at a career fair is well spent.

- **Arrive early:** When you arrive early, you save yourself time because you can find the top companies you want to visit first and will fight fewer crowds and find shorter lines.
- **Formulate a plan:** Most career fairs have a map close to the entrance that lists the organizations that are present. When you first arrive at the fair, look at this map and identify the companies you would like to visit. If a map is not available, take a quick tour of the fair and identify the booths of interest to you.
- **Do not limit yourself:** One way to make the most of a career fair is to make sure that you meet as many prospective employers as possible. Try to meet *all* of the employers related to your field.

Motivational Moment

66 Only those who will risk going too far can possibly find out how far one can go. 99

T.S. Eliot, American poet, playwright, and critic

- **Engage:** As you walk the career fair, remember to approach the booths. Do not walk in the center of the aisle between the booths, keeping a safe distance that ensures you will not have to engage anyone. Remember that the reason you are at the career fair is to get your message out; to do that, you must approach people and present your resume. Make sure to have your Verbal Career Card committed to memory so that you will know what to say when you are speaking to someone at a booth. Also, remember to be courteous and respectful.

- **Be professional:** When you greet the booth representatives, be sure that you make eye contact and keep that eye content during your conversation. If you get a mini-interview, remember to use all of the interview skills that you learned in Chapter 9, including coming prepared with some questions of your own for the representative. To maintain a professional attitude, you also should try to avoid saying anything negative during your conversation, including criticizing former employers and complaining about previous work experiences.

- **Distribute your resume:** Hand your resume to each person with whom you speak and ask for a business card in return.

- **Gather information:** In addition to collecting business cards, you should also collect brochures and other literature from the booths you visit. Such information could provide you with the name of a person you should contact or to whom you should send your resume directly after the career fair.

- **Avoid lines:** People sometimes follow a crowd and instinctively get behind other people to create a line. You can save yourself time and aggravation at a career fair by trying to look beyond the line and see whether anyone is free up at the booth. If someone is available, find a way to move through the crowd and make your way to the front of the booth without offending anyone.

- **If you must wait in line, make the most of your time:** If you grab a brochure before you get in line, you can spend your time in line scanning the brochure for information about the company. The brochure will also give you ideas for questions you might want to ask about the company. You can also spend your time in line listening to the conversations that the recruiters have with other people. Listen carefully to the questions they ask, and prepare yourself to answer these questions. Listen to how other people respond to these questions and watch the recruiters' reactions. The line can also be a networking opportunity. When you are waiting in line, talk with the people in front of you and behind you. Sharing information with others in line might help you to make the most of the rest of your time at the career fair. For example, you might learn about booths to visit or avoid. You might also make new contacts that can help you in the future. Approach these networking opportunities with the same professionalism and respect that you have when you approach a booth so that others will be willing to talk with and share information with you. And remember to swap business cards!

- **Sign up:** As you cruise the career fair, you might also find booths for professional organizations related to your interest in the health professions. If you do, sign up! By providing these organizations with your name and contact information, you make it possible for them to inform you about position openings as well as their meetings and other gatherings. These events are additional opportunities for you to network and make new contacts.

- **Follow up:** Ask each person you meet whether you can contact them in a couple days to follow up.

Contacting Staffing or Temporary Agencies

Another career search option you can use after you graduate is to contact a temporary or staffing agency. These companies offer part-time or temporary help to organizations that need such assistance due to an employee's temporary absence, understaffing, or some other reason. Organizations sometimes use temporary agencies to "test out" potential employees before hiring them. As an individual, you can register with a temporary agency for no charge, and the agency will place you to work in different offices until you are hired by one. The temporary agency generally screens and tests people before placing them. Some postsecondary educational institutions also use temporary agencies to assist students into positions after they graduate; however, most do not because these agencies typically charge them a membership fee.

One advantage of working for a staffing or temporary agency is that you have the opportunity to experience several different work settings and can add to your knowledge in the health-care field. Other advantages may include the possibility of receiving benefits and the ability to make your own schedule to a certain extent by accepting or rejecting assignments. You should not plan to reject too many assignments, though, or the agency will not want to use you.

Because of the temporary nature of the positions offered by temporary and staffing agencies, you should probably contact such an agency for work only if you have been searching for a position for 6 months or longer (6 months is the operative time period because loan payments generally start 6 months after graduation). Another important point you should know when considering a temporary agency is that you are likely to be paid less than you would if you worked for a company directly. That's because the agency takes a "cut" of the money (e.g., the agency might charge the client organization $15 per hour and pay you $8 per hour).

You can find temporary and staffing agencies in your local telephone book or on the internet. Some agencies specialize in heath-care positions. You might also find booths for temporary and staffing agencies at the career fairs you attend.

No matter what methods you employ, conducting a career search can be hard and grueling. However, once you find a position that speaks to your heart, talent, and happiness, you will be successful. See Box 12.5 for additional career search tips.

Keeping Your Career Search Organized

Once you begin to employ your career search strategies, you will find opportunities that will lead you to interviews. If you have followed the steps outlined in the previous chapters, then you are ready to start interviewing—well, almost

---

BOX 12.5 OTHER CAREER SEARCH TIPS

- Make sure that you have a working telephone message recorder or answering machine and be sure to check it every day when you arrive home. This relatively inexpensive item will help to ensure that you do not miss any important calls.
- If you are using your cell as your main number, always make sure your cell is turned on or on vibrate so that you don't miss any calls from potential employers, and be sure to check your messages regularly.
- Make sure that your prerecorded message sounds professional so that you can make a good first impression if an employer calls to schedule an interview: that means speaking clearly and properly in your message, not recording music before your message, and not having any background noise or music during your message.
- Be ready to accept a telephone interview, especially when you have just sent out your resumes.
- Do not post anything on Facebook, Twitter, a personal blog, or other places online that you would not be proud to show an employer. Employers do their research on prospective employees and will have no trouble finding items that you have posted simply by searching your name.

---

ready. Before you actually attend an interview, you need to be organized for the interviewing process. That means having a system that will help you to keep track of to whom you sent resumes and where you interview.

The best method for keeping your career search organized is to use a chart. You can create this chart in a spreadsheet program, such as Microsoft Excel, or in a word-processing program, such as Microsoft Word. You might also choose a more old-fashioned method of keeping track of your career search—creating a chart on paper. Although this method can work for you, it might be harder for you to make changes to or update your chart.

No matter which system you use, your career search organization chart should keep all of the information for one employer on one row of the chart. Therefore, you should keep the list of employer's names from top to bottom in the first column of your chart. Then you can add additional columns across the top of the chart for the following items:

- Employer contact information, including the organization's name, address, and phone and fax numbers.
- Name of the contact person for the position, as well as his or her direct phone number and e-mail address, if available.
- Date you submitted your resume.
- Position title and description, including the required education, hours, and pay, if available.

- Date you were called for an interview.
- Date and time of the first interview.
- Name and title of the person with whom you will meet for the first interview.
- Directions to the location.
- Questions you were asked on the phone.
- Comments.

If you need to, you can also add additional columns for the date, address, and time of a second interview and for the name and title of the person (or persons) with whom you will meet for that interview. See Career Search Organizing Chart

In the "Comments" column in your chart, you should include any details or information about the position that you might want to remember. For example, you might include what interested you in the position, why you are qualified, which of your skills particularly apply, and where you heard about the position. This section is a good place to keep notes about your interviews as well. For example, you might include how the interview went, including mistakes you made or questions you were asked for which you were not prepared.

You should start adding employers to this chart as soon as you start sending out your resumes. Do your best to keep it up-to-date by updating it whenever you talk with a prospective employer, schedule an interview, or go on an interview. Keeping yourself organized in this way will save you time, allow you to maintain focus during your interview, help you to keep track of the details of each interview after it is over, and help you to learn from each interview to increase your self-confidence and improve your interviewing skills as you progress through your career search.

In addition to your career search chart, you will also want to make sure that you have put in order any other information that you have. For example, once you schedule an interview you should do your homework on the employer. That means finding any information that you can. You can keep this information organized by placing it together and then keeping it in a folder. If you have a copy of the position advertisement or completed an online application, include copies of those items in your documentation as well for future reference. If you number the employers on your career search organization chart, you can also add these corresponding numbers to the documentation that you keep in your folder, which will help to further organize your career search.

Motivational Moment

66 Success means having the courage, the determination, and the will to become the person you believe you were meant to be. 99

Dr. George A. Sheehan, American author and cardiologist

Career Search Organizing Chart

Empolyer Contact Information * Name * Address * Phone number * Fax number	Contact Person * Name * Direct phone number * E-mail address	Date Resume Submitted	Position * Title * Description	Date Called for Interview	Questions Asked on Phone	Interview Details * Date * Time * Name and title of interviewer	Directions	Comments

Understanding How Employers Learn About You

One of the reasons that many people seek a career in the health professions is to be able to change their lifestyle. Depending on the person's current lifestyle, that could mean any of a number of changes:

● Making more money
● Paying off debt
● Affording a better place to live
● Owning a reliable car
● Making a fresh start

Although a new career can offer you these opportunities and you are close to reaching these goals, you bring with you the previous experiences that you have had in your life, including your financial situation and personal history. Believe it or not, these aspects of your personal life can play a role in your career search because, as you begin applying for positions, employers will also start to gather information about you as a potential employee. They sometimes look to records, such as credit reports and background checks, to find out more about potential employees.

Understanding Credit Reports

A credit report is a record of your financial history. It includes information about money you have borrowed (past and current loans and credit card debts), including your reliability in repaying this money. Also called a credit history, this document is typically used by financial lenders to determine whether your past experiences indicate that you are a "good risk" when it comes to repaying borrowed money—in other words, whether you will pay them back. However, employers also sometimes check credit reports to determine a potential employee's level of responsibility and reliability as well as his or her ability to properly handle money and finances. (See Box 12.6.)

Most of the information on your credit report comes directly from the businesses with which you have credit or outstanding loans, such as banks, mortgage lenders, credit card companies, and retail stores. These businesses report information about you, both good and bad, to credit-reporting agencies so that other lenders can research whether you are a potential borrower in good standing. (See Box 12.7 for more information on credit-reporting agencies.)

BOX 12.6 UNDERSTANDING CREDIT

Some people get themselves into a financial bind because they use credit but do not fully understand how credit works. To begin, you should know that there are two types of credit: open-ended credit and fixed credit. Lenders want to see how you handle both types.

Open-ended credit, such as that extended with credit cards, is credit that you are given that does not have a fixed number of payments. You can charge items to your credit card and carry a balance on your card up to a certain predetermined credit limit. Each time you make a charge to your credit card, the amount you owe gets added to your balance. Once a month, you are issued a bill for the balance due (the total amount of money you have charged and owe to the credit card company). The credit card company does not expect you to pay the entire amount. Instead, you are given a minimum required payment. The minimum payment is usually about 5% of your current balance, or $10, whichever is more. This amount is what you are expected to pay for the month. However, paying only the minimum payment does not help you pay off your debts because the credit card company will charge you interest on your remaining balance, and as a result, your balance will continue to climb each month.

Fixed credit has a fixed number of payments and is considered "closed" once you have paid it off. Examples of fixed credit include car loans, student loans, and mortgages. With this type of credit, you arrange for a loan from a lender for a predetermined amount of money you would like to receive. For example, if you need $2,000 dollars in order to buy a new car, a lender will determine whether you are approved for a loan, set a time frame for paying back the loan, calculate a total monthly payment, and set a monthly due date (e.g., on the first of each month). Car loans are typically short-term loans that range from 1 to 6 years, whereas mortgages are longer-term loans that are generally financed over 10 to 30 years.

The price you pay for having credit extended to you, whether it is in the form of a credit card or a loan, is known as a "finance charge." Finance charges are usually determined as a percentage of the total loan or credit extended, known as interest. Sometimes, this interest can be as high as 29%. Depending on the type of loan you agree to, your interest rate might change over the course of your loan. Therefore, you should always be aware of the current interest rate you are paying on all loans and credit cards.

To understand how your interest rate can affect the amount of money you end up paying, review this example comparison between a high-rate and low-rate fixed rate card. Suppose you charge $1,000 on a high-rate (23.99%) credit card. After that, you make no further charges and pay only the minimum payment due each month. The payments will start at $51 and slowly work their way down to $10. You will need to make 77 payments over the next 6 years and 5 months in order to pay off your debt. By then, you will have paid $573.59

BOX 12.6 (continued)

in finance charges on top of your original debt. If you charge that same $1,000 on a low-rate (9.9%) card, your minimum monthly payments will start at $50.41 and go down to $10. To pay off your debt, you will make 17 fewer payments, finishing in 5 years and paying only $176 in interest (a savings of almost $400).

When you agree to use credit, you become responsible for making monthly payments. If you miss a payment, you might be sent a reminder. However, missing payments too often or making payments too late affects your credit rating.

BOX 12.7 CREDIT-REPORTING AGENCIES

There are three main consumer credit-reporting agencies:

- Equifax: *www.equifax.com/home/en_us*
- Experian: *www.experian.com*
- TransUnion: *www.transunion.com*

Although these agencies may use different formats for their credit reports, they all gather and present the same information.

Understanding the Parts of a Credit Report

The most important component of your credit report is the credit score or rating. This score is a number between 300 and 900 that summarizes how much of a risk you are to a lender. It takes into consideration several factors:

- The total amount of credit available to you (i.e., credit limit)
- The total amount of credit you are using (i.e., money you owe on your credit cards and loans)
- Your payment history (e.g., missed payments and late payments)
- The length of time you have had open credit
- The types of credit you have (e.g., credit cards, car loans, mortgages, student loans)
- The number of new accounts you have
- Certain inquiries into your credit (i.e., when lenders request your account information)
- Collection items, such as bankruptcies, foreclosures, liens, judgments, and wage attachments

Companies are willing to offer credit and loans to individuals such as you because they assume that you will pay them back in the agreed-upon time. When you make a late payment, miss a payment completely, or do not pay the money back at all, you build up "bad credit," which registers on your credit report as a low credit score. A low credit score is like a warning to other lenders, indicating that you might not be reliable in repaying your debts. A credit score around 500 generally indicates that you have some risk and therefore might be refused credit or be given credit with an inflated interest rate. A score around 650 and over is considered good and might mean that you will have little trouble receiving credit and loans. A rating around 850 is great. It means you have almost no risk and therefore might receive better conditions when you go to borrow money, such as lower interest rates and lower down payments.

Motivational Moment

❝ Stay committed to your decisions, but stay flexible in your approach. ❞

Anthony "Tony" Robbins, American self-help author
and motivational speaker

In addition to your credit score, your credit report includes extremely sensitive personal information about you, such as your name, address, social security number, date of birth, and employment information. According to credit-reporting laws, you have the right to protect this information from being viewed by the general public. If you feel this right has been violated, you can file a lawsuit or a formal complaint with the federal government. You also have the other rights:

- The right to know who has received a copy of your credit report
- The right to dispute information contained in your credit report
- The right to "opt out" of credit card mailing lists, which ultimately prevents credit card companies and others from using your credit information for marketing purposes

See Figure 12.2 for a sample credit report.

Reviewing Your Credit Report

To ensure that the information on your credit report—and therefore the information potential employers will see when they review your credit report—is correct, you should request and review a copy of your credit report from each of the major credit-reporting agencies. You can get these copies directly from each of

CREDIT REPORT (as of 8/22/2011)

PERSONAL INFORMATION

Here you will find your personal information, including your legal name(s),
year of birth, current and previous addresses, and current previous employers.

Profile

Name:	Student Genius
(Also Know As) AKA:	
Year of Birth:	1970
Address(es):	1234 Career Path Future, USA 12345
	742 Evergreen Terrace Springfield, USA 54321
Current Employer:	ABC Dollar Store 1 Dollar Road Anyplace, USA 23456
Former Employer:	ABC Pizzeria 22 Pepperoni Place Anyplace, USA 23456

Personal Statement

This space is reserved for statements of dispute. For most consumers, no information appears in this section.

REPORT SUMMARY

This section provides you some of the most important data points on the credit report.

Summary

Accounts Listed Negative:	1
Collections Accounts:	0
Real Estate Debt:	$0.00
Installment Debt:	$3479.21
Revolving Debt:	$9892.96
% Revolving Credit Available:	51%

BANKRUPTCY & COURT JUDGEMENTS

Here you will find any court-related information, including bankruptcies, state and county court records, tax liens, monetary judgments, and in some states, overdue child support payments. Remember, bankruptcies remain on your report for 7–10 years.

Public Records

There are no Public Records on your credit report at this time.

CREDIT INQUIRIES

Here you will find the names of those who have obtained a copy of your credit report, including tenders, landlords, and employers. Remember, inquiries remain on your report for up to 2 years.

ABC Hospital

(800) 555-5555
PO Box 5445
Future, USA 12345

Business Name: ABC Hospital
Inquiry Date: 7/2/2011

ABC Bank

(888) 555-4321
49 Loan Street
Anyplace, USA 23456

Business Name: ABC Bank
Inquiry Date: 3/9/2011

ABC Retail Store

(888) 555-0000
11 Buy Stuff Blvd.
Anyplace, USA 23456

Business Name: Big Retailers of America
Inquiry Date: 12/10/2010

FIGURE 12.2 Sample credit report.

Continued

CREDIT REPORT (as of 8/22/2011)

CREDIT CARDS, LOANS, & OTHER DEBT

Here you will find specific information on each account you opened, including current status and any past due information. Positive credit information remains on your report indefinitely. Creditor contact information has been provided in order to make it easier for you to resolve any issues.

Account History

Credit Card #1

Status: Collection account $57 past due as of July 2011

Date Opened: 08/2007	**Type:** Collection	**Credit Limit:** $200
Reported Since: 08/2007	**Terms:** Collection	**High Balance:** $200
Date of Status: 01/2008	**Monthly Payment:** $0	**Recent Balance:** $57
Last Reported: 07/2011	**Responsibility:** Joint	**Recent Payment:** $0

Car Loan #1

Status: Paid, closed/never late

Date Opened: 08/2005	**Type:** Installment	**Credit Limit:** $15,459
Reported Since: 09/2005	**Terms:** 72 month	**High Balance:** N/A
Date of Status: 07/2010	**Monthly Payment:** $0	**Recent Balance:** $0
Last Reported: 07/2010	**Responsibility:** Joint	**Recent Payment:** $0

Credit Card #2

Status: Open/never late

Date Opened: 08/2001	**Type:** Revolving	**Credit Limit:** $27,000
Reported Since: 12/2002	**Terms:** N/A	**High Balance:** $24,000
Date of Status: 07/2011	**Monthly Payment:** $33	**Recent Balance:** $93
Last Reported: 07/2011	**Responsibility:** Joint	**Recent Payment:** $93

CREDIT SCORE

Your Credit Score is a numerical representation of your credit worthiness that is used by most lenders and credit card issuers. Remember, each credit agency has its own set of data in your credit file. Thats why Credit Scores may vary between bureaus.

Score: 502

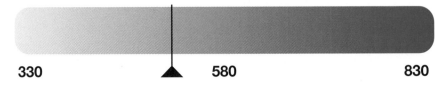

330   580   830

FIGURE 12.2—cont'd

the agencies or from a number of other websites that offer credit reports (e.g., annualcreditreport.com, www.freecreditreport.com). These other sites typically provide you with access once per year to free reports from each of the major credit-reporting agencies; however, you might not be able to see your credit score or certain details about your report unless you pay a fee. Reviewing your credit reports from all three of the credit-reporting agencies is important because they sometimes have different information.

Mentor Moment

I had heard the commercials about the importance of checking your credit report, but I thought I had good credit and always figured they were selling something so I had never bothered to do it. Then my husband and I went to refinance our home, and our bank ran our credit reports. My credit report had bad credit from two other people with similar names, and my husband's had three. We could not refinance until our credit was fixed, and it took several calls and a lot of work to get these people off our credit report.

Mary from Salt Lake City, UT

Once you receive copies of your credit report from each agency, you should carefully review them to make sure that all the information is correct. Even by reviewing free copies of your credit report, you should be able to tell whether you have any potential problems that you must address. You might also find that your credit reports have inaccuracies.

- Your personal information may be incorrect or outdated.
- They show that you were late with a payment, but you have proof that your payment was on time.
- They list accounts that you have closed as being open.
- They list accounts that are not yours.

Correcting problems such as these is important because you want to make sure that anyone who reviews your credit report has an accurate picture of your financial history.

O N   T R A C K

You are on track if you already know your credit score and can write it down here: _____.

Improving Your Credit Score

Once you find out your credit score, you can begin to take action if you find that it is not ideal. Here are some steps you can take to improve your credit score.

- **Avoid making late payments:** The later each late payment is, the more you hurt your score. Late payments not only affect your credit score, they can also make it more difficult to pay off your debts by giving your creditors cause to increase your interest rates or impose late fees. The best way—and really the only way—for you to improve your payment history is to pay your bills on time. Although you will not be able to go back and change the existing history on your credit report, you can ensure that you do not miss any more payments by finding a system to help keep track of and pay your bills. One way to do this is to put together a list of all of the bills you must pay and loans on which you owe payments, including the day of the month when they are due. This list can serve as a reminder of when payments are due, so you do not forget. You can also usually arrange for fixed payments through your bank or through the lender to ensure that the money is automatically deducted in time.

O N T R A C K

You are on track if you can make a list of all of your monthly payments and when they are due.

ITEM	DATE DUE

Mentor Moment

I usually paid my credit card on time, but then one month I missed a payment. My interest rate jumped to 26%, but I did not notice it at first. I finally did realize because, even though I was making payments on my account, my debt just kept growing. When I explored why, I found out that my interest rate had greatly increased. As a result, I was paying $100 per month on my card, but my finance charges were $300 per month. It was quite an education.

Nicole from New York City, NY

● **Pay down your debt:** Decreasing the amount of money you owe is one of the best ways to improve your credit score. Although it might be difficult to do, depending on your financial situation, you must pay more than the minimum amount due on your credit cards each month to pay off your credit card debt. Doing so will help your balances to slowly but surely decrease. Ideally, you should pay the total amount due on each account each month. The goal is not to carry debt from one month to the next, which helps you avoid paying finance charges. You can also pay down your debt on loans more quickly than scheduled by making extra payments or paying a little additional each month.

O N   T R A C K

You are on track if you can make a list of the total amount of money you owe to lenders.

ITEM	AMOUNT OWED

- **Watch your total available credit:** The total amount of money available to you from lenders, such as credit card companies, can work in your favor or it can work against you in terms of your credit score. Having debt is not necessarily bad, but having too much credit available or too much debt can be a bad thing when it comes to your credit score. If you have a lot of credit cards that you are not using, you should consider closing some. Choose to close newer accounts that you are not using first. You might want to keep some old accounts open because doing so adds to the length of your overall credit history.

- **Consolidate your debt:** Consolidating your credit debt into one account can help to make it more manageable by giving you just one payment to make each month. It can also make it easier for you to keep track of your debt and might reduce your minimum payments due each month. You should aim to consolidate the debt you owe on accounts with high interest rates or annual fees to those with lower interest rates and fees. In some cases, credit cards even offer incentives to customers who transfer balances, such as low financing rates for a specified period. If you are going to consolidate your debt, be sure to look for special offers such as this.

O N   T R A C K

You are on track if you know what the current interest rate is for each of your credit cards.

CARD	INTEREST RATE

- **Do not max out your credit cards or exceed your credit limit:** Credit issuers look at how much of your available credit you are using. For example, if you have a credit card with a $5,000 limit and have charged enough to that credit card to hit that limit, you might be considered a financial risk even if you have been keeping up with your monthly payments. This risk will be reflected in your score. In addition, if you go over your credit limit, you will likely be charged over-the-limit fees until you are able to reduce your balance. To improve this part of your score, you need to reduce the overall amount that you owe by making your payments on time and perhaps paying even more than the required monthly payment on your credit cards. Another way to correct the problem of a maxed-out credit card is to ask for an increase in your credit limit. However, if you go this route, you should keep in mind that this will affect the total credit available to you, which will also impact your credit score. You should also be careful not to use this extra line of credit, because you might overextend yourself financially.

- **Avoid opening new credit cards:** Because part of your credit rating is based on how long you have been paying back your credit, having a lot of new credit cards or opening up a lot of accounts all at once can actually lower your score, even if you are opening up those cards to consolidate debt or get lower interest rates. If you do not have any credit and want to begin building up a good history, start by opening just a couple credit cards and making sure to pay them on time.

- **Minimize inquiries on your account:** Every time you apply for a credit card or loan, the lender will inquire about your credit rating and might pull your credit report. A high number of requests for information (inquiries) can hurt your credit score because it might imply that you are preparing to go on a "borrowing binge." You can keep inquiries into your credit down by not applying for every credit card made available to you.

- **Keep open your oldest line of credit:** A long history of paying your bills on time works in your favor when it comes to your credit score because it shows financial responsibility over time.

- **Beware of being or asking for a cosigner:** Although having a cosigner can sometimes help to get you credit, you should beware of going this route because it might mean that you are being extended credit that you cannot really afford. Similarly, serving as a cosigner for other people can be risky because you become responsible for any missed payments on their accounts, and their bad credit can also affect your credit score.

Motivational Moment

66 Mistakes are part of the dues one pays for a full life. 99

Sophia Loren, Academy Award–winning actress

Understanding How Bad Credit Can Hurt Your Career Search

Believe it or not, your credit history can actually affect whether you receive a position with some employers. Although not all employers check the credit of potential candidates, they are aware that this information is available to them.

Hiring is not an easy process. It costs employers time and money in advertising, screening candidates, interviewing, and training. Therefore, some employers feel it is beneficial to protect their investments when it comes to hiring by using all possible information available to them to make an informed hiring decision. A high credit score might indicate to an employer that you possess a certain level of responsibility, which can reflect positively on you during the hiring process. Of course, if your rating is bad, the employer might interpret that you are unable to handle responsibility and lack organization. It might even lead the employer to question your ability to handle money and finances properly. Unfortunately, you are unlikely to know which employers check candidate's credit, so your best choice is to obtain and maintain the best possible credit you can.

Understanding Background Checks

As part of your employment search, you expect potential employers to check your references. These references will describe your personality, knowledge and skills you have that can benefit your future position, and your work ethics. For the most part, your references should give you some high marks. After all, you *chose* to list them as your references. However, some employers also perform background checks on prospective employees to find out additional information about their personal history. The information an employer finds about you in a background check can determine whether you get a position.

Understanding the Parts of a Background Check

A background check provides information about the following aspects of your history:

- **Court appearances**: When and why you were expected to appear in court, whether you appeared, and whether you fulfilled any court mandates or met the court requirements
- **Traffic violations:** How many traffic violations are on your record, whether you paid any resulting fines, whether you were required to go to traffic school, whether you have a consistent pattern of violations
- **Credit information:** Who are your creditors and whether you pay them on time
- **Child support and alimony payments:** Whether you are up-to-date on child support and how responsible you are in meeting any court mandates
- **Misdemeanors:** How old each offense is and how many are on your record
- **Felonies:** How many felonies are on your record and the nature of each
- **Domestic violence:** Whether you were a codefendant and whether the authorities were called

In short, any information that appears on a state or federal registry about you will appear in your background check.

Several agencies perform background checks, usually for a fee. When a cost is attached to the background check, most companies will require you to pay that fee. As a condition of employment, some states (e.g., Nevada, California) and some companies will also require you to be fingerprinted, which usually costs around $20. A drug test, which usually costs around $40.00, may also be part of the employment process.

Understanding How Your Background Check Can Hurt Your Career Search

As previously mentioned, the hiring process costs employers time and money. In addition, health-care organizations know that their employees have a lot of responsibility and are usually expected to work with the public. Therefore, employers are careful about who they hire. Most background checks are done to look at a person's criminal history, especially to look for predator-type activities and repeated offenses; however, employers might also look for more minor offenses, such as drug charges. Some offenses on a background check are considered much more negative to a potential employer than others. For example, some employers will not hire you if you have a felony on your record. For this reason, most people who have serious offenses in their history are not even accepted into health professions programs. Health professions programs generally investigate whether candidates will be employable before admitting them into their programs.

Motivational Moment

66 Failure is not fatal, but failure to change might be. 99

John Wooden, former basketball player and UCLA coach

If you do have some minor infractions in your background, you will find that honesty is the best policy when it comes to these offenses. You should work with your Campus Director, the Director of Education, and Career Services administrators to develop a strategy for how to approach this topic and present yourself during the interviewing and application process. If you have had any judgments against you in court, you might need to show the employer documentation that you met the court's requirements and were in compliance with court orders. If you have served time in jail or have been placed on probation, you might need to provide documentation that shows you were released and completed your probation. If you are still on probation, you will need to document when your probation will be completed.

Mentor Moment

When I was younger, I was hanging out with a group of people who committed a nonviolent act. Even though I did not participate, I was still written up and the incident went on my record because I was with them. Ever since, I have had to carry court documentation stating that I did not commit the crime, and every time I speak to an employer, I need to present this documentation. I was lucky enough to be admitted to a medical-assisting program, but I pray every day that I will be hired when I graduate. I have no guarantees, though, so I study really hard and try not to miss class. I have to be the very best that I can be at school to show potential employers that I am worth giving a chance.

Linda from Las Vegas, NV

Success Journal

1. Complete the sample employment application in Figure 12.1, making sure to include all of the skills you will have once you have completed your program, including those learned during your education and at your practicum.

2. Find local newspapers and employment papers for your area and determine which ones have the best information and ads for your career search. Then list them here.

   _____

   _____

3. Choose one of the job market websites mentioned in this chapter and perform a search for openings in your field. Below, list three openings that you might be interested in applying for, including the position title and company name.

   1. _____

   2. _____

   3. _____

4. Contact your career services department and ask them about upcoming career fairs. Also search the internet for upcoming career fairs in your area. Write down any career fairs that you learn about.

   _____

   _____

5. List three steps that you can take to personally improve or help maintain your credit score.

   1. _____

   2. _____

   3. _____

Survival Guide for the New Graduate

Learning Outcomes

After reading this chapter, the student will be able to:

1. Understand ways to survive a career search until acceptance of an employment offer.
2. Evaluate an employment offer.
3. List techniques for succeeding on the first day of employment.
4. Understand human resources paperwork.
5. Identify techniques for creating a good reputation at work.
6. Demonstrate knowledge of employee rights in the workplace.

Surviving Your Career Search

Congratulations! Your journey is coming to an end. Or, depending on how you look at it, your journey is just beginning. You have succeeded in your educational program and are ready to embark on a new adventure by beginning your career in the health professions. The months you spent in school now might seem like you were living a "cocoon" existence. You existed in the safe environment of your educational institution, surrounded by classmates and instructors who wanted to see you succeed. You built up your confidence and self-esteem by achieving good grades and attendance awards and earning praise from family and friends. Now that you have achieved this success, you must take the next step and enter the real world of health care. Your practicum most likely gave you a preview of what your new life will be like. However, reality is now sinking in as you hold your diploma in one hand and your portfolio in the other, ready to find your career position. Now it is up to you to show the outside world that you are ready and prepared to be a health professional.

If you started your career search early, you might have already found a position in the health-care field. Remember that finding your new position is the main reason that you work hard marketing and networking yourself before you graduate. However, if you have graduated from your program and do not have a position, you will find that your career search is your primary focus as you now enter the field. "Surviving" this career search might not be easy. In fact, you might be feeling some anxiety as you embark on this journey. This anxiety should diminish, though, as you realize the resources that are available to help you find your new place in the health professions. In addition, if you have fulfilled your responsibilities by completing your resume, networking with others, practicing your interviewing skills, and preparing for your career search, you should be ready to thrive in the search that lies ahead of you.

One very real part of surviving your career search involves getting by financially until you receive an offer. Although you will not need to make payments on any school loans you have until 6 months after you graduate, you will still need to financially support yourself (and your family, if applicable) while you conduct your search. One option that can help you to get by financially while you look for a full-time position is to acquire short-term employment through a temporary or staffing agency. Another option is to work a part-time job at night and search for career positions during the day. Continuing to work while you conduct your career search will increase the freedom you have to wait for the best possible offer from an employer. However, conducting a career search *is* a full-time job, so you might find it difficult to look for a career position while working another job. In that case, if you have school loans and have been searching for a position for almost 6 months, you might find it necessary to see if you can qualify for a deferment that would allow you to postpone your loan payments.

Mentor Moment

Everyone kept telling me how important networking was, but I didn't really start networking until after I graduated because I was so shy. Luckily, I did keep in touch with some of my former classmates. So, after I graduated, I called them to ask if they knew of any openings. It took me 3 weeks to find a position. I know if I had networked earlier I would have had a job before I graduated, like my friends did.

Stacy from Burlington, VT

Another part of surviving your career search will be enduring the well-meaning advice you receive from parents, family, and friends. People will want to share in your success by telling you how to search for your position, what to look out for when an offer is made, and even which offer to accept. Some of this advice will come from the mistakes that others have made, so listen respectfully— but listen with a critical ear. When it comes to your career search, only you can decide which position is best for you.

Motivational Moment

66 What lies behind us and what lies before us are tiny matters compared to what lies within us. 99

Ralph Waldo Emerson, American philosopher and poet

Recognizing the Right Offer

If you endure your career search for long enough, you *will* receive an employment offer. Maybe you will even receive more than one offer from different employers and will need to decide which offer is right for you. This decision is important and should be made only after taking into consideration a multitude of factors.

Depending on your experience, you might know exactly what you are looking for in a position. For example, if you are an "age-experienced" career seeker, you might have some more definite ideas about what you want in a position based on "the good, the bad, and the ugly" experiences you have previously had in the employment world. You can use your past experiences to assist you in this career search and choose the position that will work best for you. However, you must also be aware of how you judge your current career search based on your past experiences and be sure not to pass up too many offers. On the other hand, if you are seeking a position for the first time, you might not yet be aware of what your preferences are. Although this might seem like a negative thing, you may in fact be more open-minded about certain opportunities because this career position will be your first, and you may bring with you a level of enthusiasm that employers will value.

No matter what your experience, you will be looking for an *entry-level* position that will become the foundation for your career in the health-care field. Throughout this career, you will continue to develop your working style and learn about your own preferences. It is an ongoing and changing process. Employment factors that are important to you now will probably not be as important to you in 10 to 20 years. The goal is for you to select a position that meets your needs *today.*

To decide which offer is right for you, you need to balance what you want and need with what is currently being offered in the employment market. In recent years, the health-care field has been one of the fastest growing professional fields, which should work to your advantage. For example, if you find several openings in the market, then you might be able to afford to be more selective with your decision. On the other hand, if you do not see many postings in the market or you have been out of school for awhile and have not received any offers, then the first offer you receive might look really good to you. However, you should remember that your first offer will not always be your best offer. You need to make a smart employment decision based on your knowledge of the market and your own personal circumstances.

One way to decide whether an offer is right for you is to create a list of your priorities and then rank them from most important to least important. Consider how important these factors are to you in a job offer:

- Salary
- Location (proximity to home, accessibility to public transportation)
- Medical and dental benefits
- Paid time off
- Holidays
- Hours
- Schedule flexibility
- Type of office (clinic, hospital, specialty area)
- Size of office or facility (number of patients and staff)
- Multioffice practice
- Work atmosphere

- Prestige of organization
- Opportunity to gain valuable work experience
- Potential for advancement
- Stress level and pace of position
- Dress code

Mentor Moment

No matter what I need to do, I always make a list. When I need to make a major decision, I write a list of pros and cons on a sheet of paper. After I have completed my list, my decision is clear. This simple exercise just helps me clear my mind and visually see the advantages of my decision.

Kay from Decatur, IL

Unless you are extremely fortunate, no offer is likely to meet all of your needs and desires. However, the position that is right for you should meet at least 50% of your current requirements and preferences, including the ones that are most important to you. You should also remember that your first position will give you the opportunity to gain valuable experience and knowledge in your field. As this happens, you will probably have the opportunity to advance in your position or search for a new position that will help you to achieve more of your personal employment goals.

O N   T R A C K

You are on track if can you list your top three priorities in considering a job offer.

1. _____

2. _____

3. _____

Motivational Moment

❝ Your peace of mind and personal satisfaction are perhaps the most accurate guide you will ever have to doing what is right for you. **❞**

Brian Tracy, self-help author and speaker

Succeeding in Your Career

Once you find the offer that is right for you and accept it, your career search will come to an end—at least for now. You will be able to enjoy a "woo-hoo moment" that celebrates all of the hard work that you have put in throughout your education. The day you accept an offer will probably be almost as exciting as the day you graduate. You will be on top of the world because you know that your new employer wants you, and you will be filled with the confidence that you know how to perform the duties of your new position with knowledge and skill. However, you will soon need to focus your energy on getting ready for your first day in your new career and preparing to face the whole world of challenges that awaits you in your new position.

In your new career, you will have the opportunity to see how all of the knowledge you gained in the classroom, in labs, and in your practicum or clinic practice will come together in real-life practice. All of the skills that you have learned will help you to succeed in your health professions career. However, your new work environment might seem like a maze at first, as you learn office procedures, attempt to avoid office politics, and strive to create a new professional you. As the new person in the office, you will probably feel like all eyes are on you, even if they are not. Therefore, you should strive to make a good impression right from the start. The impression you create, along with your work performance, will determine whether you are able to obtain long-term success in your career.

Surviving Your First Day of Employment

The first step in succeeding in your health professions career is to survive the first day of employment. Most people are nervous on their first day at a new job because they are entering a new environment, learning lots of new information, meeting new people, and creating their first impression. However, the more you get out of your first day, the more quickly you will be able to settle in and become successful in your career.

One way to ensure that your first day in your new position goes well is to know what to expect. On your first day, certain things will probably occur:

- You will receive a tour of the office or facility.
- You will meet some or all of the office staff.
- You will be asked to fill out some paperwork from the human resources (HR) department. (See Box 13.1 and Box 13.2.)

O N T R A C K

You are on track if you can define these terms:

PPO: _____

HMO: _____

W4: _____

401K: _____

BOX 13.1 HUMAN RESOURCES PAPERWORK

This list describes some types of paperwork you might be asked to complete on your first day of work. Nowadays, much of this paperwork is done online. Be sure to pay attention to any deadlines you are given to complete this paperwork, as many insurance companies have certain windows during which you must apply for coverage. If you need help completing any of this paperwork, consult with your HR representative or your supervisor.

- **Application:** If you were not asked to complete an employment application as part of your interview process, you may need to complete one on your first day of work. (See Figure 12-1 for a sample employment application.) Take your time, and make sure to complete all sections of the application honestly and completely. If you are filling out the application by hand, be sure to print clearly, possibly printing in all uppercase letters to improve readability. In addition to some basic personal information (e.g., full name, address, social security number), the employment application will probably also ask about your education and work history. Although much of this information can be found on your resume, you will still need to complete the application in its entirety. The application may also ask about things that cannot be found on your resume, such as the reason you left each previous work position, and you might be asked to provide documentation for certain items, such as your high school diploma and discharge paperwork if you were in the military.
- **Medical insurance forms:** Depending on your employer, you might be given the option to purchase medical and dental insurance coverage, which helps to pay for any medical expenses you might incur due to illness or injury. If so, you need to be aware of the different types of insurance plans available, including the differences in your costs, coverage, copayments (i.e., copays), and deductibles (see Box 13-2). Then you must decide which insurance plan will work best for you. The cost of the insurance coverage you choose will be deducted automatically from each paycheck you receive. Note that some

(box continues on page 398)

BOX 13.1 HUMAN RESOURCES PAPERWORK (continued)

employers do not offer medical coverage until after you have been an employee for a specified period (e.g., 3 months, 6 months), and some do not offer it at all. You should find out what policies govern medical coverage by your employer *before* you accept the position. (See also Box 13.2.)

- **Life insurance forms:** Some employers also offer a type of insurance called life insurance, which pays a designated sum of money to a person of your choosing (known as a "beneficiary") upon your death. Your employer may cover the cost of some basic life insurance (e.g., $50,000) and then might also offer you an opportunity to purchase additional life insurance at your own expense. To complete your life insurance paperwork, you will need the name, address, phone number, birth date, and social security number of each person you wish to list as a beneficiary. As with medical insurance, the cost of the additional life insurance coverage you choose will be deducted automatically from each paycheck you receive.

- **Tax form:** Your employer will also ask you to complete a W-4 form from the Internal Revenue Service. This short tax form is used by your employer to calculate the amount of your earnings that are withheld from each of your paychecks to pay for such items as income tax, social security, and Medicare. For your employer to determine this information, you will need to provide information about the number of dependents for which you are responsible. For example, single people usually claim one dependent (themselves) or zero dependents. If you are married or have children, you might want to consult with a tax accountant for more detailed advice on the proper number of dependents to claim on your W-4 form. The number of dependents you claim determines the amount of money withheld by your employer, which ultimately affects whether you will receive a refund or owe money when it comes time for the next tax season. Be sure that you know how to fill out this form before you begin your first day of work, and fill out this form honestly. Providing false information on a W-4 form is considered fraud, and failure to submit a W-4 form results in the maximum withholding.

- **Retirement savings and investment forms:** A retirement savings plan is a way for you to save pretax dollars for your future. That means the amount you choose to contribute to a retirement savings plan is deducted directly from your paycheck. The most popular type of retirement savings plan is a 401K; however, depending on the type of organization you work for, you might also be given the opportunity to invest in a 403(b) plan. This type of plan is generally only available to employees of nonprofit employers, such as educational institutions, hospitals, libraries, and certain other nonprofit organizations. Some companies offer their employees matching funds to such plans, meaning that the company contributes a certain amount of money to your retirement plan up to a certain percentage (commonly 2% to 4%), based on the amount

BOX 13.1 (continued)

of money you contribute on your own. Although this is a good way to increase the total amount of money that you are technically earning in a year, most employers require you to be with the company for a certain amount of time before you can participate in their retirement savings plan. In addition, most plans require you to remain with the company for a certain number of years before you are considered to be vested for the full amount of your employer's contribution. That means that even though your employer might match your contributions up to a certain percentage of your salary, you might not receive that full amount if you leave your position too early. You should think carefully about whether to invest in a retirement savings plan. Although planning for the future is a good idea, you should make sure that you first have enough money to get by and have an emergency fund. You should also be aware that you will be forced to pay certain penalties if you try to access the money in your retirement savings before you are of age.

BOX 13.2 COMMON TYPES OF HEALTH INSURANCE PLANS

If your employer offers health insurance coverage, you will benefit from understanding a little bit about how insurance works and common plan types. For all types of insurance plans, the employer negotiates a plan for their employees with an insurance company based on the size of the company. The cost of the plan is known as the *premium*. Some companies cover a part of the premium's cost for their employees; however, in recent years companies have been putting more and more of those costs on the employees themselves. The portion of the premium that you are required to pay will come directly out of your paycheck and will be based on the type of plan that you choose.

There are two most common types of plans.

- **Health Maintenance Organization (HMO):** With an HMO, the insurance company negotiates a price for services in advance with certain medical providers. Those providers are known as the insurance company's "network," and you must stay within the network for your health care. You will likely have an out-of-pocket cost, known as a copayment or copay, for each medical visit; however, you will not have to pay the full price of what the visit would normally cost. The benefit of an HMO plan is that your costs tend to be lower. On the flip side, HMOs typically have more restrictions on who you can see and when, and you might need to get referrals to see specialists.

(box continues on page 400)

BOX 13.2 COMMON TYPES OF HEALTH INSURANCE PLANS (continued)

- **Preferred Provider Organization (PPO):** Although PPOs also have a preapproved list of providers, you have the flexibility to see almost any doctor you want at any time. The difference is that you are likely to pay more for this flexibility because PPOs are generally have higher premiums, and some have a deductible (a specified out-of-pocket expense for health care) that you must meet before your insurance company will pay for anything.

After your initial orientation, you might also be asked to follow a coworker for the morning or for an entire day so that you can learn the organization's procedures in more detail. Alternatively, you might be asked to spend a little time in a few different departments helping out so that you can see how the entire office runs. You might even be asked to begin to perform some of the duties of your new position. For example, you might be asked to spend the rest of your day completing such tasks as filing patient records, answering phones, or inputting patient information for billing. You should look at any task that you are asked to complete as an opportunity to learn how the organization functions and should learn as much as you can from this quick orientation because you will soon be expected to know all of these office procedures inside and out.

Although you will not be able to learn everything you need to know on your first day, you can make the most of that day by following certain suggestions. Here are some tips for making your first day successful:

- **Get a good night's sleep:** Be sure to get a good night's sleep the night before so that you can be refreshed to start your new health-care career.
- **Revisit your positive thinking:** Use positive thinking to calm your nerves and boost your self-confidence, and leave your stress at the door. You should tell your mind that you are going to have a fantastic first day.
- **Be friendly and courteous to everyone you meet:** Your new coworkers will be your source of information and support while you are learning the ropes in your new position, and you want to be sure that you begin to develop good relationships with your coworkers, even on your first day.
- **Learn the rules:** In addition to becoming familiar with the rules that govern office procedures and patient care, you will need to learn about office policies regarding such issues as smoking, dress code, and conduct. You might be given an official handbook or pamphlet that describes these policies. If so, be sure to review this information in detail. If not, be sure to ask the HR department any questions you have about these issues.

- **Ask questions:** Your first day is the ideal time to ask all of your basic questions because your supervisor and coworkers will not expect you to know what you are doing and will expect to provide a certain amount of guidance to you. You should ask as many questions as you need to when you first begin your position so that you can feel comfortable with all of the tasks and procedures you need to perform and can make sure that you are performing these tasks in the way that your supervisor wants them done. Remember, though, that you will not be able to get away with being the "new person" forever.
- **Take notes:** Make sure that you bring a notebook and pencil with you on your first day so that you can write down important information (e.g., fax machine, copier, and phone codes) and the answers to questions you ask. The more you write down, the easier it will be for you to function on your own until you memorize the information and the office procedures become second nature to you.

Motivational Moment

66 The only dumb question is the one you do not ask. 99

Anonymous

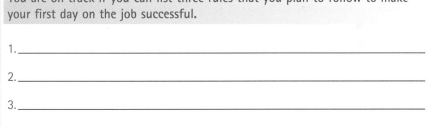

O N T R A C K

You are on track if you can list three rules that you plan to follow to make your first day on the job successful.

1. _____

2. _____

3. _____

Creating a Good Reputation at Work

The good impression that you begin to create on your first day will become the foundation for the solid reputation you are beginning to build at work. You want to make sure that others know you are reliable and dependable, have a strong work ethic, and will always behave in a professional manner on the job.

Although you should continue to build on your good reputation throughout your career, your behavior will be particularly important during your first 3 to 6 months, as many employers have probation periods that you must complete before being considered a full-time employee.

Your ability to remain professional on the job might sometimes be tested, especially when you become faced with the challenge of office politics. "Office politics" refers to the relationships that form and interactions that occur among coworkers due to the dynamic personalities within a work environment. Some of the people you work with are likely to use their positions or personalities in ways that will help them to advance in their careers, regardless of how doing so affects their customers and coworkers. For example, some coworkers use gossip to undermine or discredit other employees, whereas others use manipulation and power to control their coworkers. Although you might not notice these office politics going on around you at first, they are present in most work environments to one degree or another.

Here are some steps you can take to create a good reputation, manage office politics in your new position, and increase your chances of career success:

- **Act professionally:** Creating a good reputation begins with acting professionally at all times, including when you are on a lunch or other break. Simple steps for doing this include not eating snacks or chewing gum in front of patients or customers, filling the copy machine when you use the last sheet of paper, and making another pot of coffee when you drink the last cup. However, being a health professional involves much more. Whether you are a new employee or a veteran, it means being courteous and offering respect to and commanding the respect of others—including supervisors, coworkers, and patients—by conducting yourself in such a manner that you display grace, good etiquette, confidence, and professionalism. You should conduct yourself in this manner not only while you are at work but also when you attend social work functions, such as happy hours, office parties, and other events. (See Box 13.3.)
- **Listen to others:** Whether you are in a meeting or being given instructions on how to perform a task, you should be sure to listen carefully to others. As a new employee, you will have a lot to learn, and one of the best ways to do this is to listen to and learn from the experience of others.
- **Cultivate professional relationships:** Although you will most likely make some friends at work, you should remember that the relationships that you build there are professional relationships first. You should respect others' privacy by not becoming a part of office gossip. You should also protect your own privacy by not discussing personal matters in the workplace. A good rule to follow is to not tell anyone anything about your life that you do not want the whole workplace to know. Not everyone will respect your privacy, and "news" tends to travel fast, especially in a small office.

> **BOX 13.3**   TIPS FOR HOW TO BEHAVE AT OFFICE EVENTS
>
> Although happy hours and other company-related social functions (e.g., birthday parties, baby showers, retirement parties) might seem like a time to relax and "let your hair down," they are an extension of your professional life, and as such, you should act accordingly when you attend them. Here are some tips for making sure that you behave professionally at all office events:
>
> - Make an appearance. As a part of the team, your presence at office events matters, and people will notice if you do not attend. Plan to attend, even if only for a short time.
> - Arrive on time.
> - Dress professionally.
> - Leave office politics behind.
> - Do not drink too much. You do not want to be the next morning's gossip in the office, hospital, or clinic.

- **Do not ask for special privileges or favors:** As a new employee, you should avoid asking for time off and other special privileges until you have had an opportunity to build a strong work reputation, garner the respect of your supervisor and others, and earn these privileges. Your goal as a health professional is to help the organization increase and maintain their patients. You must understand that if you are not at work, your work does not get done. If you must ask for time off right away, be sure to offer to come in early, work late, or come in on the weekend to make up for lost time, if possible.
- **Keep busy without being asked:** You should do your best to make sure that you work a solid workday every day. That means keeping busy at all times. When you finish a project early or find yourself with extra time before your next assignment, you should look around and see where you can help. Certain tasks, such as filing, cleaning up, and restocking, almost always need to be done. Your supervisor and coworkers will admire and appreciate the initiative you show if you decide to take on these tasks without being asked. If you are not sure what tasks would be appropriate, you can always ask. Offering your help and expressing an interest in keeping busy also show initiative.

Motivational Moment

66 Giving people a little more than they expect is a good way to get back more than you'd expect. 99

Robert Half, American businessman

- **Accept that no task is too small:** Throughout your career, especially in the beginning, you might be asked to do some things that are not part of your primary job description. For example, you might be asked to make phone calls, answer phones, do data entry, or set up rooms. Helping out with such tasks and assisting other departments prepares you for being able to adapt to the demands that might be placed on you during an emergency or when the department is short-staffed. Look at these requests as opportunities for you to show your commitment to teamwork, and complete each task with a smile.

Mentor Moment

I felt so lucky when I found a position in a medical office that I really did not think much of the fact that it was a five-physician office. When I started working, I was so busy, even on my first day. I could not believe that I could work so fast. Being busy made me feel great!

Chris from Peabody, KS

- **Be tactful when presenting ideas:** Knowing how to present your ideas is very important. As a new employee, you must remember that you are still learning the policies and procedures of your office. Therefore, you should think carefully before you speak and always offer suggestions in a tactful and respectful manner. Many times, the office has good reasons for doing something a certain way. If you immediately begin to criticize existing policies and procedures, you might not learn those reasons and might quickly lose the respect of your coworkers. In addition, any good suggestions that you have might not be considered. You do not want to come off as pushy or a know-it-all before you have earned a strong work reputation.
- **Manage your time:** Managing your time means making the most of your work hours, being realistic about how long a project will take you, not procrastinating, and meeting your commitments and deadlines. Be sure to create a work schedule you know you can manage. Do not volunteer for projects unless you know you have the ability to complete them on time and at a satisfactory level. You might find that the best way to handle a project is to break it down into manageable sections and tackle a part of it each day. When you plan in this way, you are better able to manage your time and consistently perform at an optimum level. Managing your time also means making sure that you arrive at work and for scheduled meetings on time. Tardiness is not an impressive feature in a new employee.
- **Communicate professionally:** Whether in person, in writing, or via e-mail, you should make sure that all of your communications sound proper and

professional. That means making sure to proofread and spell-check everything you write, including letters, e-mails, and memos. You should check the content accuracy, check that any dates are correct, and check the spellings of people's names. In some cases, if you are composing a communication at the end of the day, you are better off waiting until the next day to send it so that you have the opportunity to proofread it again with fresh eyes.

- **Always treat patients with respect:** Depending on your position, you might encounter patients who do not feel well. This can cause some to become short-tempered, grumpy, and demanding, especially if they are in pain or are scared. Some patients require more help and attention than others. Try to be respectful, sympathetic, comforting, and reassuring at all times, and remind patients that you are there to help them.

Motivational Moment

66 Treat everyone as though they are the most important person in the world, because *to them* they are. 99

Earl Nightingale, motivational speaker and author

- **Resolve issues:** You will sometimes find yourself in situations on the job in which you experience confrontation, either with a patient or a coworker. Try your best to avoid these situations, but be sure to stand up for yourself, especially when it comes to protecting your rights as an employee or protecting the rights or safety of a patient. If you cannot avoid a situation, maintain your integrity by continuing to act professionally and focusing on solving the issue rather than attacking the other person. Find a private area (e.g., empty office or conference room) for the discussion and make sure another coworker or supervisor is present as a witness. Once a solution is found, you can shake hands and move on with your workday. Remember that resolving issues in such a manner not only maintains your professionalism but also helps you to grow as an employee.

- **Keep your enthusiasm:** Although even a new position can become dull after you have been there for a while, you need to remember how much work it took during your health professions program to get you to this point. Maintain your enthusiasm for your career by remembering the feeling of excitement you have on your first day and keeping it with you every day. Also, remind yourself of the important role you play in your patients' lives and feel excitement knowing that you are making a difference to them.

Understanding the Reasons People Get Fired

Although conducting a career search and finding a position are hard tasks, equally as hard can be the process of keeping a position once you find it. If you do not understand some of the most common reasons that people get fired, you might make mistakes that will lead you to have to begin your search all over again.

Here are some of the most common mistakes people make:

- **Unprofessional conduct:** Once you begin your new career, you should be sure to behave professionally at all times. As an entry-level health professional, this means following directives, respecting your coworkers and customers, and recognizing the authority and supervision of staff members above you. In addition to earning you a bad reputation, behaving unprofessionally in your new position could result in a verbal or written warning and possibly even dismissal.
- **Theft:** Sadly, theft in the workplace is more common than you might realize. Some people feel that employment entitles them to free access to supplies, which include drugs and equipment in the health-care field. However, most workplaces keep close inventories of such items, and personal use of the company's property is considered theft, which is grounds for immediate dismissal.
- **Dishonesty:** Dishonesty includes lying or misrepresenting yourself or others. In some cases, this deception occurs during the interview process or on the employment application, when people "stretch the truth" or falsify information about their skills or experience in order to obtain a position. However, such deceit often becomes obvious when you are placed in the health-care field and can even be dangerous when it comes to patient care. Dishonesty can also occur once a person enters the workplace, such as when a person fails to take responsibility for his or her actions or lies for another employee.
- **Poor attendance:** In the health-care field, you need to show that you are dependable, and that starts with attendance. The importance of attendance during your educational program was not only to show your commitment to graduation but also to prepare you for the reality of working in the health-care field. Unexcused absences and excessive tardiness are not accepted in a workplace and can lead to poor reviews, warnings, and even termination.
- **Poor appearance:** Your appearance needs to reveal that you respect your position in the health-care field. That begins by making sure that your scrubs, uniform, or other clothing is clean and free from stains. If you dress unprofessionally at work, you might be given a verbal or written warning before more

serious action is taken against you. Take this warning to heart and change your appearance to meet the requirements of your organization so that you do not lose your position.

- **Improper use of work time:** Your position requires all of your attention when you are on the clock. If you want 100% of your paycheck, you must put in 100% of your time. When you spend time inappropriately (e.g., talking with coworkers, making personal phone calls), you are taking time away from your patients and are effectively stealing from your employer by being paid for time for which you are not working. You must follow a higher standard in your position in the health-care field; be sure to leave personal matters out of the workplace and focus on work while you are there. If coworkers engage you while you are performing your job, you should be friendly but make it clear that you must focus on your work. You can always socialize during your breaks or at lunchtime. If your socialization interferes with your work, you might see comments about it on your review, or it could result in a verbal or written warning, probation, and possibly, termination.

- **Improper use of company equipment:** Your workspace and the equipment you use at work, including your computer, are company property. You should avoid using this company property for personal use, such as shopping online, surfing the internet, and engaging in online social networking, even on your own time (e.g., during lunch, after work hours).

- **Inefficiency:** Your supervisor will be watching to see how you handle interruptions and how well you complete your assigned tasks. Although you should always be sure to complete each task, if you work too slowly or make too many mistakes, you will call attention to yourself and people might begin to think that you are not qualified for the position. Instead of trying to just work quickly, you should work with efficiency to make sure that your work gets done quickly and correctly. When you are working with patients, inefficiency can lead you to seem inconsiderate, discourteous, or rude and might also cause you to make life-threatening mistakes that cannot be overlooked. Termination could result, depending on the seriousness of the situation.

- **Inability to get along with others:** The ability to get along with other people, including patients and coworkers, is important in the health-care field. If you are constantly starting trouble or are disrespectful to patients or coworkers, you will be reprimanded and could be terminated.

- **Refusal to follow orders:** As an employee, you must respect the rules and chain of command in the workplace. These regulations are in place to protect the rights and safety of all employees and customers. You must also be sure to follow the specific orders of your supervisor. Insubordination is unacceptable. If you have a problem with your supervisor or someone else or are asked to perform a task with which you are uncomfortable or unqualified, you should resolve the issue respectfully and follow the necessary procedures and chain of command.

- **Drug or alcohol abuse:** Although most workplaces now offer employee assistance programs to help employees who are addicted to alcohol or drugs, your employer will not tolerate any behavior that endangers the lives of patients or employees. You must be able to perform your job duties at the highest level of your ability at all times.
- **Gossiping:** Although networking with your coworkers on a professional level is important, you must be sure to avoid becoming part of the office "grapevine" that spreads rumors. Doing so is not only unprofessional, it also impinges on your work time, disrespects the rights of others, and can be grounds for dismissal. You should steer clear of people in the office who do gossip in order to avoid becoming part of or the subject of the latest rumors. If you cannot avoid office gossip, you can do your best to put it to rest by changing the subject of conversation when rumors come up.
- **Sexual harassment:** Sexual harassment is a serious offense that can result in immediate termination and possibly even legal consequences. You must be sure to be respectful of other people's rights at all times, which includes avoiding making advances toward or sexual jokes around other employees. If you become involved in a consensual relationship with a coworker, you must also be careful to keep your relationship professional in the office because displays of affection in the workplace can also be considered sexual harassment to other employees. If you are unsure what constitutes sexual harassment, check your employee handbook or HR paperwork. In addition, most employers conduct sexual harassment training for new employees. You might even be asked to sign a form when you first start working that acknowledges that you understand the organization's policies regarding sexual harassment. Be sure to ask any questions about the policy before signing the form.

By avoiding these common mistakes, you can increase your chances of remaining successfully employed in your new position.

Mentor Moment

When I graduated from health professions school and got a position as a surgical technologist, I had to fill out real HR paperwork for the first time. I was so excited about accepting an offer that I never even thought about the paperwork I would need to complete. I was kind of embarrassed to ask so many questions, but I was really lucky that the person in HR did not mind and was willing to help. And I was glad when all of that paperwork was done.

Jimmy from Framington, NM

Understanding Your Rights in the Workplace

One aspect of employment that most employees do not think about—and hope they never *have* to think about—is their rights in the workplace. Just as employers are entitled to expect certain things from an employee and can terminate that employee if those expectations are not met, as an employee you also have rights to which you are entitled and that your employer must uphold. Unfortunately, most employees do not understand their rights under the law.

Here are some common legal terms and issues that might affect you at work:

- **At-will employment:** Technically, the term "at-will employment" means that either you or your employer can end your working relationship at any time for any reason or for *no* reason at all. This means that, if you have not signed a contract for a specified length of employment, you may be laid off or fired from your position even if you are a good employee. Although some laws exist that limit an employer's ability to terminate employees without reason (e.g., unlawful discrimination), in some cases such terminations are justifiable from the employer's perspective (e.g., downsizing). At-will employment also means that you are able to quit your position without notice for any reason; however, most employers require 2 weeks notice, and giving notice is a form of professional courtesy that will benefit you, especially if you want to use that employer as a future reference.

- **Equal pay:** Equal pay refers to an employee's right to receive the same pay for the same position. Although you want to make sure that your employer is treating you and paying you fairly, as an entry-level employee you should focus first on meeting the requirements of your position. During an evaluation or review, you can take the opportunity to ask questions concerning pay scales. You should keep in mind, however, that your employer is not allowed to and will not discuss with you how much other employees make. In addition, the equal pay concept applies only to people with the exact education who care for the same type of clients in the exact region and have the exact responsibilities. Because of these firm guidelines, companies usually do not have trouble justifying differences in pay for similar positions.

- **Privacy:** As previously mentioned, your workspace and the equipment you use at work, including your computer, are company property. Therefore, they are rightfully subject to inspection at any time. In some cases, your company will monitor your use of this equipment without you even knowing it. For example, most companies have the ability to tap into an employee's computer to review e-mails and see what internet sites have been visited. For this reason, you should avoid using company property for personal use at all times.

- **Unemployment compensation:** Most people assume that they will receive unemployment benefits if they are let go, laid off, or fired from a position. However, if you are let go for being disobedient, not following orders, or engaging in misconduct of any kind, you might not be eligible for unemployment. The rights governing unemployment vary by state, so be sure to find out the rules that apply in your state, if necessary.

By better understanding some of these basic legal concepts, you can begin to protect yourself as an employee. Your employee handbook should also outline some of the rights you have as an employee. You might even receive special rights and protection due to unions, employee contracts, and collective bargaining agreements. Consult with your HR department and read your employee handbook to see if and when you are eligible for this special type of protection.

Success Journal

1. What would your ideal work environment be like? Write a brief description.

_____

_____

_____

_____

2. Complete the chart below to help you determine which items your job offer *must* include, which items you would *like to have,* and which items you *do not want.*

	Must have	Like to have	Do not want
Flexible hours			
Large medical office (more than 5 physicians)			
Large hospital			
Small clinic			
Multioffice practice			
Low-income area office			
Paid time off			
Sick time			
Paid holidays			
Medical benefits			
Dental benefits			
Specialty office			
Access to public transportation			

(continues on page 412)

Success Journal (continued)

	Must have	Like to have	Do not want
Close proximity to home			
More than 25 staff members			
Opportunity for advancement			
Social work atmosphere			
Fast-paced environment			
Slow-paced environment			
Low-stress position			
Dress code			
Organization with good reputation			

3. Now, using the chart you just completed, list by priority the top five items your employment offer needs to include to be right for you.

1. _____

2. _____

3. _____

4. _____

5. _____

4. List three mistakes that you want to work hard to avoid in order to succeed in your new career.

1. _____

2. _____

3. _____

Epilogue

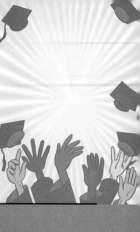

Congratulations! At this point in your journey, you have completed your transformation and are ready to embark on your own in your new career. As a new health professional, you should be sure to celebrate your success and carry with you the new confidence you have acquired.

Salute your courage! Throughout your health professions program, you have shown that you had the courage and strength to change old habits, learn new information, and work hard. You now have the courage to walk tall as an example to your family and friends. Celebrate that courage and maintain it as you take your diploma and face the world in your new career.

Salute the new professional you! Your journey has armed you with the qualities you need to become a health professional. Realize how you have transformed yourself throughout your program. Your knowledge and skills have increased as you read this book and worked your way through your program. Have confidence in those new skills, and allow your new self-confidence and professional look to boost your self-esteem and to show in all you do.

Salute all you have achieved! You kept a positive outlook, maintained your focus on your goals, and overcame your brick walls with determination. By attending class and getting good grades, you made it to graduation. You have achieved a new you, and a new career position is in your sights—one that will continue to make a difference in your life and in the world. You can now look ahead and follow the path of opportunity toward a new future.

Motivational Moment

66 It's all about dreams. If I had to attribute my success in life to any one thing it is this: I believed in my dreams, even when no one else did. 99

Oprah Winfrey, talk show host, founder of O.W.N. television network

Resources and References

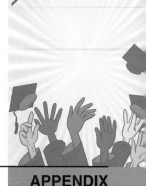

WEBSITES

Achieve! 60-Second Nuggets of Inspiration
www.achieveezine.com/nuggets/
This family-friendly website is a resource for personal development and motivational materials that offers quick, inspirational thoughts to make you feel happy, stop and think, smile, or answer a perplexing problem. The site also offers access to a free subscription to *Achieve! Ezine,* a weekly online publication that inspires and motivates people to achieve their goals.

Association for Applied and Therapeutic Humor
www.aath.org
The Association for Applied and Therapeutic Humor is a nonprofit organization dedicated to providing evidence-based information about the practical applications of using humor to enhance work performance, support learning, and improve health and healing. The website provides information about the organization, including details on membership and its annual conference as well as an extensive humor resources page with suggested readings and humorous articles.

Dr. Wayne W. Dyer
www.drwaynedyer.com/
Dr. Wayne W. Dyer, who is referred to as the "father of motivation" by his fans, is an internationally renowned motivational author and speaker. He has authored many books about how to change your life, thoughts, and outcomes. His website offers information on his books, seminars, and other products. It also offers daily inspirations, podcasts, and a blog that focus on offering great tips to get you moving in a positive direction.

Health Career Web

www.healthcareerweb.com/

This user-friendly site offers the ability to search for health professions jobs by local area. It also offers a forum for discussions on health-related topics, user groups, and a blog on which users can post information about themselves, including their current situation and skills.

Hire Health

http://www.hirehealth.net/

This site offers a job search engine dedicated to the health-care professions. The home page features a list of health-care jobs across the country, but users can also easily search for jobs in their area. Users can also send job postings to their e-mail addresses.

Inspiration Peak

www.inspirationpeak.com/

Also known as "The Peak," this fun and user-friendly website is a great place to find inspiring quotes, poems, stories, essays, and speeches. In addition, the website offers forums, subscription to a free mailing list, and a store to shop for items with inspirational themes.

Oprah.com

www.oprah.com/index.html

Oprah Winfrey is one of the most influential women in television history. Her website offers information on everything from finding happiness to cooking and gardening. It also features video clips from her show, audio clips from her satellite radio show *Oprah Radio*, details about Oprah's favorite motivational speakers and authors, and much more.

World Laughter Tour

www.worldlaughtertour.com

If you believe that laughter is good for the soul and can help to make the world a better place, you might want to visit the World Laughter Tour website. This site provides a clearinghouse of information, ideas, and news about the importance of laughter in healing and life and also provides information about how to start a laughter club and become a "Certified Laughter Leader."

BOOKS

Byrne, R. (2006). *The Secret.* New York: Atria Books.

Carnegie, D. (1936). *How to Win Friends and Influence People.* New York: Simon & Schuster.

Dyer, W.W. (1987). *How to Be a No-Limit Person.* Chicago: Nightingale-Conant.

Dyer, W.W. (2006). *Inspiration: Your Ultimate Calling.* Carlsbad, CA: Hay House.

Dyer, W.W. (2007). *Change Your Thoughts, Change Your Life: Living the Wisdom of the Tao.* Carlsbad, CA: Hay House.

Dyer, W.W. (2009). *Excuses Begone: How to Change Lifelong, Self-Defeating Thinking Habits.* Carlsbad, CA: Hay House.

Fallon, B. (1982). *Two Hundred Tips to Students on How to Study,* 2nd edition. Danville, IL: Interstate Publishers.

Johnson, S. (1998). *Who Moved My Cheese? An Amazing Way to Deal with Change in Your Work and in Your Life.* New York: Putnam.

Johnson, S. (2003). *The Present: The Gift That Makes You Happy and Successful at Work and in Life.* New York: Doubleday.

Johnson, S. (2009). *Peaks and Valleys: Making Good and Bad Times Work for You.* New York: Atria Books.

Lattanzi, J.B., & Purnell, L.D. (2006). *Developing Cultural Competence in Physical Therapy Practice.* Philadelphia: F.A. Davis.

Nugent, P.M., & Vitale, B.A. (2008). *Test Success: Test-Taking Techniques for Beginning Nursing Students,* 5th edition. Philadelphia: F.A. Davis.

Pausch, R., with Zaslow, J. (2008). *The Last Lecture.* New York: Hyperion.

Purnell, L. (2009). *A Guide to Culturally Competent Health Care,* 2nd edition. Philadelphia: F.A. Davis.

Ziglar, Z. (1994). *Over the Top.* Nashville, TN: Nelson Publishers.

Ziglar, Z. (1997). *Something Else to Smile About: Encouragement and Inspiration for Life's Ups and Downs.* Nashville, TN: Nelson Publishers.

Ziglar, Z. (2005). *Conversations with My Dog.* Nashville, TN: Broadman & Holman Publishers.

Ziglar, Z. (2006). *Better Than Good: Creating a Life You Can't Wait to Live.* Nashville, TN: Integrity Publishers.

Index

Note: Page numbers followed by "b," "f," and "t" indicate boxes, figures, and tables, respectively.